"Must We All Die?"

"Must We All Die?"

Alaska's Enduring Struggle with Tuberculosis

Robert Fortuine

UNIVERSITY OF ALASKA PRESS :: FAIRBANKS

© 2005 University of Alaska Press

Published by University of Alaska Press
An imprint of University Press of Colorado
1580 North Logan Street, Suite 660
PMB 39883
Denver, Colorado 80203–1942

 The University Press of Colorado is a proud member of
Association of University Presses.

The University Press of Colorado is a cooperative publishing enterprise supported, in part,
by Adams State University, Colorado State University, Fort Lewis College, Metropolitan State
University of Denver, University of Alaska Fairbanks, University of Colorado, University of Denver,
University of Northern Colorado, University of Wyoming, Utah State University, and Western
Colorado University.

ISBN: 978-1-889963-69-3 (hardcover)
ISBN: 978-1-64642-679-9 (paperback)

Library of Congress Cataloging-in-Publication Data

Fortuine, Robert.
    "Must we all die?": Alaska's enduring struggle with tuberculosis / Robert Fortuine.
        p. cm.
Includes bibliographical references and index.
ISBN-10: 1-889963-69-0 (ISBN-10: 10 (hardcover) : alk. paper)
ISBN-13: 978-1-889963-69-3 (ISBN-10: 13 (hardcover) : alk. paper)
ISBN-13: 978-1-64642-679-9 (paperback : alk. paper)

1. Tuberculosis—Alaska—History. I. Title.
RC313.A63F67 2005
614.5'42'09798—dc22

                            2004028620

Cover: Boys viewing x-rays hung out to dry, ADH mobile truck unit, 1940s (*Courtesy of Alaska State
Library, Alaska Department of Health and Social Services Collection, PCA 143-999*)

Cover design by Dixon J. Jones, Rasmuson Library Graphics
Text design by Rachel Fudge

This book is dedicated
to those Alaskans
whose lives were changed forever by tuberculosis

:: Contents

:: Illustrations

:: Preface

IN THE FALL OF 1946 a mobile x-ray survey team visited a small Native village in interior Alaska. This village of seventy persons comprised about twenty households, each with two to eight members. Although most lived in one-room cabins, a few families had only tents for shelter. During their brief stay in the village, the team identified ten active cases of tuberculosis and several other individuals with x-rays suspicious for active disease. Because of the lack of sanatorium beds and other treatment resources at that time, only two of the newly discovered cases could be hospitalized.

When the team returned the following summer, they found that seven children and at least two adults in the village had died, each of whom had documented evidence of tuberculosis. Those who had not been hospitalized showed ominous progression of their disease, while many of the suspicious cases from the previous year were now suffering full-blown tuberculosis. Two such individuals were near death. There were no infants and no pregnant women left in the community.

One of the villagers asked the physician to come and see his nine-year-old son. The boy was lying in a tent on a few dirty blankets, within three feet of another son who had recently become very thin, was coughing constantly, and had occasionally spit up blood. The child was too weak to move and showed no interest in his surroundings. His father watched helplessly as the doctor examined the child. When he was told that his son had far advanced pulmonary tuberculosis and would die soon, the father pleaded, "Five of my children die this way—I don't want my other kids to go. Must we all die of the TB?"*

This poignant story illustrates the extent and impact of the tuberculosis problem in rural Alaska around the end of World War II. It would, in fact, be reasonable to suggest that this tuberculosis epidemic, with all its tragic personal, social, and economic consequences, was the most devastating event affecting the lives of Alaska Natives in the twentieth century. Few families in the past one hundred years have not been touched by this baleful disease. Many individuals did not live

---

* Leo J. Gehrig and Elaine A. Schwinge, "Must We All Die of the TB?" *Alaska's Health* 6, no. 10 (1947).

to grow up, or they escaped with damaged lungs; a crippled spine, knee, or hip; a scarred neck; or an irreparably impaired brain. Nearly everyone who survived lost a grandparent, parent, child, sibling, or friend. Although Alaska Natives bore and continue to bear the heaviest burden, tuberculosis also assaulted many foreign cannery workers, some Caucasians, and a few African Americans. In more recent years the disease has also ravaged new Alaska residents from Asia, the Pacific Islands, and Latin America and has laid a special curse upon individuals infected with HIV and AIDS.

This book tells the story of tuberculosis in Alaska—its likely origins, its relentless spread to the far corners of the land, and its grim impact on individuals, families, and society. It tells of the determined efforts to understand tuberculosis and to control the havoc it caused. The story unfolds from the point of view of the physicians, nurses, government officials, elected leaders, teachers, and missionaries who fought against it with every skill available to them, but also from the viewpoint of those—predominantly Alaska Natives—who suffered from the disease. The narrative contains elements of frustration and despair, but it also demonstrates extraordinary outcomes resulting from the hard work and determination of those afflicted, the health workers and their agencies, and the people of the territory and state.

At one level, this is the story of a remarkable success—one of the great triumphs of public health anywhere. As a result of the concentrated efforts of many agencies and individuals over about twenty-five years, the greatest killer in Alaska was brought into subjection. Yet the story has a darker side. The disease claimed many victims and changed the lives of the survivors and their families forever. Its ravages left especially deep and abiding scars on the outlook of Alaska Native people, and undoubtedly have hastened destructive changes in their cultures. The disease, moreover, has by no means been eradicated. Because of the many previously infected Alaskans at risk, changing socioeconomic conditions, the emergence of HIV/AIDS, immigration, and public indifference reflected in legislative withdrawal of program funds, the embers of this disease still smolder in the ashes, flaming up from time to time in cities and villages—a constant reminder that we have not quenched it.

The story of tuberculosis in Alaska is a microcosm of the havoc that the disease has wreaked worldwide for thousands of years. Few if any populations have had a more savage encounter with the disease than Alaskans, but in a sense what happened in Alaska was a late replay of what many groups of Europeans have suffered since the eighteenth century, and what the nations of the developing world continue to suffer today. What makes the Alaska experience notable is that it took place in a relatively small and defined population about a generation after the disease was coming under acceptable control elsewhere. While tuberculosis was declining rather rapidly elsewhere in the United States, it actually increased in Alaska, until public demand for action finally brought to bear control measures that were already standard elsewhere. Once the process began in earnest, tuberculosis retreated rapidly, although its threat persists.

In a broader sense, this book is the biography of a disease and how it has affected life, politics, and history in the state. Most histories of Alaska are part of a grand tapestry of the region's exploration, settlements, population shifts, economic trends, resource extraction, and political leaders. This history follows one thread in that vast tapestry—perhaps a white one to symbolize the "White Plague." The people in this story are rarely mentioned in standard histories of Alaska. They include doctors, teachers, public health nurses, x-ray technicians, citizen volunteers, and a few far-seeing politicians, but they also include the many individuals and families from all walks of life who carried the burden of tuberculosis.

This book is written for the public at large—especially the people of Alaska—but most of all for Alaska Natives, since the story intersects their lives again and again in real and moving ways. I have tried to document the story as fully as possible, with the hope that it can be a starting point for further studies in this neglected corner of Alaska history—the health of its people.

R.F.
Wasilla, Alaska
September 2004

:: Acknowledgments

THE IDEA FOR THIS BOOK, and indeed the impetus to complete it rather late in life, I owe to many colleagues and friends over the years, including some of those who played an important part in the story itself. It would be perilous to try to list everyone who has been helpful, but I cannot avoid naming some, at least, who gave me inspiration, encouragement, and information and freely shared documentary materials that would probably have not been otherwise available.

One of the first to set me on my course was Dr. George W. Comstock, an almost legendary figure in American epidemiology, who personally supervised the individual and community INH prophylaxis trials during the 1950s and 1960s. Dr. Comstock, whom I had met in Bethel in the mid-1960s, some years ago sent me a box of personal books and papers on tuberculosis in Alaska with the pointed suggestion that I should write the full story sometime. Dr. M. Walter Johnson, of Homer and Anchorage, has been a friend and colleague for nearly forty years. His office as clinical director at the Alaska Native Medical Center adjoined mine for several years during the early 1970s, while he served as tuberculosis control officer for the Alaska Area Native Health Service. His long-standing interest in Alaskan history, and tuberculosis in particular, has helped in ways too numerous to mention. Elfrida Nord, RN, has been a constant source of encouragement, not only personally and by pointing me to materials, but through her own excellent historical writings. Marge Larson of the American Lung Association of Alaska made available on a long-term loan important archival materials from the early days of the Alaska Tuberculosis Association. Dr. Robert Wainwright, formerly of the Arctic Investigations Program of the Centers for Disease Control and Prevention, steered me to neglected archival materials from the Arctic Health Research Center. Dr. Robert Fraser, the state director of tuberculosis control for over twenty years, read several chapters in draft and offered his encouragement. Dr. Beth Funk, the current tuberculosis control officer for the Alaska Division of Public Health, provided help and encouragement, and shared unpublished tuberculosis documents from the Alaska Department of Health and Social Services. Margery Albrecht, widow of Dr. C. Earl Albrecht, the leader of the struggle against tuberculosis in Alaska, generously made available many photographs and documents from her husband's papers. Dr. Arthur

C. Aufderheide, an eminent paleopathologist from the University of Northern Minnesota at Duluth, has been promptly and unfailingly helpful on several occasions, as has Professor Linda Green of the anthropology department of the University of Arizona, who has given me much encouragement. Professor Terrence Cole of the history department at the University of Alaska Fairbanks helped me obtain a number of old tuberculosis manuals and textbooks. Lisa and Max Dolchok of the Traditional Medicine Program of the Southcentral Foundation, Robert Sam of the Sitka Tlingit Tribe, and Harold Napoleon, a noted Yup'ik writer, have all been very supportive of the project. Most of these individuals have also read in draft one or more chapters of the book and have been helpful in other ways.

I am especially grateful to Don E. Dumond and Joan Braddock for reading the entire manuscript and making many valuable and constructive suggestions. Erica Hill of the University of Alaska Press devoted many hours to the manuscript and left it better in countless ways. In the few instances where I did not accept the suggestions of these individuals, I take full responsibility.

Librarians and archivists are of course indispensable to the historian. Here I would give special recognition to a longtime friend and helper Loretta G. Andress, formerly at the Alaska Health Sciences Library; Dennis F. Walle, archivist at the University of Alaska Anchorage, and his staff; Bruce Merrell, librarian of the Alaska Collection at the Z. J. Loussac Library in Anchorage; Dianne Brenner, formerly of the Anchorage Museum of History and Art; Bruce Parham of the National Archives and Records Administration, Pacific Alaska Region, in Anchorage; Anne Laura Wood and Kay Shelton at the Alaska State Historical Library in Juneau; and Ron Inouye and Rose Speranza of the Alaska and Polar Regions Department at Rasmuson Library, University of Alaska Fairbanks.

One of the pleasures of delving into this topic was that I was reintroduced to the contributions of those who have played an important part in the story itself. A number of the individuals who make an appearance in the book I have known personally, among them:

Alaska Department of Health: C. Earl Albrecht, Dorothy Craig, Milo Fritz, Leo Gehrig, Lois Jund, Mildred Mantle, Frank Pauls, Francis Phillips, Elaine Schwinge

Alaska Native Service/Indian Health Service: Richard Chao, Joseph Gallagher, M. Walter Johnson, Kazumi Kasuga, Martha and Joe Wilson, E. S. Rabeau, David W. Templin

Alaska Division of Public Health: Michael Beller, Arne Beltz, Robert I. Fraser, Elizabeth Funk, John Middaugh, Elfrida Nord

Arctic Health Research Center: A. B. Colyar, Catherine E. Haley, Mary Lou Hanson, Margaret Lantis, Theresa Overfield, Merilys E. Porter

Centers for Disease Control: George W. Comstock and David Sencer

Finally, I would like to give special thanks to my wife, Sheila, who has helped in ways too numerous to mention. She has been unceasingly caring, encouraging, and patient (indeed, long-suffering), and has repeatedly reminded me of the significance of the story and why it should be told. She also reviewed the entire book in draft form and with her sharp editorial eye offered many cogent suggestions on style and content.

:: Abbreviations

Agencies, Organizations, Health Workers, and Drugs

AANHS   Alaska Area Native Health Service (USPHS)

ACCA   Alaska Crippled Children's Association

ADH   Alaska Department of Health (territorial)

ADHW   Alaska Department of Health and Welfare (state)

ADHSS   Alaska Department of Health and Social Services (state)

AHRC   Arctic Health Research Center (USPHS)

AMA   American Medical Association

ANMC   Alaska Native Medical Center

ANS   Alaska Native Service (the Alaska Area Office of BIA)

ANHS   Alaska Native Health Service (USPHS)

ATA   Alaska Tuberculosis Association

BIA   Bureau of Indian Affairs (same as Office of Indian Affairs)

BoE   Bureau of Education

CDC   Communicable Disease Center, *later* Centers for Disease Control and Prevention (USPHS)

DIH   Division of Indian Health (USPHS)

DPH   Division of Public Health, a component of the ADHSS

IHS   Indian Health Service (USPHS)

INH   Isoniazid hydrochloride

NTA   National Tuberculosis Association

OIA   Office of Indian Affairs (see BIA)

PAS   Para-amino salicylic acid

PHS   (United States) Public Health Service

PPD   Purified Protein Derivative (used in tuberculin testing)

USCG   United States Coast Guard

USPHS   United States Public Health Service

USMHS   United States Marine-Hospital Service

USRCS   United States Revenue-Cutter Service

VA   Veterans Administration

Citations

ADN   *Anchorage Daily News*

ADT   *Anchorage Daily Times*

AH   *Alaska's Health*, published by the Alaska Department of Health (territorial)

AHW   *Alaska's Health and Welfare*, published by the Alaska Department of Health and Welfare

AHRC   Arctic Health Research Center papers, Robert Fortuine Collection,
Papers   Archives and Manuscripts Department, University of Alaska Anchorage

Albrecht   C. Earl Albrecht Collection, Archives and Manuscripts Department,
Collection   University of Alaska Anchorage

ATA   Alaska Tuberculosis Association Collection, American Lung
Collection   Association of Alaska

BIA   US Department of the Interior, Bureau of Indian Affairs, Alaska
Correspondence   Division, Correspondence, 1908–35, National Archives and Records Administration, RG 75

EB   *Epidemiology Bulletin*, published by the Epidemiology Section, Division of Public Health, Alaska Department of Health and Social Services

FDNM   *Fairbanks Daily News-Miner*

Governor   Alaska, Territorial Government. Governor, General
Correspondence   Correspondence, 1909–58, National Archives and Record Administration RG 80-14

GPO   Government Printing Office

JAE   *Juneau Alaska Empire*

MMWR   *Morbidity and Mortality Weekly Reports,* published by the Centers for Disease Control and Prevention, Public Health Service, US Department of Health and Human Services

:: Introduction

Tuberculosis: An Ancient Affliction

Tuberculosis Today—A Very Present Danger

Nearly 8.8 million new cases of tuberculosis were reported worldwide in 2002, and approximately 1.8 million people died of the disease. One-third of the world's population is already infected with the organism that causes tuberculosis; in fact, somewhere in the world someone is newly infected every second. Five to ten percent of those infected will develop active tuberculosis during their lifetimes. Left untreated, each person with active tuberculosis will infect from ten to fifteen people annually.[1]

In sub-Saharan Africa over two million new cases of tuberculosis are occurring annually as a result of the HIV/AIDS epidemic. Tuberculosis is a leading cause of death among those who are harboring HIV, accounting for some 13 percent of global AIDS deaths. Other factors increasing the spread of tuberculosis are wars and economic hardship, which lead to increased numbers of refugees, displaced persons, emigrants, and migrant laborers. In industrialized countries, urban homeless and prison populations are significant reservoirs of tuberculosis. In addition, the incidence of multidrug-resistant (MDR) strains of the tuberculosis organism is increasing worldwide, causing many infected individuals, even with modern treatment, to die of the disease.[2]

In the United States the number of reported tuberculosis cases rose nearly 20 percent in the period from 1985 to 1992, due in large part to declining funding for tuberculosis control, the spread of HIV/AIDS, large-scale immigration from countries where the disease is prevalent, increased transmission of the disease in institutional settings, and the development of MDR strains. Fortunately, the situation has improved somewhat since that time because of increased attention to treatment and prevention.[3] By 2003 the number of new active cases reported in the United States had declined for the twelfth straight year to an all-time low of 14,874, giving an overall incidence rate of 5.1 per 100,000. The highest incidence rates have remained in those aged sixty-five years and older, and the lowest in children under fifteen, although rates continue to decline in both groups.[4] The ethnic groups with the highest rates are Asians/Pacific Islanders (27.8 per 100,000), followed by black non-Hispanics (12.6 per 100,000), Hispanics (10.4 per 100,000), American Indians/Alaska Natives (6.8 per 100,000), and finally white non-Hispanics (1.5 per 100,000).

Nearly 51 percent of new cases reported in 2002 occurred in those born outside the United States.[5]

In Alaska, the State Division of Public Health reported that in 2002, the last year for which complete data are available, forty-nine cases of active tuberculosis were identified. Only two years before, the figure was 109 cases, or 17.4 per 100,000, the highest rate in the nation. Southwestern and northern Alaska, where the population includes large numbers of Alaska Natives, generally have the highest rates within the state. Over the five-year period from 1997 to 2002, 61 percent of all reported cases of tuberculosis occurred among Alaska Natives, who make up only 17 percent of the population. Many of the remainder were Asians or Pacific Islanders, who accounted for an additional 21 percent of the total cases, while making up only 5 percent of the state's population.[6]

Tuberculosis, the Disease

What is tuberculosis? A modern medical dictionary defines it as:

> a specific disease caused by the presence of *Mycobacterium tuberculosis*, which may affect almost any tissue or organ of the body, the most common seat of the disease being the lungs; the anatomical lesion is the tubercle . . . ; local symptoms vary according to the part affected; general symptoms are those of sepsis: hectic fever, sweats, and emaciation; often progressive with high mortality if not treated.[7]

The immediate cause of tuberculosis is the microorganism known as *Mycobacterium tuberculosis*, a rather slow-growing bacterium with a high fatty content in its cell wall. With a few exceptions, the susceptible individual acquires the organism through the respiratory tract by inhaling droplet nuclei, or tiny aerosol droplets containing live bacteria. Infected persons may produce these infectious droplets by coughing, sneezing, or even talking and singing.

Tuberculosis is spread almost exclusively from one person directly to another, with those most at risk being family and household members, or even coworkers in close proximity to the infected individual in a poorly ventilated work space. Despite widespread fears and traditional misapprehensions, tuberculosis is not spread by shaking hands or by contact with contaminated furniture, dishes, clothing, bedsheets, or house dust. Nor is it spread by food, with the exception of unpasteurized milk from cows infected with a related organism, *Mycobacterium bovis*, which may cause human disease.

The likelihood of disease transmission is enhanced by the virulence of the bacterial strain, the concentration of droplet nuclei in the environment, the proximity and length of exposure, and the genetic or immunological susceptibility of the person exposed. Good ventilation, with frequent air exchange, obviously limits the opportunity for spread. The tubercle bacillus is also acutely sensitive to the effects of ultraviolet light, both from natural sunlight and lamps.

With sufficient exposure, the susceptible individual inhales airborne droplets containing live bacteria into the lungs, where they initially settle in the tiny terminal air spaces, or alveoli, of the lower lung fields, causing what is known as a primary infection. The first line of defense by the body are the cells known as macrophages, which line the walls of the alveoli. These cells ingest the bacteria and immobilize them while the body begins to develop a protective immunological reaction known as cell-mediated immunity. The tubercle bacilli in the macrophages may multiply slowly, killing the host cells and spreading first to surrounding tissues and then to local lymph nodes, occasionally even seeding the bloodstream. After four to six weeks, however, the growing tissue immunity causes the bacteria in most people to be walled off by fibrous tissue and sometimes destroyed. This complex immune reaction may be demonstrated by the so-called tuberculin test (or Mantoux test), in which a derivative of the tubercle bacillus called PPD (purified protein derivative) is injected into the layers of the skin, leading to a reaction of localized swelling and firmness. A positive PPD test demonstrates that the individual has been infected with the tubercle bacillus.

About 90 to 95 percent of those who convert their skin reaction from negative to positive are able to isolate and contain the tubercle bacilli within their bodies and thus remain well. Their chest x-rays may remain normal, or they may show small areas of scar tissue or calcification, often in the hilar, or root region, of the lungs. A few in whom the disease progresses somewhat further before becoming inactive may show on x-ray the so-called Ghon complex, a combination of a scar (often with calcification) in the periphery of the lower lung field, together with enlarged hilar lymph nodes. Most of these individuals remain healthy for the remainder of their lives, although their PPD skin test will remain positive.

In about 5 to 10 percent of infected individuals, the body's immunological response is insufficient and the tuberculosis bacteria gain a foothold, continuing to multiply in the tissues and causing a low-grade destructive inflammatory reaction known as a tubercle. Some tubercles contain live bacteria, usually within the phagocytes. The local tissue is gradually destroyed, causing structural or functional disability. Individuals with a reduced immunologic response or a genetic susceptibility develop the progressive disease called tuberculosis. The bacteria seed the bloodstream and may be carried to any organ of the body, although the upper lung fields, or apices, seem to be a favored destination because of the higher oxygen concentrations found there.[8]

In the lungs, tuberculosis causes an intense inflammatory response manifested by liquefaction of the tissues and sometimes the formation of cavities teeming with proliferating bacteria. Tissue destruction with damage to the walls of the

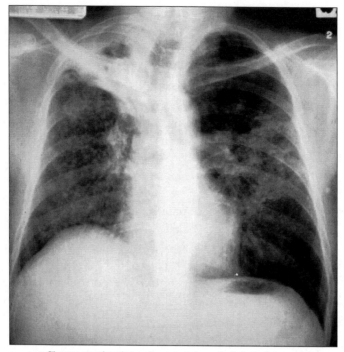

:: Chest x-ray showing pulmonary tuberculosis in both lungs. ::
(Courtesy Beth Funk, Alaska Division of Public Health)

bronchi leads to cough and sputum production, and, when a blood vessel is eroded, to hemoptysis, or the spitting of blood. Such patients usually have a rapid downhill course if not treated promptly and appropriately. Other less common sites of tuberculous infection include the pleurae (layers covering the lungs), pericardium (a fibrous covering of the heart), peritoneum (lining of the abdominal cavity), spine, the ends of long bones, the kidneys, or the fallopian tubes. Tuberculosis of the pleurae, pericardium, and peritoneum may be associated with the accumulation of inflammatory fluid, called an effusion. Tuberculosis of the spine, known as Pott's disease, leads to the collapse of one or more vertebral bodies, often with a sharp angulation of the affected segment of the spine. Other individuals develop infection and destruction of some of the larger joints, especially the knee, hip, ankle, and wrist. Before the modern era of treatment, a particularly widespread form of tuberculosis was scrofula, which involved the lymph nodes of the neck, especially in children, and was characterized by swelling of the glands, chronic foul drainage, and residual scarring of the skin.

A few primary cases rapidly progress to one of three severe and, before the development of effective anti-tuberculosis drugs, nearly uniformly fatal forms of the disease. The first type is progressive tuberculous pneumonia, once colorfully known as galloping consumption. The second is caused by a rapid blood-borne dissemination of the organism throughout the body, causing overwhelming infection and tiny tubercles in many different organs. The similarity in appearance of these lesions to millet seeds led to the name miliary tuberculosis. The third type of rapidly progressive tuberculosis is tuberculous meningitis, in which the organisms infect the cerebrospinal fluid and the brain coverings called meninges. All of these forms are more common in children, the aged, or those with impaired immunity.

Latent foci of the tubercle bacillus may sometimes reactivate, usually because of some change in the status of the immune system. Some individuals were infected with the organism as children or young adults, when their body defenses effectively neutralized the disease. Others may once have had active disease and received, for whatever reason, an inadequate course of treatment. Most reactivations involve the lungs, but other sites can also be affected. The lesions cause local tissue death, which in the lungs may lead to cavity formation and erosion of blood vessels. Such patients may be very infectious to others, since they usually cough up large numbers of organisms in the form of aerosol droplets. Reactivation disease is frequently progressive, leading to fever, weight loss, and in many cases, if untreated, to death.

Pulmonary tuberculosis is diagnosed principally by examination of the sputum for tubercle bacilli, either by direct stained smear or by culture, or both. Less definitive but also widely used is the chest x-ray, which may show characteristic patterns in the lungs, such as cavities, fibrosis, and calcifications. The PPD test is still widely used to identify those who have been infected with the organism and are thus at special risk of developing the disease.[9]

Tuberculosis, the Illness

While tuberculosis the disease may be studied through objective methods, tuberculosis the illness is more subtle and subjective. The doctor, scientist, and technician study the disease; the patient (and to some extent his or her family) experiences the illness. Since few physicians today are familiar with the late stages of the disease, I turn to the descriptions from tuberculosis manuals of fifty to a hundred years ago.

Not everyone with tuberculosis felt sick, especially those with primary tuberculosis, or in the earlier stages of pulmonary tuberculosis. Since they were able to carry out their normal daily activities and obligations without any apparent impairment, many such individuals were unwilling to accept their diagnosis and the rigorous and often ineffective treatment that followed. In fact, the body's natural immunity or defense mechanisms often caused spontaneous healing, with the result that "victims" never really knew that they had been sick at all until the telltale x-ray revealed the scars, sometimes many years later.

For the less fortunate individual with the disease, however, symptoms inevitably appeared as the disease progressed. Individuals often remembered frequent "colds," manifested by general malaise and a slight fever, although without the runny noses and sore throats characteristic of a viral illness.

Unexplained lassitude or weariness was often the first symptom of pulmonary tuberculosis. This was gradual in onset and frequently attributed to overwork, especially since the disease was widespread among the working classes. Tiredness was first noticed in the latter part of the day and might be relieved by a short rest or by a few days off from work. Soon, however, the fatigue returned and began appearing earlier in the day. Every daily task, at home or at work, became a burden. As the disease progressed, tiredness progressed to total physical exhaustion, with simple tasks such as eating or talking taking a dreadful energy toll. The patient would fall into bed only to find no rest during the night.[10]

Fever was a common finding, manifested as a slight elevation of temperature of perhaps a half degree Fahrenheit in the late afternoon. As the disease progressed, however, temperature changes became more pronounced, often with normal morning temperatures and an elevation to 100–101°F in the late afternoon. In the late stages of the disease, the temperature might peak at 103–104°F every evening for months at a time and never fall to normal during the twenty-four-hour period, a pattern formerly known as a hectic fever.[11] An accompanying increase in the pulse rate was often perceived by the patient as a rapid, pounding heartbeat after minimal exertion. Another consequence of the fever was flushing of the face—the so-called hectic flush of the tuberculous made famous by the Romantic writers of the nineteenth century.[12] The redness was particularly prominent in the cheeks and contrasted with the general pallor of the skin.[13]

So-called night sweats—the patient waking in the night drenched in perspiration—were probably less common than the public was led to believe. A subtler type of sweating was more common, namely, increased moisture of the palms and armpits, probably due to a low-grade fever.

Some cases presented with vague digestive disturbances. These might begin as excessive gas, or a feeling of fullness after eating. Loss of appetite usually followed, together with a reluctance to make the effort to eat, perhaps from feelings of depression. Weight loss was the inevitable consequence. Few patients with progressive disease failed to show a loss of at least a few pounds, and some literally wasted away as their disease developed.[14]

The most prominent symptom of pulmonary tuberculosis, however, and present in virtually every case, was a cough, generally most noticeable upon awakening in the morning and at bedtime. Sometimes coughing spells could be provoked by talking, laughing, exertion, or a change in the temperature of the ambient environment. The cough could be paroxysmal, occurring in violent fits lasting several minutes, and often ending in a bout of vomiting. These spells, although exhausting, could be productive of virtually no sputum, or at best a little clear mucus. In the terminal stages of the disease, coughing could be painful, severe, and incessant, exhausting the patient's energy reserves.[15]

With cavity formation in the lungs, the cough became productive of a copious amount of sputum, which was highly infectious. Posture sometimes influenced the amount of coughing, as secretions drained from the cavity into the nearby bronchi. The sputum itself varied with the stage of the disease. In the early stage it might be mucoid with gray or yellowish flecks. As the disease progressed into cavity formation, more of the material became solid or semisolid. In the last stages, with significant tissue destruction, the sputum could become simply liquid pus.[16]

Spitting of blood, or hemoptysis, became the hallmark sign of tuberculosis, at least in the public imagination, although by no means all persons with tuberculosis manifested it. Caused by an erosion of a blood vessel in the lung, it was certainly the most alarming symptom, especially if the quantity of blood was substantial. In a few cases it was the presenting symptom, when after a tickle in the throat the person tasted blood or noted a slight pinkish tinge to the sputum. Initially the blood was usually bright red, frothy, and minimal in quantity, but as the disease developed, larger hemoptyses could occur, including a massive arterial hemorrhage resulting in the sufferer drowning in his own blood.

Shortness of breath, or dyspnea, usually paralleled the amount of lung tissue affected, and was particularly frequent in cases in which fibrosis was prominent. Sometimes breathlessness resulted from a spontaneous collapse of the lung, called a pneumothorax, or from a pleural effusion, in which inflammatory fluid in the pleural cavity compressed the lung. Dyspnea could also be due to chest pain, either from pleurisy or from a muscle strained from excess coughing.

All these symptoms and signs could be exaggerated and exacerbated in individuals suffering from tuberculous pneumonia, or galloping consumption. The onset in such cases might be a sudden chill, associated with chest pain, breathlessness, and a productive cough, much the same picture as with a bacterial pneumonia from other causes. With miliary spread, manifestations of the disease could be nonspecific, an unexplained fever with weakness and prostration being typical. Tuberculous meningitis presented most often in children, and usually began with fussiness, drowsiness, loss of appetite, restlessness, and weight loss. Headache was a prominent feature, but since many small patients could not localize their pain, its manifestation was inconsolable screaming. Fever and vomiting followed, and not infrequently seizures. Without modern treatment the disease progressed rapidly to coma and death.[17]

Chronic extrapulmonary tuberculosis might be quite subtle, with few symptoms unless there was local tissue destruction leading to impaired function. Tuberculosis of the brain, kidney, adrenal glands, fallopian tubes, seminal vesicles, or intestinal tract might not give any clear clinical picture until irreparable damage had occurred. The only signs and symptoms in scrofula might be nontender, swollen glands in the neck. Initially these glands were freely movable and clearly distinguishable under the skin, although as the disease progressed the glands tended to mat together, became adherent to the skin, and ultimately formed an abscess, with chronic drainage and scarring.[18]

Tuberculous pleurisy might begin with malaise, a low-grade fever, slight to moderate breathlessness, and either a sharp one-sided chest pain or a dull central chest pain made worse by deep breathing or coughing. The pain diminished as the pleurisy progressed because inflammatory fluid accumulated between the layers of the pleurae separating the inflamed surfaces. This same fluid, however, caused gradual compression of the adjacent lung tissue and increased shortness of breath. In pericarditis, fluid accumulating between the pericardial layers would lead to compression of the heart through a process known as cardiac tamponade. In chronic cases, the pericardium became scarred and rigid, restricting the contractions of the heart and leading to congestive heart failure. In peritonitis, the symptoms might vary considerably, from none at all to acute fever, abdominal pain, and fluid accumulation in the abdominal cavity.

Bone and joint tuberculosis began insidiously and typically caused pain and swellings, known as cold abscesses, near the larger joints, such as the hip, knee, or ankle. In long-standing cases bone and joint destruction resulted, often with persistent draining sinuses. Those with chronic tuberculosis of the spine, or Pott's disease, sometimes developed paralysis of the lower extremities or loss of bladder or bowel control due to pressure on spinal nerves. In advanced cases, the wedging of vertebrae and consequent telescoping of the rib cage could lead to breathlessness, due to an inability to expand the lungs fully.

Psychologically, the diagnosis of tuberculosis could be a devastating blow, especially in the days before effective drugs. Often it meant a death sentence, or at the very least a lifetime of illness, disability, isolation, and poverty. If institutional treatment were available at all, the "cure" sometimes took years, without guaranteeing a favorable outcome. Furthermore, family members were separated for long periods and with uncertain economic consequences. Many of those who survived were not able to support themselves in their previous work, if they were able to find work at all. The stigma of tuberculosis clung to a consumptive, even if the disease process was arrested. Yet, curiously, many patients with tuberculosis had an optimistic view of life, especially in the latter stages of the disease when their bodies were wasted and their lives were ebbing away. This "hope of the tuberculous," known in the Latin phrase as *spes phthisicorum* (or *spes phthisica*), doubtless eased many to their graves.

Tuberculosis in History

The origin of tuberculosis in humans has been the subject of great speculation. All authorities concede that the disease in humans is very old and predates written records. One widely held view is that *M. tuberculosis,* the organism affecting humans, evolved from a more ancient but closely related organism, *M. bovis*, which infects a wide variety of warm-blooded animals, including rodents, deer, and livestock. An argument in favor of such a view is that the bovine strain can cause disease in humans, whereas the human strain is greatly attenuated in cattle.[19] Initial human contact with the bovine organism was probably sporadic and resulted from eating raw or inadequately cooked meat. About 8,000 to 10,000 years ago, however, humans began to domesticate cattle and supplement their diets with milk and cheese, another means of spreading the bacteria. As human contact with cattle intensified, a cow or steer with infected lungs might have transmitted the disease to the respiratory tracts of humans.[20] Over the generations, the organisms infecting humans became more dependent on oxygen (aerophilic) and evolved the ability to spread from person to person via the respiratory tract.[21]

Tuberculosis in humans remained sporadic for many centuries, especially when primarily transmitted by the ingestion of contaminated meat or milk products. It was only after the respiratory tract became the primary mode of transmission that it could spread widely in a susceptible population, especially when crowding occurred. Initially the disease infected primarily children and young adults, but gradually it began to attack older individuals.

Although tuberculosis, at least in modern times, most often affects the lungs, the earliest physical evidence of tuberculosis in most areas of the world is limited to skeletal remains, which represent a relatively uncommon form of the disease. Many of the changes in bones affected by tuberculosis are quite distinctive, both grossly and microscopically, but absolute certainty in a specific instance may remain elusive unless findings are confirmed by DNA techniques. One of the earliest examples of tuberculosis determined by sequencing a DNA fragment of the organism comes from a skeleton with signs of Pott's disease found in Egypt and dating to some 5,400 years ago.[22] Other skeletal remains in Egypt have demonstrated the characteristic changes of spinal tuberculosis, including those of a priest of Amen, dating from around 1000 BC, with a sharply angled hunchback, destruction of vertebral bodies, and even evidence of a psoas abscess, a collection of pus along the sides of the lower spine.[23] One mummy of a five-year-old child showed recent pulmonary hemorrhage, tuberculosis of the lung and vertebrae, and even acid-fast bacilli.[24] Skeletal remains with presumptive spinal tuberculosis have been found from as early as 6,000 years ago in archeological sites in Italy, Germany, and Denmark.[25]

Ancient records from throughout the ancient Middle East, including Babylonian spells, Old Testament writings, and the epics of Homer, describe a constellation of symptoms, signs, and clinical course that could point to pulmonary tuberculosis. Early Hindu and Chinese records also seem to point to the presence of tuberculosis.[26]

The Greek physician Hippocrates and his followers in the fifth and fourth centuries BC described in detail several types of a disease known as *phthisis*, from a verb meaning "to waste away" or "decay." One form, which must have been fairly common, was characterized by a protracted course, a productive cough, malodorous sputum, sweats, and severe weight loss. When diagnosed at a late stage, the accounts say, the outlook was hopeless. Another form of consumption had a more favorable prognosis, with the victim sometimes surviving seven or nine years if treated with special diets and botanical remedies. A rather remarkable description of a disease of the spine—almost certainly Pott's disease—may be found in the Hippocratic treatise called *Joints*. This account mentions the characteristic hunchback, the presence of tubercles, bladder complications, and the occurrence of abscesses along the lower spine.[27]

Medieval and Renaissance physicians advanced our understanding of tuberculosis very little, instead accepting rather uncritically the beliefs of the physicians of antiquity. Scrofula was sometimes mentioned, particularly within the context of the supposed ability of kings to cure it by the laying on of royal hands. Presumably tuberculosis continued to smolder in Europe and elsewhere, but no one yet had a clear concept of the disease, nor did they relate in any way phthisis, spinal tuberculosis, and scrofula.[28] The rising prevalence of phthisis (or, in English, consumption) in seventeenth-century Europe is suggested by its frequent mention in literary works, including those by Shakespeare, Milton, and in the famous line by John Bunyan, "The captain of all these men of death that came against him to take him away, was the consumption...."[29] The seventeenth-century Dutch physician François de le Boë (Franciscus Sylvius) was the first to describe "tubercles" in the lungs.[30]

As the Industrial Revolution progressed in Great Britain and on the continent, many rural people flocked to the cities, where they lived in crowded, decaying, poorly heated, and poorly ventilated tenements. Consumption became the leading cause of death in Europe, claiming its victims predominantly among the urban poor. The disease found favorable conditions among the malnourished, exhausted, and spiritually depleted factory workers and their children. By the end of the eighteenth century, consumption was epidemic in Europe, affecting not only the poor but also the more economically favored.

The clinicians and scientists of the period, however, viewed consumption as a constitutional, not an infectious, disease. Those affected were said to have inherited a predisposition (or diathesis) to tuberculosis, which became manifest in their manner of living, with poverty, alcohol abuse, and moral depravity usually the precipitating factors. Those susceptible to the disease were thought to have certain inherited physical characteristics, especially a narrow (or "phthisic") chest.

By the end of the eighteenth century, consumption was becoming more widespread in its distribution, involving the middle class and even the well-to-do. A curious new attitude began to develop that the disease was associated with an increased sensitivity to life and beauty. Poets, musicians, and artists seemed particularly affected and people speculated that the disease itself played some part in the creative process, perhaps as a result of the persistent fever.[31]

It wasn't until 1868 that a French researcher, Jean Antoine Villemin, demonstrated that tuberculosis was contagious through a series of elegant experiments involving injecting extracts of tuberculous lesions into rabbits, which then developed the classic manifestations of tuberculosis. He was also able to show that tuberculosis, a word first used in English in 1860,[32] flourished where population density was high, while it was rare in scattered populations.[33]

A German physician, Robert Koch, made the discovery that forever changed thinking about tuberculosis, announcing in 1882 that he had identified microscopically the organism causing the disease, and that he had cultured it from sputum and then reinfected laboratory animals. Despite the apparent conclusiveness of his findings, it was years before the infectiousness of tuberculosis was widely accepted. In 1890 Koch announced that he had discovered a "cure" for tuberculosis in the form of tuberculin, an extract he had prepared from the tuberculosis organism. Although this substance proved worthless as a mode of treatment, it turned out to have another valuable property. A purified form, called PPD (purified protein derivative), is still employed today as an essential tool for tuberculosis case finding.[34] The identification of Koch's bacillus, either in smear or in culture, remains the gold standard for the diagnosis of tuberculosis.

The next diagnostic advance in tuberculosis came from the German physicist Wilhelm Konrad Röntgen, who in 1895 announced his discovery of x-rays. Now, for the first time, doctors could actually look "inside" the living patient. As techniques improved and equipment became safer, radiographic images were routinely used not only to diagnose individual patients but also to screen large populations for tuberculosis.

As diagnostic methods improved, the true extent of tuberculosis became even more painfully clear. In city slums, especially among immigrants and minority populations, the disease was the principal cause of death both in Europe and America through the first quarter of the twentieth century, although for reasons that are unclear, mortality and prevalence seemed to decline gradually after the middle of the nineteenth century. In the latter part of the nineteenth century, the death rate from tuberculosis in Boston was 400 per 100,000, and tuberculosis accounted for nearly one-quarter of the deaths in New York and Philadelphia. European rates were at least as high, with Budapest recording a rate of 800 per 100,000 in 1876.[35] Economic factors are clearly indicated by the fact that in 1890, some of the poorer sections of Lower Manhattan in New York City had a tuberculosis death rate of 776 per 100,000, while in the prosperous Upper West Side the rate was only 49.[36] At the end of World War I, the great Spanish flu epidemic selectively ravaged the tuberculous, while many who recovered developed tuberculosis in their weakened state.[37]

By the 1930s, tuberculosis still claimed more than 200 lives per 100,000 in most cities of Europe and North America, with much higher rates in South America. Manila's rate was 650 per 100,000; other Asian cities probably had comparable mortality.

At the end of World War II, nearly all developed nations were experiencing significant decreases in tuberculosis mortality, with rates between 20 and 30 per 100,000 for northern Europe. The reasons for this decline are largely unknown, although a general improvement in housing, nutrition, and economic conditions, especially among the working classes, probably played a part. Methods of treatment were still at a primitive level throughout this period and had little effect, although efforts to isolate those with active disease likely contributed to the decline. In North America the worst conditions continued among minorities, especially African Americans and Native Americans, and among the urban poor.

Evolution of Treatment in Tuberculosis

An aphorism of medicine is that if a disease has many treatments, then none is effective. Since antiquity, almost every therapeutic option available to physicians or quacks has been tried for tuberculosis. Without knowledge of the true cause and mode of spread of the disease, all treatment was necessarily empirical.

Early Chinese and Egyptian remedies were largely derived from plants, but also included animal matter such as urine and dung, as well as mineral substances.[38] For the worst types of phthisis, with its inexorable downhill course, Hippocrates advised no treatment at all, whereas for those with a better prognosis, he prescribed a decoction of lentils, hellebore, a nutritious diet, vomiting after meals, and walks out of the wind and sun.[39] The Roman physician Galen stressed the value of baths, oil rubs, diet, and especially milk—human milk where possible, but otherwise that of goats and asses.[40]

As early as the medieval period, kings were widely believed to heal scrofula, known as the king's evil, by touching the afflicted person. The practice was first recorded in the fifth century among the Franks and persisted as late as the coronation of King Charles X of France in 1824. For centuries, physicians in Renaissance Europe tried various measures, including harsh drugs, purges, enemas, bleeding, leeches, and blistering, in the hope of arresting the relentless march of the disease. There were advocates of gentler remedies as well, such as plasters, poultices, coffee, tea, or tobacco. The great seventeenth-century English clinician Thomas Sydenham advocated horseback riding in the country.[41]

Towards the end of the eighteenth century, it became fashionable for those suffering from tuberculosis, at least in northern countries, to seek a change of air in a sunny climate. The sea voyage itself was considered salubrious and Italy was among the most popular destinations.[42] Treatment became less aggressive in the nineteenth century, although there remained fierce advocates of bleeding and purging, notably Dr. Benjamin Rush, one of the signers of the Declaration of Independence.

A new approach for treating tuberculosis seems to have originated in England in 1836 with George Bodington, who advocated fresh, cold air, light and progressive exercise, a good dinner accompanied by wine, and an opium pill for rest. For these revolutionary and eminently sensible ideas, he was bitterly attacked in the medical press.[43] In 1859 a young German medical graduate named Hermann Brehmer established an institution for the treatment of tuberculosis in the mountains of Silesia, recommending a regimen of fresh air, moderate exercise, a liberal diet, and water treatments. One of his patients and pupils, Peter Dettweiler, modified this regimen by insisting that his patients rest for extended periods on open-air porches. Soon the idea was prevalent throughout Europe that rest and fresh mountain air were beneficial to the tuberculous, and many consumptives flocked to facilities in Switzerland and elsewhere.[44] In America the idea of fresh-air treatment is particularly associated with Dr. Edward Livingston Trudeau, who as a young medical graduate developed tuberculosis. His disease progressed rapidly and he resolved to spend his last days in his beloved Adirondacks. Relaxing at Saranac Lake, he found that his condition rapidly improved; his fever went down and he began to gain weight. Finally, in 1884, he built a cottage hospital at Saranac, New York, which over the years grew into the Trudeau Sanatorium, once the foremost center for treating tuberculosis in North America.[45]

Most of those who suffered from tuberculosis in America in the late nineteenth century sought a change of climate if they could afford it. Many went west, including a large number to the mountains of Colorado and a substantial contingent to the desert southwest. Still others moved south, to the seashore, or to the bracing air of the northern forests. None of these moves had any scientific merit, of course, other than perhaps getting the patient out of the city and into the fresh air.

The poor—those most affected by the disease—had no such options. A few terminal cases were treated in city hospitals, but the majority died in crowded tenements. In Philadelphia, Dr. Lawrence Flick, who like Trudeau suffered from the disease, not only established tuberculosis hospitals and dispensaries for the urban poor but also founded a major sanatorium in the Pennsylvania countryside.[46]

The details of sanatorium treatment remained basically the same for both rich and poor, although the quality of the surroundings and the amenities favored the paying patients. Most early sanatoriums were not large institutional buildings, but rather a series of small cottages with room for six to eight patients. Treatment first of all was bed rest—sometimes for months, or until the fever was gone. Most patients were expected to sleep out of doors, or at least in a room open to the outside air. Much of the day they spent wrapped in blankets in lounging chairs on the porches of their cottages. Progress was largely measured by weight gain, and to this end the patients were force-fed milk and raw eggs—sometimes gallons of the former and over a dozen of the latter each day. If patients improved, they were gradually allowed to increase their activity by walking on the grounds. Few if any drugs were used, except for laxatives.

The essence of the treatment was discipline. Patients were presented with a detailed rule book upon their admission, and they were responsible for obeying every article. They were told what and when to eat, when to get up in the morning and when to go to bed at night. An almost inviolable rule was the two-hour rest period in the afternoon, from two until four. The idea of discipline was that the patients would totally give up direction of their lives to their physician, and invest their faith in his ministrations. Unwavering nurses, often ex-tuberculosis patients themselves, managed the institutions on a sterile and rigid schedule, whereas the physician might visit on a weekly basis.[47]

Surgical treatment for tuberculosis, particularly the partial collapse of an infected lung, dates back at least to the late eighteenth century. The notion that a lung "put at rest" would be better able to heal led to the concept of therapeutic pneumothorax, or the introduction of air into the pleural cavity, a technique that became a standard form of treatment between approximately 1915 and World War II.[48] Pneumothorax was a harrowing procedure for the patient, despite morphine and local anesthetic. Moreover, the procedure could be technically difficult, especially when scar tissue in the lungs and pleurae prevented the needle from entering the pleural space. Several dangerous complications could ensue, including air embolism, leading to breathlessness, seizures, and even sudden death.[49] In about 1933 a related and somewhat safer procedure called pneumoperitoneum was introduced, in which air was injected into the abdominal cavity to prevent full aeration of the lungs by interfering with the downward movement of the diaphragm. Both techniques, however, had to be repeated every six weeks or so, since with time the air in the cavities was reabsorbed, leading to re-expansion of the lungs. Pneumothorax and pneumoperitoneum could be performed in the sanatorium, whereas more invasive surgical procedures required a full operating suite in a general hospital.

Another idea for minimizing the expansion of a diseased lung was phrenicectomy, or cutting the phrenic nerve at the base of the neck, causing paralysis of half the diaphragm and thus greatly diminishing respiratory excursions on that side. A later, less permanent modification was merely to crush the nerve, a procedure that caused partial paralysis of the diaphragm but that had to be repeated every six months or so.

For those with scarred pleurae unsuitable for pneumothorax, another briefly popular technique for permanently collapsing the apex of the lung involved stripping or dissecting the parietal pleurae from inside the chest wall and inserting an inert material outside the lung to prevent it from expanding completely. Initially a wad of paraffin was used, a procedure known as plombage. Liquid fat was also used for this purpose, as were small hollow Lucite spheres not unlike Ping-Pong balls. A far more mutilating procedure called thoracoplasty involved the removal of several of the upper ribs on the affected side, causing permanent collapse of the upper segment of the lung. This operation was particularly designed for those who had a tuberculous cavity in the upper lobes of the lung. Besides being subject to more complications, particularly surgical sepsis, the procedure also left a distorted and unsightly chest wall. Thoracoplasty originated in the nineteenth century and reached its peak in the 1930s and 1940s.[50]

Surgical removal of diseased lobules, lobes, and even entire lungs became common procedures by the mid-1930s, although the complication rate was high. One of the major difficulties was the so-called bronchopleural fistula, a chronic tuberculous infection of the area of bronchial closure, which often led to death. This problem was not solved until the advent of effective anti-tuberculosis drugs, when, for a short period, the more heroic surgical procedures staged a revival. Surgery had largely disappeared as a treatment for tuberculosis by about 1960, when its benefits were largely outweighed by its risks.[51]

The ultimate dream of physicians has always been to cure this stubborn disease by a specific and effective drug, the fabled magic bullet. The first such drug was streptomycin, developed by Albert Schatz and Selman Waksman in 1944 from a strain of soil fungi. After suitable animal experiments, clinical trials were undertaken. Although a few miliary tuberculosis and tuberculous meningitis cases were actually cured, it soon became apparent that the organism rapidly became resistant to the drug. Other problems were that the drug had to be administered by a painful injection, and that some individuals developed a severe balance disorder due to toxic effects on the vestibular portion of the inner ear.[52]

In 1946 a Danish researcher, Jorgen Lehmann, reported on a second effective anti-tuberculosis agent, para-aminosalicylic acid (PAS), a chemical cousin of aspirin. Although initial clinical trials were encouraging, PAS had significant limitations. The tuberculosis organism again rapidly adapted itself to the drug when it was used alone. Patients also found the drug difficult to take, since it might involve a dosage of up to 15 grams, or thirty large pills, a day.

The third drug to be synthesized, isoniazid (INH), remains the mainstay of tuberculosis treatment. Known chemically since 1912, the drug was first manufactured and tested clinically in 1951 by three pharmaceutical firms—Squibb, Hoffman-La Roche, and Bayer—based in part on Gerhard Domagk's work on thiosemicarbazones. After extensive trials, the drug was finally released for general use in 1952.[53] INH had all the virtues that scientists had been searching for in an anti-tuberculosis medication: it was inexpensive to make, required only a small daily dosage, and had relatively few side effects. Its use alone, however, also led to resistance on the part of the tubercle bacillus.

A Scottish scientist, John Crofton, proposed a solution to the problem of drug resistance: cases should be treated not with one drug, but with a combination of drugs. Over the next decade, for the first time in history, even advanced cases of tuberculosis could be cured. Sanatoriums and surgery were found to be largely superfluous.[54]

Since the advent of INH, several new anti-tuberculosis drugs have been developed, the most important of which are ethambutol (1962) and rifampin (1966), which largely replaced streptomycin and PAS in the routine treatment of the disease. INH itself remains the single most useful drug because of its low cost, relative lack of toxicity, and value in both treatment and prevention. The anti-tuberculosis drugs brought tuberculosis into the medical mainstream, with the result that patients are generally treated in the hospital for only brief periods, if at all.[55]

The federal Centers for Disease Control and Prevention periodically publishes recommended treatment guidelines for tuberculosis, based on the twin goals of curing the individual patient and minimizing the spread of the disease to others. All cases should be treated with a comprehensive approach to both medical and social issues, and treatment should follow the principles of directly observed therapy (DOT), in which a health worker observes the patient take each prescribed dose of medication. The current recommendation provides a four-drug regimen in the initial phase of treatment, at least until the results of drug sensitivity have been reported. The details of treatment depend on many individual factors, but for most patients the recommended initial drugs include INH, rifampin, pyrazinamide, and ethambutol for a two-month period. Assuming the organism is found to be sensitive to standard drugs, pyrazinamide and ethambutol are discontinued after eight weeks, while INH and rifampin are continued for a total of twenty-six weeks.[56]

Tuberculosis is a complex and ancient enemy of mankind and may be with us always, despite our best efforts. It is a chronic, infectious disease that, without appropriate treatment, can cause death, disability, and deformity. Anyone is susceptible, whether rich or poor, young or old. Until modern times the diagnosis of tuberculosis, like AIDS today, seemed like a death sentence, with the sufferer harboring little hope of ever returning to home, family, or work. The consumptive was often shunned by society, and many of the afflicted were condemned to die miserably in filthy tenements. Despite the antiquity of the disease, effective treatments were developed only around the middle of the twentieth century. Although tuberculosis has faded somewhat from the consciousness of both health officials and the general public, especially in the United States, it remains a serious threat worldwide.

This book is about the story of tuberculosis in Alaska—one distant corner of the world where this disease has had a profound and lasting impact on its people and their history.

Notes

1. World Health Organization, Geneva, Fact Sheet No. 104, rev. March 2004.

2. World Health Organization, Geneva, Fact Sheet No. 104, rev. August 2002; World Health Organization, Geneva, Press Release WHO/31, 23 April 1993.

3. "World TB Day—March 24, 2002," USDHHS, CDC, MMWR 51 (March 22, 2002): 229.

4. "Reported Tuberculosis in the United States, 2003," CDC, US Department of Health and Human Services, September 2004.

5. "Reported Tuberculosis in the United States, 2002," CDC, US Department of Health and Human Services, September 2003.

6. Personal communication from Beth Funk, ADHSS, DPH, Section of Epidemiology.

7. *Stedman's Medical Dictionary*, 26th ed. (Baltimore: Williams and Wilkins, 1996).

8. Lloyd N. Friedman, *Tuberculosis: Current Concepts and Treatment*, 2nd ed. (Boca Raton, FL: CRC Press, 2001), 20.

9. A modern discussion of these issues may be found in recent textbooks such as Michael D. Iseman, *A Clinician's Guide to Tuberculosis* (Philadelphia: Lippincott Williams & Wilkins, 2000); Friedman, *Tuberculosis*; and William N. Rom and Stuart M. Garay, *Tuberculosis* (Boston: Little Brown and Company, 1996).

10. R. Y. Keers and B. G. Rigden, *Pulmonary Tuberculosis: A Handbook for Students and Practitioners*, 3rd ed. (Edinburgh: E. & S. Livingstone Ltd., 1953), 72–73.

11. Maurice Fishberg, *Pulmonary Tuberculosis* (Philadelphia and New York: Lea & Febiger, 1916), 178–79.

12. Note, for example, Thoreau's *Journal* entry for June 11, 1852, "Decay and disease are often beautiful, like the pearly tear of the shellfish and the hectic glow of consumption."

13. Keers and Rigden, *Pulmonary Tuberculosis*, 78.

14. Compare the line of John Keats, who died of tuberculosis, in "Ode to a Nightingale": "Where youth grows pale, and spectre-thin, and dies."

15. Fishberg, *Pulmonary Tuberculosis*, 150–56.

16. Fishberg, *Pulmonary Tuberculosis*, 157; Keers and Rigden, *Pulmonary Tuberculosis*, 80–81.

17. William Osler, *The Principles and Practice of Medicine*, 7th ed. (New York and London: D. Appleton and Company, 1909), 302–3.

18. Osler, *Principles and Practice*, 304–7.

19. George A. Clark, Marc A. Kelley, John M. Grange, and M. Cassandra Hill, "The Evolution of Mycobacterial Disease in Human Populations: A Reevaluation," *Current Anthropology* 28, no. 1 (1987): 45–62.

20. William W. Stead, "The Origin and Erratic Global Spread of Tuberculosis: How the Past Explains the Present and Is the Key to the Future," *Clinics in Chest Medicine* 18, no. 1 (March 1997): 65–77.

21. François Haas and Sheila Sperber Haas, "The Origins of *Mycobacterium tuberculosis* and the Notion of Its Contagiousness," in *Tuberculosis*, ed. William N. Rom and Stuart M. Garay (Boston: Little, Brown and Company, 1996), 4.

22. Charles W. Henderson, "Egyptian who lived 5,400 years ago may have had TB," *Tuberculosis & Airborne Disease Weekly*, January 18, 1999.

23. Haas and Haas, "Origins of *Mycobacterium tuberculosis*," 4–5.

24. Michael R. Zimmerman, "The Mummies of the Tomb of Nebwenenef: Paleopathology and Archaeology," *Journal of the American Research Center in Egypt* 14 (1977): 33–36.

25. Arthur C. Aufderheide and Conrado Rodríguez-Martín, *The Cambridge Encyclopedia of Human Paleopathology* (Cambridge: Cambridge University Press, 1998), 126–27.

26. Ralph H. Major, *A History of Medicine*, 2 vols. (Springfield, IL: Charles C. Thomas, 1954), vol. 1: 70; Erwin H. Ackerknecht, *History and Geography of the Most Important Diseases* (New York: Hafner Publishing Company, 1965), 102.

27. *Hippocrates*, vol. 5, trans. Paul Potter (Cambridge, MA: Harvard University Press, 1988), 277–85; *Hippocrates*, vol. 3, trans. E. T. Withington (Cambridge, MA: Harvard University Press, 1948), 279–83.

28. Sanford A. Rubin, "Tuberculosis: Captain of All These Men of Death," *Radiologic Clinics of North America* 33, no. 4 (1955): 619–39.

29. Maurice B. Strauss, ed., *Familiar Medical Quotations* (Boston: Little, Brown and Company, 1968), 642.

30. For the original account, see Ralph H. Major, ed., *Classic Descriptions of Disease, with Biographical Sketches of the Authors*, 3rd ed. (Springfield, IL: Charles C. Thomas, Publisher, 1945), 59–60, 62–63.

31. For an extended discussion of this idea, see Susan Sontag, *Illness as Metaphor* (New York: Farrar, Straus and Giroux, 1978), and Rene Dubos and Jean Dubos, *The White Plague: Tuberculosis, Man and Society* (Boston: Little, Brown and Company, 1952), especially chapters 2–5. A more symbolic treatment of the topic may be seen in Thomas Mann's *The Magic Mountain*.

32. *Oxford English Dictionary*, 2nd ed. (Oxford: Oxford University Press, 1994). The term "tuberculous consumption" is recorded from 1799. The Swiss physician Johann Lucas Schönlein had coined the term *"Tuberkulose"* in 1839.

33. Michael E. Teller, *The Tuberculosis Movement: A Public Health Campaign in the Progressive Era* (New York: Greenwood Press, 1988), 16.

34. Thomas Dormandy, *The White Death: A History of Tuberculosis* (New York: New York University Press, 2000), chapters 12 and 13.

35. Paul Dufault, *The Diagnosis and Treatment of Pulmonary Tuberculosis* (Philadelphia: Lea and Febiger, 1957), 12.

36. Sheila M. Rothman, "Seek and Hide: Public Health Departments and Persons with Tuberculosis, 1890–1940," *The Journal of Law, Medicine and Ethics* 21, no. 3–4 (1993): 289–95.

37. Dormandy, *White Death*, 235.

38. Rubin, "Tuberculosis: Captain."

39. *Hippocrates*, vol. 5: 103–15.

40. Milton B. Rosenblatt, "Pulmonary Tuberculosis: Evolution of Modern Therapy," *Bulletin of the New York Academy of Medicine* 49, no. 3 (1973): 161–96.

41. Dormandy, *White Death*, 6.

42. Dubos and Dubos, *White Plague*, chapter 3.

43. Dormandy, *White Death*, 57–59.

44. Barbara Bates, *Bargaining for Life: A Social History of Tuberculosis, 1876–1938* (Philadelphia: University of Pennsylvania Press, 1992), 38–39.

45. Edward Livingston Trudeau, *An Autobiography* (1915; repr. Garden City, NY: Doubleday, Doran & Company, 1936); Robert Taylor, *Saranac: America's Magic Mountain* (New York: Paragon House Publishers, 1988). The facility was originally called the Trudeau Sanitarium, an older word derived from the Latin word *sanitas*, meaning health. Shortly after the turn of the century, "sanatorium," from the Latin *sanare*, meaning "to heal," was generally adopted. A hybrid form, "sanitorium," is also commonly seen, but this word has no official standing.

46. For an excellent recent study of Flick and the sanatorium movement, see Bates, *Bargaining for Life*.

47. For a humorous but grimly realistic view of sanatorium life, see Betty MacDonald, *The Plague and I* (1948; repr. Pleasantville, NY: Akadine Press, 1997).

48. Iseman, *Clinician's Guide*, 13.

49. Dormandy, *White Death*, chapter 22.

50. Rosenblatt, "Pulmonary Tuberculosis," 177–79; Dormandy, *White Death*, chapter 31.

51. Rubin, "Tuberculosis: Captain"; Frederick C. Warring, Jr., "A Brief History of Tuberculosis," *Connecticut Medicine* 45, no. 3 (1981): 177–85; John A. Meyer, "Tuberculosis, the Adirondacks, and Coming of Age for Thoracic Surgery," *Annals of Thoracic Surgery* 52 (1991): 881–85.

52. Selman A. Waksman, *The Conquest of Tuberculosis* (Berkeley and Los Angeles: University of California Press, 1964).

53. Frank Ryan, *Tuberculosis: The Greatest Story Never Told* (Bromsgrove, UK: Swift Publishers, 1992), 349–53.

54. For an extended discussion of the history of anti-tuberculosis chemotherapy, see Ryan, *Tuberculosis*.

55. For a modern discussion of chemotherapy for tuberculosis, see Michael H. Cynamon, "Chemotherapeutic Agents for Mycobacterial Infections," in Friedman, *Tuberculosis*.

56. "Treatment of Tuberculosis," the American Thoracic Society, CDC, and the Infectious Diseases Society of America, *MMWR* 52, no. RR-11 (2003): 1–12. This document, which is regularly updated, gives a comprehensive view of the state of the art in tuberculosis therapy.

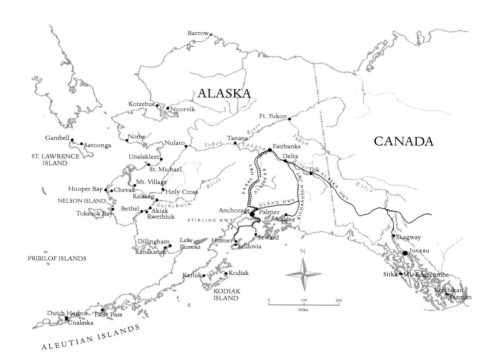

:: Map of Alaska ::

: 1 : Whence the Scourge?

Origin and Spread of Tuberculosis in Alaska

Tuberculosis in the Americas

Conventional wisdom has it that tuberculosis, like so many other destructive diseases, was introduced among the inhabitants of the Americas by European explorers and settlers. The archeological evidence of the past twenty years or so casts doubt on this hypothesis, although experts are not in full agreement on all the issues.

In the early part of the twentieth century, Alĕs Hrdlička, a physician and anthropologist, was one of the first to state on the basis of extensive fieldwork among the Indians in North America that tuberculosis, if it existed at all in the New World, must have been very rare, since he knew of no bones of pre-Columbian origin with typical tuberculous lesions, nor had he found any from the early contact period.[1] New evidence for the antiquity of tuberculosis has recently emerged. Six skeletons with lesions consistent with spinal tuberculosis have been recovered from Ohio, with carbon dating from AD 1125 to 1425.[2] The skeletal remains of 457 burials from around 1500, found in an Iroquois ossuary in Ontario, revealed some twenty-six skeletons, or 5.7 percent, with bone lesions characteristic of tuberculosis.[3] Skeletal specimens showing presumptive Pott's disease have also been recovered in New York, Illinois, and Tennessee.[4]

More substantial proof of New World tuberculosis came in 1973 with the report by Allison and others of their examination of a mummified Indian child from southern Peru, dating from approximately AD 700. Examination showed tubercles suggestive of miliary tuberculosis in the pleurae, lung, liver, pericardium, heart, and kidneys, with acid-fast bacilli in the lung, kidney, and liver. Three lumbar vertebrae showed lesions characteristic of Pott's disease, and there was evidence of a psoas abscess along the spine.[5] The same authors later reported on a study of 330 mummies from Peru and northern Chile, in which they identified eleven additional cases of possible tuberculosis. In two of these they demonstrated acid-fast bacilli in lung cavities, whereas the remainder had bone lesions consistent with tuberculosis.[6]

Even more persuasive is the 1994 report of the recovery of DNA unique to *M. tuberculosis* from a lung lesion from the thousand-year-old mummified remains of a woman forty to forty-five years old in southern Peru. Neither a 1.5 cm nodule with a cavity from the right upper lobe nor two calcified peribronchial lymph nodes revealed intact acid-fast organisms, but samples subjected to a polymerase chain reaction (PCR) amplification technique resulted in the identification of a DNA sequence also found in the modern M. tuberculosis organism.[7] In response to these findings, however, another group of experts was quick to note that the DNA fragment identified in the mummy was present not only in M. tuberculosis but also in the related species M. bovis, M. africanum, and M. microti, all of which can cause disease in animals as well as humans.[8] What seems certain is that a clinical disease indistinguishable from modern tuberculosis occurred among the indigenous peoples of the New World prior to European contact, and that this disease was associated with acid-fast bacteria with an exact match of certain DNA characteristics found in the M. tuberculosis organism today.[9]

In the mid-1970s, Zimmerman and Smith autopsied the frozen remains of a postmenopausal woman from St. Lawrence Island, Alaska, dated to AD 400. They found fibrous adhesions between the lungs and the chest wall and diaphragm, and small healed granulomas in the spleen and meninges. Their most important finding, however, was a single lymph node located at the bifurcation of the trachea. This node contained "numerous concentric areas of fibrosis with central calcification" and was interpreted as a "healed granuloma." Stains for acid-fast bacilli were negative, as were specialized tests for Histoplasma capsulatum, the causative agent for the fungus disease histoplasmosis. The authors concluded that the lesions were most likely caused by the fungus rather than tuberculosis, on the grounds that tuberculosis "is considered to have been nonexistent in Alaska prior to its introduction by the Russians in the early 18th century."[10]

An entire frozen family, with radiocarbon dating of circa AD 1500, was discovered near Barrow in the early 1980s. Two of the bodies, both females who died of crush injuries to the chest, were preserved well enough to permit a detailed examination, this time by Zimmerman and Aufderheide. In the younger of the two, they found calcified, apparently healed granulomas in the middle lobe of the right lung and calcified lymph nodes near the junction of the main bronchi. Again they attributed their findings "probably" to histoplasmosis rather than to tuberculosis, once more on the basis that tuberculosis was supposedly introduced by Europeans.[11]

The case for histoplasmosis in the Arctic, however, seems quite weak. Histoplasmosis is a fungal disease with a worldwide distribution, although it is most common in tropical and temperate zones. In North America it is endemic in the major river basins of the central United States. Most human cases are thought to be acquired from contact with caves, hollow trees, or old barns contaminated by bird or bat droppings, or from areas of recent soil excavation. Although some human cases are progressive, more often the disease is self-limiting, leading to granuloma formation, caseation necrosis, fibrosis, and calcification of lymph nodes, as in tuberculosis.[12] I am not aware that a single clinical case of histoplasmosis in an Alaska Native has ever been diagnosed in life or by autopsy, a finding confirmed by four infectious-disease specialists with a long experience in the state.[13]

If tuberculosis indeed occurred in Alaska prior to contact with Europeans, it presumably arrived with those hardy souls who crossed the Bering land bridge beginning approximately 12,000 years ago and remained in the Arctic and subarctic. The disease probably continued to be endemic and sporadic in its manifestations for several thousand years. The total population was small, as were their scattered villages and fishing and hunting camps. Moreover, the number of individuals living in each household remained small, except perhaps among the Aleuts and the Indian cultures of Southeast Alaska. The people spent much of their time outdoors traveling, fishing, or following the hunt. They moved their camps frequently and built new dwellings when the old ones became unusable. Tuberculosis was probably sporadic in these people, since cultural practices limited opportunities for spread. Furthermore, their long experience with the organism, which in any case may have been of low virulence, allowed most of those affected to heal their lesions spontaneously through fibrosis and calcification.[14]

Alaska Native Traditional Healing Practices for Tuberculosis

A second type of evidence—healing practices—can provide additional information on the health status of an aboriginal population. Unfortunately, most healing techniques known to us today date from the twentieth century and have probably been modified by the disease patterns of the past century.

Traditional healing practices among Alaska Native cultures, as they are preserved today, are of two principal types: shamanic and empirical.[15] Shamanic healing survives in a very modified and limited form among Alaska Natives today. Shamans carried in their minds much of the cultural knowledge of their people, including stories, myths, taboos, and knowledge of the spirits. As intermediaries between the spirit world and the human world, they had many functions, only one of which was healing. Their healing techniques were directed toward finding and removing the spiritual causes of illness as they understood them. Shamans were generally employed to heal life-threatening and mysterious diseases, not, for example, simple colds, digestive disturbances, or minor injuries. For example, the Tlingit Indians of Southeast Alaska believed that tuberculosis was caused by sorcery and was therefore appropriate for treatment by a shaman.[16]

Perhaps easier to understand in the modern world is what may be called "empirical" healing, based on the use of plant, animal, or inorganic substances, surgery, massage, or manipulation. All Alaska cultures had such healers, who were often women. The prominent place of traditional practices in the treatment of tuberculosis, or at least of symptoms related to tuberculosis, may mean that the disease was endemic in Alaska, or it may simply reflect that tuberculosis was a common and familiar disease among the past few generations. Some of the treatments described below for nonspecific symptoms and signs, such as cough, spitting blood, wasting, and breathlessness, could have been directed to diseases other than tuberculosis.

In broad outline, the southern cultures in Alaska, such as the Tlingit, Haida, Aleut, and Alutiiq, used plant remedies more frequently than the northern cultures, such as the Yup'it, Inupiat, and Athabascans. Not only did more species of plants flourish in the milder climates, but the plants themselves were accessible for longer periods during the year.[17]

The Tlingit had numerous plant remedies for tuberculosis. For pulmonary phthisis and pains in the chest they used an infusion, or tea, made from a member of the buttercup family, and a decoction from the dogwood family. Pleurisy required drinking a tea made from mugwort or inhaling a vapor produced by suspending the plant over hot stones and pouring hot water on it.[18] According to Emmons, the Tlingit used infusions of the dried leaves and stems of Labrador tea, the maidenhead fern, and a certain berry bush. They also treated the milder forms of tuberculosis by boiling spruce and hemlock gum in fresh water.[19] Traditional remedies from the Yakutat area included an infusion made from the bark and pitch of a hemlock tree, or prepared from the roots of the mountain ash. An infusion derived from the leaves and stem of the thimbleberry was also popular, as was an infusion derived from the leaves and stems of the fetid, or skunk, currant. Another tuberculosis treatment from Yakutat was derived from goatsbeard, the roots of which were boiled fresh in the spring.[20]

No plant was more important or had a wider range of uses for healing than devil's club. The Tlingit dried and ground the inner bark, mixed it with oil, and applied it to the skin over scrofulous glands,[21] or scraped the bark, boiled it in saltwater, and drank it as a tea for the treatment of consumption.[22] The Haida, southern neighbors of the Tlingit, made an infusion of the bark to treat tuberculosis of the bone.[23]

At least two nonplant treatments for tuberculosis have been described for this region. The first, to prevent spitting blood, involved drinking the slime made from dissolving slugs in water,[24] and the other was the inunction of the whole body with the oil of the candlefish, or ooligan.[25]

The Aleuts were the first Alaska Natives to have close and extended contacts with the Russians and explorers from other countries. Father Veniaminov, a Russian Orthodox missionary to the Aleuts between 1824 and 1834, described a disease known to the Aleuts as *chakhotka*, a Russian word meaning phthisis, or consumption. The Natives considered the disease incurable, but treated it nonetheless with various herbs. If hemoptysis was prominent, they would let out the "bad blood" and "foul air" by puncturing the patient below the ribs with a stone lancet.[26]

The Alutiiq peoples of the North Pacific Rim, like the Aleuts, were in close contact with the Russians as early as the eighteenth century. On Kodiak Island, Labrador tea was thought to have medicinal value for chest ailments of any kind, including tuberculosis, and an infusion made from the leaves of the nettle may have been used specifically for tuberculosis. Geranium roots were sometimes chewed as a tuberculosis remedy,[27] and an infusion of yarrow leaves was used for hemoptysis.[28] The people of Prince William Sound prepared a tea from the bark or the soft young branch tips of the Sitka spruce for tuberculosis; at Port Graham and English Bay (now called Nanwalek), they used an infusion of mountain ash or meadow rue for much the same purpose.[29]

The Dena'ina Indians,[30] an Athabascan people living mainly around the shores of Cook Inlet, used devil's club for colds, cough, and tuberculosis. They also drank the spring sap or chewed the pitch gum of the spruce tree for tuberculosis, and made a tea from the needles to treat illnesses, including tuberculosis. The inland Dena'ina used an infusion from the lady fern and the related wood fern for several illnesses, including breathing troubles and tuberculosis.[31] The inner bark and fresh berries of the mountain ash were also used for tuberculosis, as well as for several other complaints.[32] The Dena'ina also drank a tea prepared by boiling the inner bark of the alder.[33]

Kari described a traditional use of low-bush cranberries for the treatment of tuberculosis among the Dena'ina: "Place a beargut raincoat on the floor of the steambath and put cooked or raw, crushed cranberries on the coat. Have the ailing person lay [sic] on the berries, and place more berries on top of him. Continue this treatment for three months."[34] Another popular remedy for respiratory infections, including tuberculosis, was a tea made from the outer bark of the roots of the red-berried elder. The Dena'ina also soaked the root of the coltsfoot in hot water and drank the infusion for tuberculosis and other chest troubles, made an infusion from the berries as a cough medicine, and chewed the roots as a remedy for blood in the sputum.[35] They boiled the leaves and drank the tea of the sweet gale for tuberculosis, and chewed the berries or made a tea from the roots and leaves of the timberberry as a remedy for tuberculosis, sore throat, or stomach trouble. An infusion from the roots of the larkspur was drunk for tuberculosis, or, alternatively, the boiled roots were applied externally as a poultice.[36]

The Athabascans of the Upper Tanana River prepared an infusion made from juniper sprigs for tuberculosis, raw gums, or toothache. Another tuberculosis remedy from this region involved boiling and drinking the ashes from burning wood punk.[37] People around Tetlin chewed raw spruce cambium and the Gwich'in took spruce pitch internally for cough or tuberculosis.[38]

The Yup'it of Nunivak Island, in southwestern Alaska, ate the flowers of the roseroot as a treatment for tuberculosis.[39] Another remedy reported was "sugar of urine," the white precipitate scraped from the bottom of urine pots.[40] The people of the lower Kuskokwim and Nelson Island regions used several different plants to treat blood in the sputum, among them Labrador tea, an infusion prepared from the leaves and bark of various willows, and the raw tops of the wild chamomile plant.[41] In an account dating from the 1830s, Baron F. P. von Wrangell stated that shamans and old women used castor, obtained from beavers, for the treatment of chest pains and spitting blood.[42]

The northern Eskimos, or Inupiat, also used Labrador tea for chronic cough.[43] In the Noatak River region, an infusion prepared from the leaves of the stinkweed (*Artemisia tilesii*) was considered helpful for hemoptysis.[44]

The existence of many traditional remedies for tuberculosis and for the symptoms of tuberculosis does not prove that tuberculosis existed in Alaska prior to European contact, but it does demonstrate that tuberculosis was a long-standing and ubiquitous problem in the region.

The Russian Era in Alaska (1741–1867)

The first Europeans to reach Alaska probably came to the Diomede Islands as early as 1732, but traditionally credit for "discovery" goes to the men of the second Bering expedition, who visited several sites in 1741. Although crew members of both the *St. Peter*, under Vitus Bering, and the *St. Paul*, under the command of Alexei Chirikov, saw Alaska Natives, these encounters were brief. Over the next half century, the Russians had numerous close contacts with the Aleuts and the Alutiiq people of Kodiak Island. Not only did many trading ships ply these waters, but after about 1770 a few permanent settlements were established, notably at Unalaska and at Three Saints Bay on Kodiak Island. Furthermore, the Russians fought with the Natives, took them prisoner, held them hostage, and required them to hunt and perform domestic chores for them. Many Russian men also cohabited with Alaska Native women, sometimes forcibly and sometimes as husband and wife. Elsewhere in Alaska, European explorers or traders from England, Spanish Mexico, France, or the fledgling United States had only brief and rather remote encounters with Natives during this period.

Most of the crew members of European trading ships during the second half of the eighteenth century came from social groups that suffered high rates of tuberculosis. Many sailors were from urban areas where living conditions were crowded and noisome. Often they had been recruited from bars and taverns, and more than a few were impressed into service against their will. Voyages were long, the food terrible, and the discipline severe. The seamen lived in cramped, unventilated quarters in the forecastle, sleeping in crude hammocks stacked almost on top of each other. Any individual who suffered from tuberculosis was almost certain to put his shipmates at risk, and it is likely that the disease was spread from one to another on shipboard. Conditions were only marginally better on the major exploring vessels of this era. These were generally naval ships, with a large complement of men and frequently a surgeon, or even a university-trained physician, on board. Officers were generally from "good" families, in contrast to the poverty and low estate of the sailors.

William Anderson, Capt. James Cook's young surgeon and friend on the *Resolution*, was one of the first documented victims of tuberculosis in Alaska. Only thirty at the time of his death, he had been sick for at least a year, even before the ship left England. He was a full participant in the expedition until the ships reached Cook's River (Cook Inlet), when his illness forced him to give up his work. He died quite emaciated on August 3, 1778, while the ship was in the Bering Sea, and was buried at sea the following day. Cook, who was very fond of the young man, named the land he sighted three hours after his friend's death Anderson Island, but it later proved to be the eastern end of St. Lawrence Island, already discovered and named by Bering in 1728.[45]

On his return south through the Bering Strait in September 1778, Cook sighted land that he named Clerke's Island in honor of his second-in-command, Capt. Charles Clerke, apparently failing to recognize that this time it was the western end of the same St. Lawrence Island. Clerke, who was appointed to command the expedition after Cook's death in Hawaii that winter, had also been ill with consumption since the ships left England. He took the vessels north again, but, "reduced to almost an absolute skeleton," he died at the age of thirty-eight at Avacha Bay, on the Kamchatka Peninsula, in August 1779.[46] Both Anderson and Clerke, like other members of the expedition, had brief contact with several groups of Natives, usually outdoors, but they would have had little opportunity to spread their disease to others ashore. Much greater would have been the risk to their shipmates in the extended close contact on board.

Other known victims of the disease among the early explorers included Alexei Chirikov and Khristian Bering, grandson of Vitus, but their deaths occurred long after their brief sojourns in Alaska.[47] If such prominent naval officers of good families were dying of tuberculosis, it goes without saying that the rank-and-file sailors also did, either at sea or upon their return home. In fact, two sailors on the Kotzebue expedition in 1816–17 were reported to be spitting blood during the voyage, but both apparently remained well.[48]

The first tenuous report of tuberculosis in Alaska Natives seems to be that of two Aleuts from Akutan, Alexei Soloviev and Boris Ocheredin, who were taken to Russia in 1770 by the Russian trader Afanassii Ocheredin. Both were said to have died from consumption on the long trek across Siberia.[49] Even assuming the validity of the diagnosis, these individuals may well have contracted the disease in Siberia rather than in Alaska.

After 1799, when the Russian-American Company was established, most Russians in Alaska lived in fixed settlements, although some continued to travel widely for trade and exploration. Most of the settlements, such as New Archangel (Sitka), Unalaska, Atka, and St. Paul Harbor (on Kodiak Island), had a nucleus of Russians in residence, including company officials, a few soldiers, and perhaps an Orthodox priest. At any given moment, one or more ships might be in the harbor with their Russian or Siberian crews moving freely ashore. Each of these settlements also had a resident Native population, mostly Aleuts or Alutiit employed by the company as hunters or workers. Natives from the surrounding regions frequently came to the settlement to trade.

It seems likely that some of the rank-and-file settlers in the larger villages suffered from tuberculosis. Shortly before his arrival in Alaska in August 1804, Count Rezanov lost a member of his crew, a cook, to consumption.[50] During their visit to St. Paul Island, Rezanov's traveling companion and physician, Georg H. von Langsdorff, remarked, "It was striking to see how much weight those thin, consumptive men [of the ship's crew]...gained in a few days on a diet of fur seal meat." At Sitka he was appalled by the living conditions of the workers, who were crowded into "damp, dirty barracks filled with poisonous, stuffy air," with the windows nailed shut.[51]

Other records of tuberculosis from this period are scarce and unreliable. Around 1805 Capt. Lisianskii noted that the most common diseases of the people were venereal diseases, colds, consumption, itch, and ulcers.[52] In 1824 the Russian Orthodox missionary Veniaminov gave last rites to the wife of a Russian living in Unalaska; she had been bedridden for seven months and suffering from "consumption."[53] The Creole[54] missionary Netsvetov described an Aleut man at Atka in 1834, a woman in 1837, and a "spinster" in 1839 who died of consumption. In his later years on the Lower Yukon, he reported performing burial services for victims of consumption in 1857 and 1859.[55] Around 1830 Baron von Wrangell noted that humpbacks seemed unusually common among the Kenaitze Indians, a possible reference to spinal tuberculosis.[56]

In 1842 Dr. Eduard Blaschke, a former Russian-American Company physician, published his medical thesis in St. Petersburg, based on his five years' experience at New Archangel between 1835 and 1840. By the time Blaschke arrived in the colonies, the company had maintained a hospital at Sitka, staffed by one or two physicians, for approximately fifteen years. The population of Sitka at the time included Russian military officers and company officials, Russian workers and enlisted men, Creoles of mixed heritage, "Aleut" hunters (including both Alutiit from Kodiak and people from the Aleutian Islands), and a few Tlingit hostages from the adjacent hostile Tlingit village. While Blaschke challenged the accuracy of the broad diagnoses entered on official death records begun at Sitka in 1821, he observed that "phthisis" was one of those frequently listed. His own death records for 1836 to 1840 included "hectic fever," tumor of the joints associated with hectic fever (probably tuberculosis of the joints), and tuberculosis of the larynx. Since physician services were available only at New Archangel, many sick people, he explained, arrived there with "chronic diseases, often incurable." Creoles and Aleuts were especially afflicted with hemoptysis and "tuberculous phthisis," while the Russians often suffered from phthisis of the "pituitary" kind—*"phthisis pituitosa"*—that is, associated with mucus or phlegm. Both hemoptysis and phthisis seemed particularly to affect the women, especially after childbirth. When phthisis occurred, it was usually in a florid form, causing the physician to stand helplessly by while the disease ran its rapid course. Prepubertal children often spit blood, leading to a later fatal outcome from phthisis. Other diseases afflicting children included "lymphatic and scrofulous tumors" and tuberculous joints. Nearly every year an epidemic of acute respiratory disease occurred in the Aleutians and Kodiak Island, leaving in its wake phthisis, "hectic fevers," and a predisposition to hemoptysis, especially among the children from five to ten years old.[57]

By 1841 the hospital in Sitka had expanded to about forty beds. Sir George Simpson, chief factor of the Hudson's Bay Company, noted on a visit there that year that most of the Native people looked "sallow and unhealthy," and at the hospital "continued fevers, pulmonary complaints," and "haemoptysis" were among the most common illnesses being treated.[58]

The Finnish physician Alexander Friedrich Frankenhaeuser, stationed at New Archangel from 1841 through 1852, provides us with great insight into the status of tuberculosis in Alaska during the 1840s. In 1846 he reported that ten out of fifty-one total deaths in Sitka were due to consumption, including eight of the eleven women who died that year. In this era most women at the settlement were either Creoles or Aleuts, although a few of the company officers had brought their wives from Russia. Frankenhaeuser noted that Creoles were especially susceptible to the disease, partly through heredity and partly because of their way of life. The females, he felt, developed the disease early in life chiefly because of all the immorality around them. Approximately 20 percent of the deaths in Sitka from 1845 to 1847 were due to consumption, while in 1847–48 the figure reached almost 30 percent.

The situation was much the same or worse at Kodiak, where the Russians had also established a small hospital staffed by a *feldsher*, a kind of physician's assistant. In 1846 some five of thirteen deaths (39 percent) at St. Paul Harbor were attributed to consumption. The climate was thought to have a particularly harmful effect on the children, who were subject to recurrent colds. The doctor felt that the seeds of consumption were sown early, citing as proof the fact that Europeans, despite many years in the colonies, had arrived when they were already "mature," and thus were able to resist the noxious effects of the climate. He was puzzled, however, by the observation that Creoles seemed to be as susceptible to the disease as full-blooded Natives, whereas he expected a physical improvement by intermarriage.[59]

That the disease was not confined to major Russian settlements during this period is shown by the report of Lt. Lavrentiy Zagoskin, who traveled widely in the Yukon-Kuskokwim region between 1842 and 1844, noting that the most common diseases among the Natives were abscesses, eye disease, and consumption. On the Middle Kuskokwim he asserted that it was an exceptional Native who did not cough blood by the age of twenty.[60] Farther north, the surgeon of the British exploring vessel *Plover* described the case of a ten-year-old Eskimo girl he treated while the ship wintered over in Port Clarence on the Seward Peninsula in 1851–52.

The child was taken into the sick bay for three weeks before she died of consumption "too far advanced before she came."[61] In 1851 Capt. Richard Collinson of the HMS *Enterprise* had reported discharging a sailor at Port Clarence with "decided symptoms of pulmonary disease," almost surely a reference to consumption.[62]

Another view is that of Dr. Z. Govorlivyi, a Russian physician working in Sitka in the 1860s, who found that although as many as 60 percent of adult Indians suffered from hemoptysis, he never once encountered a case of pulmonary consumption among them. He was unable to perform any autopsies on his Tlingit patients, but he never found tubercles in the lungs of Aleuts with the same clinical picture.[63] The phenomenon of benign hemoptysis among the Tlingit had been previously noted by Blaschke, Simpson, and Frankenhaeuser, and remains unexplained. It would also be noted frequently in the decades to follow.[64]

In his comprehensive report on the Russian-American Company in 1861–62, P. N. Golovin noted with concern that "nearly all" the Creoles, who were playing an increasing role in the administration of the colonies, began to suffer in their early thirties from a chest disorder that often developed into full-blown consumption. He felt that their undisciplined life and excessive use of alcohol were major factors in the development of the disease. The Aleuts were particularly subject to respiratory diseases and often fell sick and died when they moved to Sitka. Despite living in adequate quarters and receiving enough to eat, they suffered from the change of diet and loss of their accustomed freedoms.[65]

Tuberculosis, of course, did not remain solely a problem of the Natives. At the time of Golovin's visit, the chief manager was Johan Hampus Furuhjelm, whose younger sister Constance had come to visit Sitka in 1859 and died of tuberculosis there two years later. During her journey to Alaska, Constance had traveled with Prince Makutsov, the new assistant chief manager, and his bride Anna. The princess herself delivered three children in Sitka, but during her final pregnancy friends noted that she seemed to be much thinner. She died of what was said to be "galloping consumption" about three months after giving birth.[66]

Diagnostic techniques in the period were quite primitive, and the label of consumption was freely bestowed on anyone with a chronic cough and weight loss. As an example of the diagnostic hazards, an American, George Adams, was working at Nulato in 1865 when the Russian commandant asked him to treat his Indian wife, who was very ill. The girl was already known to Adams, who, because of her wasted appearance, thought she was consumptive. All he had in his kit was some castor oil, which he administered to her in a generous two-ounce dose. The next morning Adams was summoned excitedly by the commandant, who showed him a tapeworm she had passed, which measured thirteen and a half feet.[67]

In summary, during the Russian era tuberculosis was probably no more common in Alaska than it was among the lower classes in Mother Russia. There was little evidence of tuberculosis in Alaska during the eighteenth century, except for a few reports of the disease on the ships that explored the coastline. With the first shore settlements of the Russian-American Company at the beginning of the nineteenth century came a period of harsh living conditions, near starvation, and warfare, all of which were conducive to the development of tuberculosis among rank-and-file Russian workers, many of whom may have arrived in Alaska with the disease. Within a few decades, living conditions had improved considerably in the colony and basic medical services were available. By mid-century, consumption was recorded as the main cause of death at Sitka and Kodiak, particularly among the Creoles and Aleut women, both groups living in close and sometimes intimate contact with the Russians. Other types of tuberculous disease were also recorded, including scrofula, bone and joint involvement, meningitis, and hectic fevers. Based on available evidence, there was little tuberculosis among the Tlingit living in their own village in Sitka, with whom the Russians had limited contact. No information is available on the tuberculosis status of Natives living in villages away from the Russian settlements.

The United States Acquires Alaska (1867–1906)

After the purchase of Alaska by the United States in 1867, the earliest clinical observations on tuberculosis came from travelers, government officials, lay missionaries, and a few physicians of the military and revenue cutter services. In 1869 Gen. George H. Thomas noted that many Aleuts suffered from scrofula, which he attributed to contact with the "stronger-willed Americans."[68] The same year, army Lt. Charles Raymond found the Eskimos of the lower Yukon River to be generally vigorous and healthy, although consumption and other respiratory diseases were "by no means uncommon."[69] Assistant Surgeon John Brooke, assigned to the old Russian Hospital in Sitka, by then a US Army hospital, wrote in 1875 that "pulmonary phthisis is not uncommon" and formed a large percentage of the cases of disease among the Indians.[70] Around the same time a visiting physician in Southeast Alaska found tubercular diseases prevalent among both Natives and whites, but most common among those of mixed blood, noting that "phthisis pulmonalis runs a fearfully rapid course."[71] The Russian Orthodox Hieromonk Nikita noted that tuberculosis was one of several diseases prevalent among the Kenaitze Indians around this time.[72]

In 1879 Dr. Robert White of the US Marine Hospital Service sailed Alaskan waters as the medical officer of the US Revenue Cutter (USRC) *Richard Rush*. In his report of the voyage he noted that in Southeast Alaska "chronic catarrhal affections [*sic*] of the lungs are common, and often terminate fatally in pneumonic forms of phthisis." At Kazan Bay he encountered a few cases of advanced phthisis, and found "phthisical affections" common at Fort Wrangell. On Kodiak Island he related the prevalence of scrofula and tubercular diseases of the lung to recurrent colds and to living in close, unventilated huts. Among the Aleuts west of Unalaska he observed the swellings and scars of scrofula to be the cause of "much disfigure-ment in the old and young." In the Pribilof Islands, he found that pneumonic forms of phthisis and bronchitis caused a large proportion of the deaths.[73]

Another early report from the Revenue Cutter Service was that of Dr. Irving C. Rosse, who served on the cutter *Thomas Corwin* during its voyage to the Arctic Ocean in 1881. Among the crews of the arctic whaling fleet he found "consumption and constitutional syphilis" to be the most notable diseases, and that one of the two deaths he personally attended was due to consumption. On the Pribilofs he learned that three of the six deaths in a recent year were from scrofula, and at St. Michael pulmonary troubles "prevailed to an alarming extent." Rosse's report is one of the more detailed medical surveys of the period, yet he seems to have encountered little tuberculosis himself on his travels, except among the whalers.[74]

Ivan Petroff, a Russian employed to gather information throughout Alaska for the Tenth United States Census in 1880, is a rather controversial figure among Alaska historians because of his tendency to inflate the facts, but there is no reason to doubt the accuracy of his assessment of tuberculosis among the Native popula-tion, allowing for his lack of medical training:

> Exposed as [the Native children] are in their manner of living to draughts, to insuf-ficient covering, and cold nooks for slumber, they naturally at the outset of their rude lives lay the foundation for pulmonic troubles in all their varied degrees. Consump-tion is therefore the simple and comprehensive title for that disease which destroys the greatest number throughout Alaska. The Aleut, the Indian, and the Eskimo suffer from it alike; and they all exhibit the same stolid indifference to its stealthy but fatal advancement....
>
> After consumption, perhaps the largest number of deaths may be ascribed to scrofulous diseases, which, taking the form of malignant ulcers, eat into the vitals and destroy them, rendering the people of whole settlements sometimes lepers in the eyes of the civilized visitor; and it is hard to find a settlement in the whole coun-try where at least one or two of the families therein has not had the singularly promi-nent scars peculiar to the disease.[75]

In a footnote, Petroff refers to a supposedly widespread habit among the Natives of "devoted wives" gathering up the sputum of their consumptive husbands and swallowing it. Whatever the truth of this statement, Father Veniaminov, a much more reliable observer, mentions a similar practice among the Aleuts in which fathers and uncles gathered up the saliva of healthy old men known for their achievements and gave it to their children to ward off contagious diseases.[76]

Dr. Will F. Arnold, a naval surgeon, reported to the governor in 1890 on his expe-rience with the Native population around Sitka. A high mortality of approximately 60 per 1,000, he found, was almost wholly attributable to tuberculosis, due to the poor living conditions.[77] Over the next decade, others made passing comments on the extent of tuberculosis. A woman visiting Southeast Alaska in the 1880s remarked that consumption "is the common ailment and carries them [the Tlingit] away in numbers."[78] Another visitor to Southeast Alaska found "nearly all" of the children tainted with marks of scrofula.[79] In Prince William Sound in 1884, army Capt. William Abercrombie explained that the "exceedingly common pulmonary disease" among the Chugach Eskimos was the result of constant exposure to cold and wet and their unvaried diet and scanty clothing, combined with a hereditary tendency to the disease. Few, he said, reached the age of fifty.[80] In 1894 Dr. James White attended a woman dying of consumption at Nuchek, in Prince William Sound; at Karluk, on Kodiak Island, a few days later he noted that "consumption prevails among the women.[81] The living conditions of drunkenness, filth, and "lewdness" of the Aleuts at the huge canneries at Karluk, according to an 1898 report by an Orthodox priest, led to "degeneration, sickness, pulmonary troubles, syphilis, scrofula, tuberculosis, epidemics, etc.," a situation made worse by the influx of Asian workers.[82]

The early Moravian missionaries on the Kuskokwim cared for patients in the advanced stages of consumption, even though the area until that time had had little contact with whites.[83] On the Pribilof Islands, "varying forms of consumption and bronchitis" were the principal cause of death, according to Henry W. Elliott, "greatly aggravated by that inherited scrofulous taint or stain of blood."[84] Isabel S. Shepard, traveling on the USRC *Rush* in 1889, was struck by the prevalence of scrofula in the Aleutians, especially at Belkofski. "The physical condition of most of the Aleutes [*sic*] is dreadful...," she wrote. "Many die of pneumonia and consumption is very general."[85]

Around Cook Inlet, where the Russians had been active even before 1800, the problem seemed especially bad. A geologist visiting Tyonek in 1898 estimated that half of all deaths there were preceded by pulmonary hemorrhage, and at Susitna Station he found that "most of them die of tuberculosis."[86] Another visitor to the Susitna Valley around this time reported that the Natives were dying from pulmonary diseases, a situation he attributed to the introduction of the Russian steam bath, which had become popular among the Natives. After becoming overheated in the bath, a Native might rush out naked into the snow, "after which he is on the high road to consumption."[87] A report from Prince William Sound described a group of children as "a mass of sores and running ulcers" as the result of scrofula.[88] At St. Michael, Dr. H. M. W. Edmonds remarked in 1899 that among a couple dozen Eskimos crouched by the dock awaiting the steamer, few, if any, were not constantly coughing.[89] In 1898 the teacher on St. Lawrence Island reported that bleeding from the lungs was very prevalent among the Eskimos and that pulmonary diseases were nearly always fatal.[90]

During the summer of 1900, a terrible epidemic of influenza and measles swept through western Alaska, causing a high mortality throughout the Seward Peninsula,

Lower Yukon, Lower Kuskokwim, Bristol Bay, and the Aleutian Islands. In the following months, many of the survivors either reactivated a dormant tuberculous infection in their weakened state or developed the disease for the first time. A physician-miner at Nome wrote, "The diseases which are carrying them [the Eskimos] off are consumption and pneumonia; before these their constitution seems to be helpless.... Whole families, and even tribes, have died off; and there is more than one case where children have been left without parents or a single relative to look after them."[91] Lanier McKee, another miner in Nome, recalled the poignant image of a sick Eskimo family coughing in the attic above his room while a man across the street was yelling to exhort people to visit the dance hall and see the "most beautiful women in the world."[92] Dr. P. H. J. Lerrigo, a teacher and physician on St. Lawrence Island, wrote that at Gambell forty-six individuals were actually carried off by influenza, but many others who survived died the following year from tuberculosis.[93]

Civil government finally came to Alaska in 1884, and the following year President Cleveland appointed Alfred P. Swineford, the first of several governors who took a special interest in health matters. During his first full year in office, Swineford asked Dr. Zina Pitcher, a physician, to make a report on health conditions in the Native village at Sitka. In his 1886 report Pitcher discussed a range of health issues, including scrofula and consumption, describing the latter as "the natural enemy of the Alaskan Indian." Pitcher recommended the establishment of an Indian hospital, although not specifically for tuberculosis. The governor himself warmly endorsed the idea of a hospital as "absolutely indispensable, if it be the desire of the Government to arrest the progress of diseases which threaten their complete extinction." Warming to his subject with missionary zeal, he went on: "The appeals for help from these poor suffering people are incessant, and I see them dying almost daily for the want of the medical care.... Shall it continue to be said that our free and enlightened Government is less regardful of the imperative needs of this helpless, suffering people than was despotic Russia?"[94]

Swineford's successor, Governor Lyman E. Knapp, took up the theme. In his first report, after only a few months in office, he asserted that "consumption and pneumonia prevail to an alarming extent, with terribly fatal results."[95] He favored the establishment of Native hospitals, and continued to press for them in his last two *Annual Reports*. In 1892 he wrote, with evident sincerity but with the patronizing attitude typical of the period:

> I am profoundly impressed with the idea that, as a nation, we owe it to ourselves and to the natives of Alaska that we build, equip, and support hospitals in various parts of the Territory for the care of the sick and chronically diseased. Humanity demands it, treaty obligations require it, and self-interest ought to prompt it. These hospitals...should be the most potent agencies of civilization in the land. They should teach proper ways of living, the principles of ventilation, habits of cleanliness, care

of the young and the old, true relations with one another, and various ideas of life belonging with our American civilization.[96]

Governor John G. Brady, a former missionary, took up the theme in 1901 following the severe epidemics that had swept through western Alaska the previous summer. Noting that consumption caused more deaths among Natives than all other diseases combined, he wrote, "It is truly sad to see how many people are dying from it month by month. In view of the fact that these people have never been a charge to the Government, . . . it would be a gracious thing for the Government to step in and assist them to combat this deadly malady." He proposed that this task be assigned to the Marine Hospital Service, later to become the US Public Health Service. The idea had first been suggested by Dr. Carroll Fox, a Marine Hospital Service physician assigned to Southeast Alaska in May 1901 to investigate the outbreak of a smallpox epidemic. Fox saw tuberculosis as a greater threat than smallpox, observing not only pulmonary disease but also scrofula and bone and joint tuberculosis among the Indians of the region.[97]

By the end of the nineteenth century, tuberculosis—particularly in the form of chest disease and scrofula—was known to be a serious health problem among the Alaska Natives. The full scope of the disease, however, had not yet been defined, nor had a plan of action been formulated. In the view of most observers, tuberculosis was still a constitutional or hereditary disease, attributable in large measure to the Native way of life. Government officials were beginning to recognize their obligation to face this growing problem squarely. It was partly for humanitarian reasons, partly for economic reasons, and partly because they saw it as "the white man's burden" that they set out to change this way of life.

Notes

1. Aleš Hrdlička, *Tuberculosis among Certain Indian Tribes of the United States,* Bulletin 42, Smithsonian Institution, Bureau of American Ethnology (Washington, DC: GPO, 1909), 1.

2. Hans L. Rieder, "Notes on the History of an Epidemic. Tuberculosis among North American Indians," *The IHS Primary Care Provider* 14, no. 5 (May 1989): 45–50. For detailed discussions of the question of tuberculosis in the New World, see Jane E. Buikstra, ed., *Prehistoric Tuberculosis in the Americas* (Evanston, IL: Northwestern University Archeological Program, 1981).

3. S. Pfeiffer, "Paleopathology in an Iroquoian Ossuary, with Special Reference to Tuberculosis," *American Journal of Physical Anthropology* 65, no. 2 (October 1984): 181–89.

4. Arthur C. Aufderheide and Conrado Rodríguez-Martín, *The Cambridge Encyclopedia of Human Paleopathology* (Cambridge: Cambridge University Press, 1998), 127.

5. Marvin J. Allison, D. Mendoza, and A. Pezzia, "Documentation of a Case of Tuberculosis in Pre-Columbian America," *American Review of Respiratory Disease* 107, suppl. 6 (June 1973): 985–91.

6. Marvin J. Allison, Enrique Gerszten, Juan Munizaga, Calogero Santoro, and Daniel Mendoza, "Tuberculosis in Pre-Columbian Andean Populations," in Buikstra, *Prehistoric Tuberculosis,* 49–61.

7. W. Salo, A. C. Aufderheide, J. Buikstra, and T. A. Holcomb, "Identification of *Mycobacterium tuberculosis* DNA in a Pre-Columbian Peruvian Mummy," *Proceedings of the National Academy of Sciences USA* 91 (1994): 2091–94.

8. W. W. Stead, K. D. Eisenach, M. D. Cave, M. L. Beggs, G. L. Templeton, Charles O. Thoen, and J. H. Bates, "When Did *Mycobacterium tuberculosis* First Occur in the New World?" *American Journal of Respiratory & Critical Care Medicine* 151 (1995): 1267–68.

9. Kapur et al. have speculated that speciation and global dissemination of *M. tuberculosis* may have occurred from 15,300 to 20,400 years ago, based on the organism's unusual lack of nucleotide diversity. This range fits in broadly with the presumed dates of the first human migrations into the New World, and is also consistent with the theory that *M. tuberculosis* may have evolved from *M. bovis*. See Vivek Kapur, Thomas S. Whittam, and James M. Musser, "Is *Mycobacterium tuberculosis* 15,000 Years Old?" *Journal of Infectious Diseases* 170 (November 1994): 1348–49.

10. Michael R. Zimmerman and George S. Smith, "A Probable Case of Accidental Inhumation of 1600 Years Ago," *Bulletin of the New York Academy of Medicine* 51, 2nd series (1975): 828–37.

11. Michael R. Zimmerman and Arthur C. Aufderheide, "The Frozen Family of Utqiagvik: The Autopsy Findings," *Arctic Anthropology* 21, no. 1 (1984): 53–64.

12. Lee Goldman and J. Claude Bennett, eds., *Cecil Textbook of Medicine*, 21st ed. (Philadelphia: W. B. Saunders, 2000), chapter 394.

13. The only evidence suggesting histoplasmosis in Alaska comes from three older epidemiological studies. In the earliest of these, a group of 356 Aleuts of the Pribilof Islands were skin tested in 1946 with both a 1:1000 and 1:100 dilution of histoplasmin, an antigen derived from the fungus. A single thirty-one-year-old woman reacted (3+) to the antigen, her only experience outside the islands being a sojourn in Funter Bay in Southeast Alaska during World War II. In 1957 Gentles applied histoplasmin tests to Native and Caucasian patients with tuberculosis at the Seward Sanatorium. He found no positive reactors among about a hundred Natives tested, none of whom had traveled outside Alaska, whereas some non-Native patients who had come from outside the territory did react. That same year Comstock carried out a much larger survey along the lower Yukon and southeastern shore of Norton Sound. Only 3 out of 509 individuals tested (0.6 percent) showed induration of the skin of more than five millimeters, usually considered a positive reaction. The only significant response was thought to be a recording error, because the same individual had a negative tuberculin test on the other arm. Comstock concluded that "there is reason to believe that there is no specific histoplasmin sensitivity in this population." Schaefer, in a study of Canadian Inuit, reached the same conclusion. See R. L. Sexton, J. R. Ewan, and R. C. Payne, "Determination of the Specificity of Histoplasmin and Coccidioidin as Tested on 356 Aleuts of the Pribilof Islands," *Journal of Allergy* 20 (1949): 133–35; E. W. Gentles, "Tuberculosis in Alaska," *Alaska Medicine* 1 (June 1959): 53–54; George W. Comstock, "Histoplasmin Sensitivity in Alaskan Natives," *American Review of Tuberculosis and Pulmonary Diseases* 79 (1959): 542; Otto Schaefer, "Pulmonary Miliary Calcification and Histoplasmin Sensitivity in Canadian Eskimos," *Canadian Journal of Public Health* 57, no. 9 (1966): 410–12. Dr. Aufderheide, in a personal communication to the author on October 14, 2002, feels in retrospect that the lesions found in the Barrow body are fully compatible with and most likely represent tuberculosis rather than histoplasmosis, which he concurs is rare in the Arctic.

14. For a further discussion of these issues, see the epilogue to this book.

15. For an extended account of traditional healing among Alaskan cultures, see Robert Fortuine, *Traditional Health and Healing Practices of the Alaska Natives, Based on Early Sources* (unpublished monograph, 1986). A copy is available in the Robert Fortuine Collection, University of Alaska Anchorage Archives.

16. George T. Emmons, *The Tlingit Indians*, ed. Frederica De Laguna (Seattle: University of Washington Press; New York: American Museum of Natural History, 1991), 363–64.

17. For further reference on Alaska Native healing plants, two detailed illustrated monographs have recently been published. The first, by the present author, is "The Use of Medicinal Plants by the Alaska Natives," published as a special issue of *Alaska Medicine* 30, no. 6 (November/December 1988): 185–226. The second work is Ann Garibaldi's fine compendium *Medicinal*

Flora of the Alaska (Alaska Natural Heritage Program, Environmental and Natural Resources Institute, University of Alaska Anchorage, 1999).

18. Eduard Blaschke, *Topographia Medica Portus Novi-Archangelscensis, Sedis Principalis Coloniarum Rossicarum in Septentrionali America* (St. Petersburg, Russia: K. Wienhoeber and Son, 1842), 71.

19. Emmons, *Tlingit Indians,* 364.

20. Frederica De Laguna, *Under Mount Saint Elias: The History and Culture of the Yakutat Tlingit,* Smithsonian Contributions to Anthropology, vol. 7, pt. I (Washington, DC: Smithsonian Institution Press, 1972), 657.

21. Livingston F. Jones, *A Study of the Thlingets of Alaska* (London and Edinburgh: Fleming H. Revell, 1914).

22. Emmons, *Tlingit Indians,* 364.

23. Nancy J. Turner, "Traditional Use of Devil's-Club (*Oplopanax horridus;* Araliaceae) by Native Peoples in Western North America," *Journal of Ethnobiology* 2, no. 1 (1982): 17–38.

24. John R. Swanton, *Social Condition, Beliefs, and Linguistic Relationship of the Tlingit Indians* (1908; repr., New York: Johnson Reprint Corporation, 1970), 448.

25. Robert White, "Notes on the Physical Condition of the Inhabitants of Alaska," in George W. Bailey, United States Revenue-Cutter Service, *Report upon Alaska and its People* (Washington, DC: GPO, 1880), 141–49.

26. Ivan Veniaminov, *Notes on the Islands of the Unalashka District,* trans. Lydia T. Black and R. H. Geoghegan (Kingston, Ontario: Limestone Press, 1984), 291–92.

27. Eudora M. Preston, "Medicine Women," *Alaska Sportsman* 27, no. 11 (1961): 26–29.

28. Frances Kelso Graham, *Plant Lore of an Alaskan Island* (Anchorage: Alaska Northwest Publishing Company, 1985), 29, 38, 49.

29. Alix Jane Wennekens, *Traditional Plant Usage by Chugach Natives Around Prince William Sound and on the Lower Kenai Peninsula, Alaska* (master's thesis, University of Alaska Anchorage, 1985), 41–42, 46; see also Priscilla Kari, in Ann Garibaldi, *Medicinal Flora of the Alaska Natives* (Anchorage: Alaska Natural Heritage Program, Environmental and Natural Resources Institute, University of Alaska Anchorage, 1999), 175.

30. This is now the preferred name for this group, formerly known as Taniana.

31. Priscilla Russell Kari, *Tanaina Plantlore, Dena'ina K'et'una,* 2nd ed. (Anchorage: National Park Service, Alaska Region, 1987), 34, 38, 86,131; see also Cornelius Osgood, *The Ethnography of the Tanaina* (New Haven: Yale University Publications in Anthropology no. 16, 1937), 11.

32. Joan B. Townsend, *Ethnohistory and Culture Change of the Iliamna Tanaina* (PhD dissertation, 1965, UCLA; Ann Arbor, MI: University Microfilms, 1965), 346.

33. Townsend, *Ethnohistory and Culture Change,* 345–46; Kari, *Tanaina Plantlore,* 20, 22.

34. Kari, *Tanaina Plantlore,* 67.

35. Kari, *Tanaina Plantlore,* 90, 148; see also Osgood, *Ethnography of Tanaina,* 116.

36. Kari, *Tanaina Plantlore,* 57, 91, 96, 110, 116, 145, 147.

37. Robert A. McKennan, *The Upper Tanana Indians* (New Haven: Yale University Publications in Anthropology no. 55, 1959), 109.

38. Kari, quoted in Garibaldi, *Medicinal Flora,* 30; Richard K. Nelson, *Hunters of the Northern Forest: Designs for Survival among the Alaskan Kutchin* (Chicago: University of Chicago Press, 1973), 37.

39. Margaret Lantis, "Folk Medicine and Hygiene: Lower Kuskokwim and Nunivak-Nelson Island Areas," *Anthropological Papers of the University of Alaska* 8, no. 1 (1959): 1–75.

40. Edward S. Curtis, *The Alaskan Eskimo,* ed. Frederick Webb Hodge (Norwood, MA: Plimpton Press, 1930), 44.

41. Lantis, "Folk Medicine"; T. A. Ager and L. P. Ager, "Ethnobotany of the Eskimos of Nelson Island, Alaska," *Arctic Anthropology* 17, no. 1 (1980): 27–47; Wendell H. Oswalt, "A Western Eskimo Ethnobotany," *Anthropological Papers of the University of Alaska* 6, no. 1 (1957): 16–36.

42. Ferdinand Petrovich von Wrangell, "The Inhabitants of the Northwest Coast of America," *Arctic Anthropology* 6, no. 2 (1970): 5–20.

43. Mauneluk Cultural Heritage Program, *Timimun Mamirrutit* (Kotzebue: Mauneluk Cultural Heritage Program, 1976), 51.

44. Charles V. Lucier, James W. VanStone, and Della Keats, "Medical Practices and Human Anatomical Knowledge among the Noatak Eskimos," *Ethnology* 10, no. 3 (1971): 251–64.

45. Richard A. Pierce, *Russian America: A Biographical Dictionary* (Kingston, Ontario: Limestone Press, 1990), 7; David Samwell, in James Cook, *The Journals of Captain James Cook on His Voyages of Discovery*, ed. J. C. Beaglehole, vol. 3, *The Voyage of the* Resolution *and* Discovery *1776–1780* (Cambridge, UK: Hakluyt Society, 1967), vol. 3, pt. 2: 1130. See also Lt. King's touching memorial to Dr. Anderson in the same volume, 1427–28.

46. Pierce, *Russian America*, 94; Samwell, *Journals of Captain Cook*, vol. 3, pt. 1: 699fn1; vol. 3, pt. 2: 1243, 1271.

47. Pierce, *Russian America*, 53.

48. Frederick Eschscholtz, "On the Diseases of the Crew During the Three Years of the Voyage," in Kotzebue, *Voyage of Discovery*, vol. 2: 315–37.

49. Quoted in Hubert Howe Bancroft, *History of Alaska, 1730–1885* (1886; repr., New York: Antiquarian Press, 1959), 154fn41. The source is said to be pp. 162–63 of *Neue Nachrichten*, a book published in German in 1776, by an author identified simply as "J. L. S."

50. Petr Aleksandrovich Tikhmenev, *A History of the Russian American Company, Vol. 2, Documents, Period 1783–1807*, trans. Dmitri Krenov and ed. Richard A. Pierce and Alton S. Donnelly (Kingston, Ontario: Limestone Press, 1979), 145–46.

51. Georg Heinrich von Langsdorff, *Remarks and Observations on a Voyage Around the World from 1803 to 1807*, 2 vols., trans. Victoria Joan Moessner and ed. Richard A. Pierce (Kingston, Ontario: The Limestone Press, 1993), vol. 2: 9, 35, 43, 54.

52. Urey Lisiansky, *A Voyage Round the World in the Years 1803, 4, 5, and 6; Performed by Order of His Imperial Majesty Alexander the First, Emperor of Russia, in the Ship* Neva (London: John Booth, Longman, Hurst, Rees, Orme, and Brown, 1814), 206.

53. Ioann Veniaminov, *Journals of the Priest Ioann Veniaminov in Alaska, 1823–1836*, trans. Jerome Kisslinger (Fairbanks: University of Alaska Press, 1993), 17.

54. Creoles belonged to a distinct social class in Russian America, and were usually the offspring of a Russian father and a Native mother. Many Creoles were trained by the Russians to work as traders, ship captains, navigators, priests, and *feldshers*, or medical practitioners.

55. Iakov Netsvetov, *The Journals of Iakov Netsvetov: The Atkha Years, 1828–1844*, trans. Lydia Black (Kingston, Ontario: Limestone Press, 1980), 117, 145, 183; *The Journals of Iakov Netsvetov: The Yukon Years, 1845–1863*, trans. Lydia Black (Kingston, Ontario: Limestone Press, 1984), 366, 395.

56. Wrangell, "Inhabitants of the Northwest Coast."

57. Blaschke, *Topographia Medica*, 74.

58. George Simpson, *Narrative of a Journey Round the World During the Years 1841 and 1842*, 2 vols. in one (Philadelphia: Lea and Blanchard, 1847), vol. 2: 79.

59. Aleksandr Romanovskii and Alexander Frankenhaeuser, "Five years of medical observations in the colonies of the Russian-American Company (1843–1848), by (Doctors) Romanovskii and Frankenhaeuser," trans. Richard A. Pierce (Juneau: Alaska Division of State Libraries, 1974), 2, 26, 27–28, 29.

60. Lavrentiy Zagoskin, *Lieutenant Zagoskin's Travels in Russian America 1842–1844*, ed. Henry Michael and published for the Arctic Institute of North America (University of Toronto Press, 1967), 110, 255.

61. Quoted in Dorothy Jean Ray, *The Eskimos of Bering Strait, 1650–1898* (Seattle and London: University of Washington Press, 1975), 147.

62. Richard Collinson, *Journal of H.M.S. Enterprise, on the Expedition in Search of Sir John Franklin's Ships by Behring Strait 1850–1855* (London: Sampson Lowe, Marston, Searle, and Rivington, 1889), 134.

63. Z. Govorlivyi, "Diseases prevalent among the Kolosh Indian inhabitants of the Island of Sitka" (unpublished typescript, trans. Tanya DeMarsh), 7–9.

64. Simpson, *Narrative of a Journey*, 2: 79; Frankenhaeuser, "Five years of Medical Observations," 27–28; Blaschke, *Topographia Medica*, 72. Several later observers noted this predilection for pulmonary hemorrhage among the Natives; Milton H. Foster, "Reports of Dr. Milton H. Foster," in *Report on Education of Natives, 1910–11*, 72; P. J. Mahone, "Report of the United States Hospital for Natives at Juneau," in "Report on the Work of the Bureau of Education for the Natives of Alaska, 1911–12," US Department of the Interior, Bureau of Education, Bureau of Education Bulletin, no. 36, whole number 546 (Washington, DC: GPO, 1913), 34; L. H. French, "Report of Dr. L. H. French, Kanakanak," in "Report on the work of the Bureau of Education for the Natives of Alaska, 1913–14," US Department of the Interior, Bureau of Education, Bureau of Education Bulletin, no. 48 (Washington, DC: GPO, 1915), 39.

65. P. N. Golovin, *The End of Russian America. Captain P. N. Golovin's Last Report 1862*, trans. Basil Dmytryshyn and E. A. P. Crownhart-Vaughan (Portland: Oregon Historical Society, 1979), 17, 63, 65.

66. Pierce, *Russian America*, 328; personal communication with Richard A. Pierce, September 3, 1995.

67. George R. Adams, *Life on the Yukon 1865–1867*, ed. Richard A. Pierce (Kingston, Ontario: Limestone Press, 1982), 70.

68. Robert G. Athearn, ed., "An Army Officer's Trip to Alaska in 1869," *Pacific Northwest Quarterly* 40, no. 1 (1949): 44–64.

69. Charles P. Raymond, "Reconnoissance [sic] of the Yukon River, 1869," in *Compilation of Narratives of Explorations in Alaska*, 56th Congress, 1st Sess., Senate Rep. no. 1023 (Washington, DC: GPO, 1900), 33.

70. John Brooke, "Sitka, Alaska," in *A Report on the Hygiene of the United States Army, with Description of Medical Posts*, circular no. 8, War Department, Surgeon General's Office, May 1, 1875 (Washington, DC: GPO, 1875), 483.

71. W. T. Wythe, "Medical Notes on Alaska," *Pacific Medical and Surgical Journal* 4, no. 44 (January 1871): 337–42.

72. *Documents Relative to the History of Alaska* (typescript, 15 vols., Fairbanks: Alaska History Research Project, University of Alaska, 1936–1938), vol. 2: 63.

73. White, "Notes on the Inhabitants of Alaska," 33–35, 37–39.

74. Irving C. Rosse, "Medical and Anthropological Notes of Alaska," in *Cruise of the Revenue Steamer* Corwin *in Alaska and the N. W. Arctic Ocean in 1881. . . . : Notes and Memoranda . . .* US Dept. of the Treasury, Revenue-Cutter Service, Treasury Document no. 429 (Washington, DC: GPO, 1883), 17–18, 21.

75. Ivan Petroff, *Report on the Population, Industries, and Resources of Alaska*, US Bureau of the Census, 10th Census, 1880 (Washington, DC: GPO, 1882), 43.

76. Veniaminov, *Notes on the Unalashka District*, 224.

77. Lyman E. Knapp, *Report of the Governor of Alaska for the Fiscal Year 1890* (Washington, DC: GPO, 1890), 24, 31.

78. Eliza Ruhamah Scidmore, *Alaska, its Southern Coast and the Sitkan Archipelago* (Boston: D. Lothrop and Co, 1885), 89.

79. Septima M. Collis, *A Woman's Trip to Alaska: Being an Account of a Voyage through the Inland Seas of the Sitkan Archipelago in 1890* (New York: Cassell Publishing Company, 1890), 104.

80. William R. Abercrombie, in Edwin F. Glenn and W. R. Abercrombie, *Reports of Explorations in the Territory of Alaska (Cooks Inlet, Sushitna, Copper, and Tanana Rivers) 1898. Made under*

the Direction of the Secretary of War, United States Adjutant-General's Office, Military Information Division, War Department Doc. no. 102 (Washington, DC: GPO, 1899), 399.

81. James T. White, "James Taylor White diary of cruise of US Revenue Steamer *Bear,* 1894," typescript, copy in John Wesley White–James Taylor White Collection, Alaska and Polar Regions Collection, Rasmuson Library, University of Alaska Fairbanks, box VII, folder 42.

82. "Travel journal of Priest Tikhon Shalamov," *Documents Relative to History of Alaska,* vol. 2: 87.

83. Ann Fienup-Riordan, *The Real People and the Children of Thunder: The Yup'ik Eskimo Encounter with Moravian Missionaries John and Edith Kilbuck* (Norman: University of Oklahoma Press, 1991), 322, 332.

84. Henry W. Elliott, *Our Arctic Province: Alaska and the Seal Islands* (New York: Charles Scribner, 1886), 238, 110.

85. Isabel S. Shepard, *The Cruise of the US Steamer* Rush *in Behring Sea: Summer of 1889* (San Francisco: Bancroft Company, 1889), 44, 84.

86. George B. Thomas, "From Middle Fork of Sushitna River to Indian Creek," in *Compilation of Narratives,* 735.

87. H. G. Learnard, "A trip from Portage Bay to Turnagain Arm and up the Sushitna," in *Compilation of Narratives,* 666–67.

88. Frank C. Schrader, "A Reconnaissance of a Part of Prince William Sound and the Copper River District, Alaska, in 1898," in *Twentieth Annual Report of the US Geological Survey to the Secretary of the Interior 1898–99,* part VII, "Explorations in Alaska in 1898" (Washington, DC: GPO, 1899), 367.

89. H. M. W. Edmonds, "The Eskimos of St. Michael and Vicinity, as Related by H. M. W. Edmonds," ed. Dorothy Jean Ray, *Anthropological Papers of the University of Alaska* 13, no. 2 (1966): 29.

90. V. C. Gambell, in Sheldon Jackson, *Report on Introduction of Domestic Reindeer into Alaska. 1898,* 55th Cong., 3rd Sess., S. Doc. 34 (Washington, DC: GPO, 1898), 144.

91. L. H. French, *Nome Nuggets: Some of the Experiences of a Party of Gold Seekers in Northwestern Alaska in 1900* (New York: Montross, Clarke, and Emmons, 1901), 59–60.

92. Lanier McKee, *The Land of Nome* (New York: Grafton Press, 1902), 37.

93. P. H. J. Lerrigo, "Annual Report of the Presbyterian Reindeer Station, Gambell," in Sheldon Jackson, *Eleventh Annual Report on Introduction of Domestic Reindeer into Alaska. 1901,* 57th Cong., 1st Sess, S. Doc. 98 (Washington, DC: GPO, 1902), 92.

94. Alfred P. Swineford, *Report of the Governor of Alaska for the Fiscal Year 1886* (Washington, DC: GPO, 1886), 28–29.

95. Lyman E. Knapp, *Report of the Governor of Alaska for the Fiscal Year 1889* (Washington, DC: GPO, 1889), 22.

96. Lyman E. Knapp, *Report of the Governor of Alaska for the Fiscal Year 1892* (Washington, DC: GPO, 1892), 57–58.

97. John G. Brady, *Report of the Governor of Alaska. 1901* (Washington, DC: GPO, 1901), 50; Carroll Fox, "Tuberculosis among the Indians of Southeast Alaska," *Public Health Reports* 16 (1902): 1615–16.

: 2 : **An Enemy Stalks the Land**

Tuberculosis Ascendant

The Alaska Native Health Program

A necessary background for understanding the history of tuberculosis in Alaska is some knowledge of the beginnings of federal health services for Alaska Natives, for without the testimony of the many government teachers, nurses, and doctors who provided basic health care to Natives during the first half of the twentieth century, we would have little factual information on this disease and its consequences.

Federal health services for Indians in the United States began in the early nineteenth century, as military physicians at frontier posts helped prevent the spread of communicable disease among the groups in their vicinity. Between 1832 and 1871 the government concluded at least two dozen treaties with Indian tribes that provided some sort of medical care, usually the services of a physician, in exchange for the cession of land and other rights. After 1849 the Bureau of Indian Affairs gradually expanded the medical services available to Indians beyond the minimal requirements of the treaties because of the wretched health conditions on the reservations.[1]

In Alaska, however, federal responsibility for Native health began with a different agency, the Bureau of Education, another component of the Department of the Interior. The Alaska School Service traced its origins to the efforts of Rev. Sheldon Jackson, a Presbyterian clergyman who by his persistence and forceful personality became the advocate of Alaska in the nation's capital. Appointed General Agent for Education in Alaska in 1885, Jackson showed interest in the health of the Alaska Natives. Beginning in 1890 he made several trips to the Arctic on the USRC *Bear*, reporting on his first trip that "the prevailing diseases among the Eskimo are scrofula, diphtheria, pneumonia, and consumption, and the death rate is large."[2] Jackson recognized that Native children in poor health could not benefit properly from their schools, and during his later years as commissioner attempted whenever possible to recruit teachers with some medical knowledge to serve in the more remote schools. A few of these recruits were actually physicians, as were several teachers in the mission stations.[3] Before the turn of the century, there were missionary physicians at Point Hope, Sitka, Barrow, Anvik, Bethel, Circle City, Unalaska, Unalakleet, and several other locations.

Harlan Updegraff succeeded Jackson in 1907, when he was appointed the new head of the Alaska Division of the Bureau of Education on May 1, 1907. Recognizing that widespread disease interfered with economic productivity, Updegraff proposed that the bureau develop an enforceable sanitary code for Native villages, hire physicians and nurses, and build hospitals. These latter would "serve as centers for relieving disease and destitution," furnish instruction for Native girls in nursing, and "promote the health of white people in Alaska by lessening the danger of contagious diseases." Updegraff laid the foundations for his health program by providing medical texts for the teachers in eleven village schools, together with a kit containing basic supplies and remedies.[4]

The next year the bureau initiated contracts with missionary and private physicians for the care of destitute Natives in their vicinity, the first of these at Nome, Barrow, and Nushagak. The School Service also hired its own full-time physicians—Drs. A. C. Muller and Henry (Harry) Carlos De Vighne—to provide direct medical care to Alaska Natives in the Cook Inlet region and Southeast Alaska, respectively.[5] Updegraff also appealed to Washington to establish small hospitals in some of the larger Native villages to control contagious diseases, noting that there was a particular need for facilities for the isolation of tubercular patients beyond hope of recovery, and a separate place for those who might recover with treatment. The latter could be built at small cost in conjunction with village hospitals.[6]

The commissioner of education's statement for 1909 broke out for the first time a line item in the record of Alaska school expenditures called "Sanitation and Medical Relief," amounting to some $7,523, less than 4 percent of the total education budget. That year the bureau had nine physicians on the payroll, each of whom was required to make tours through his district to provide medical relief, introduce sanitary methods in the villages, and collect vital statistics. Teachers in sixty of the seventy-eight school stations were now provided with medical supplies and textbooks.[7]

Although many government officials—and certainly the missionaries—saw the need for health services for Natives as a humanitarian undertaking, there were other motives, particularly the fear that the white population was in danger from exposure to the diseases of the Natives. Governor Clark in his 1910 *Report* pointed to the menace of infection for the white population, "for there are Indian, Eskimo, or Aleut villages in the immediate neighborhood of nearly all the principal towns, and the natives mingle freely among the whites in public places."[8] His successor, Governor Strong, picked up this refrain in 1917. After an earnest appeal for additional funding for medical care and hospitals for the Natives, Strong felt compelled to add, ominously, "Equally important is the consideration for the white population, as the physical deficiencies of the natives, unless promptly attended to, become a menace to their white neighbors."[9] The governors' motives are not completely clear in such statements, but they may have thought such an approach would increase the chances of passage of favorable legislation.

Fiscal year (FY) 1910 saw the Alaska School Service employing ten physicians, no fewer than five of whom also served as teachers or regional school administrators.[10] That year the bureau first employed three nurses as "teachers of sanitation and hygiene," stationed in Hoonah, Kake, and Seward. They were to assist the doctors in the care of the sick, give instruction in the classrooms on health subjects, and conduct physical training for the students. They were also expected to visit homes and give instruction in healthful living and sanitation in their own communities and in the surrounding districts.[11]

In November 1910 the bureau opened its first Native hospital in Juneau in a rented building, under the direction of Dr. Charles Slightam.[12] In his first report, the doctor expressed great enthusiasm for and pride in his new work, stating, "We aim to treat all natives with the same deference we would show white people in a hospital for whites.... They [the Natives] seem to feel a certain pride in the establishment, knowing that it is for them alone, and named the United States Native Hospital."[13] A second Native hospital opened in September 1911 in the old Moravian Carmel Mission buildings at Nushagak, under Dr. L. H. French, to serve about 2,000 Natives in the Bristol Bay area.[14] In these early years the bureau was permitted to spend school appropriations for its "emergency" medical program, but could not use them to build new hospitals.[15]

As the health work in Alaska rapidly expanded, the Interior Department asked the US Public Health and Marine Hospital Service to conduct a survey of Native health problems. This was carried out in the summer of 1911 by Dr. Milton H. Foster, who limited his investigations largely to the communities of Southeast Alaska and the Pacific Rim. Foster's principal recommendations were that the bureau request an officer of the Public Health and Marine Hospital Service be detailed as commissioner of public health for Alaska, and that facilities for medical work in village schools be improved.[16] In response, Dr. Emil Krulish was assigned to the Bureau of Education in Alaska in March 1912 and immediately began a series of extended trips around the territory seeking reliable data on the health problems of the Natives.[17] Over the following year he collaborated with Dr. Neuman of Nome to revise and extend the latter's draft medical manual for teachers. Their efforts resulted in 1913 in a detailed *Medical Handbook* for the Alaska School Service that was enthusiastically received and widely used for many years by teachers in the villages.[18]

The next few years saw the establishment of new hospitals in school buildings in Kotzebue and Nulato and additional new doctors and nurses.[19] The superintendent's appeals for increased health funding became ever more strident.[20]

In FY1916 repeated humanitarian appeals were finally successful in persuading Congress to include money earmarked for medical care. With the special appropriation the bureau was able to build a new two-story, twenty-bed hospital in Juneau, which opened May 9, 1916.[21] In the summer of 1917 a ten-bed hospital was constructed at Akiak, a Yup'ik community that was the center of the reindeer industry on the Lower Kuskokwim, and in 1921 a twelve-bed hospital was built at Noorvik, another reindeer center, on the Kobuk River.[22]

The great Spanish influenza epidemic of 1918–19 caused an estimated 2,000 deaths among the Native population and over the next few years left many survivors an easy prey for tuberculosis. The bureau established several orphanages in the Aleutians, Bristol Bay, and Seward Peninsula regions, where the epidemic had taken its greatest toll.[23] The following year Governor Riggs noted that tuberculosis was beginning to be detected among the white population as a result of the influenza epidemic.[24]

Teachers continued to play an essential role in providing "first responder" medical care to the Natives. When teachers were hired for Alaskan schools, they were urged to read Dr. Krulish's handbook carefully, giving particular attention to the sections on ventilation, quarantine, disinfection, and self-protection. The bureau also provided a detailed hygiene curriculum for the students, beginning in the first grade with the importance of cleanliness of hands, opening windows, airing bedding, the dangers of the common drinking cup, and the proper use of handkerchiefs. Over the next few grades, the curriculum enlarged upon these dictums, but oddly did not mention such obvious anti-tuberculosis practices as proper disposal of sputum or avoiding close contact with a sick person.[25]

In FY1926 the US Public Health Service inaugurated a system of inspecting and vaccinating all cannery employees embarking to Alaska for the summer season.[26] As early as 1915 the school superintendent in Bristol Bay (who happened to be a physician) had complained that the "law cannot protect the amiable Eskimo of southwestern Alaska from the scum of San Francisco's Chinatown which the canneries ship up here."[27] Although figures are unavailable, it is likely that many cannery workers—often recent immigrants from China, Japan, and the Philippines—were suffering from active tuberculosis and may have played a role in spreading the disease among the Alaska Natives. This new program for screening cannery workers continued for a couple of decades and undoubtedly reduced the number of individuals with active tuberculosis entering Alaska.

In FY1930, the last year of the bureau's medical program, expenditures were only $137,000, considerably below the budgeted figure of $171,780, for the maintenance of hospitals, a Yukon River health boat, and the employment of some sixty-one physicians, dentists, and nurses.[28] The Bureau of Education had made a beginning, at least, in recognizing the serious health problems of the Alaska Natives, and in setting up a health program to address them. Despite the enthusiastic and devoted efforts of many doctors, nurses, and teachers, however, the scanty budgets, the small, isolated health facilities, and the state of medical knowledge during this period ensured that little real progress could be made, especially against the greatest threat of all—tuberculosis.

The Spreading Threat of Tuberculosis: Seeking the Numbers

The extent of tuberculosis in Alaska at the beginning of the twentieth century is unknown. Moreover, the diagnosis of tuberculosis in this period was primarily a clinical one: that is, the observer made the determination on the basis of findings such as wasting, a prolonged fever, and a chronic cough, often with bloody sputum. Standard diagnostic methods such as x-rays, microscopic examination or culture of the sputum, and the tuberculin skin test were not widely available in Alaska until the mid-1930s. Some—perhaps many—cases were incorrectly diagnosed as tuberculosis; likewise, many mild, early, or atypical cases of tuberculosis were probably overlooked. Decennial census figures in Alaska were also unreliable, particularly in the more isolated areas, making the determination of mortality and morbidity rates difficult or impossible.

An early attempt at a tuberculosis survey of a specific population was that of army Capt. Paul C. Hutton, stationed at Fort Seward in Haines. He based his estimates, published in 1908, partly upon the number of Tlingit Indians who reported to the army hospital for treatment and partly on a house-to-house survey he conducted of every Indian home in the area near the fort. Persons with weight loss, cough, and purulent sputum he considered "suspicious" cases, whereas those with a history of hemoptysis he regarded as "positive." Of the 117 adults he examined, twenty-four, or 21 percent, were considered positive for pulmonary tuberculosis and another fourteen (12 percent) were considered suspicious. An additional nineteen among the group had scrofula, joint disease, or some other tuberculous manifestation, making a total of fifty-seven, or nearly half, who probably had tuberculosis in some form.[29] Around the same time Dr. Henry C. De Vighne reported on a survey he conducted in twenty villages in Southeast Alaska, comprising a population of 4,739. Between November 1908 and April 1909 he examined 1,161 Natives with symptoms of the disease, of whom he considered 418 (36 percent) to be tuberculous.[30]

In the summer of 1910 Dr. H. E. Hasseltine, a Public Health and Marine Hospital Service physician on the USRC *Rush*, visited most of the communities of Southeast Alaska and the Alaska Peninsula region from Kodiak Island to the head of Bristol Bay. Although he did not personally conduct a survey, he asked each of the physicians he met what percentage of the Natives suffered from tuberculosis. Their answers ranged from 25 to 60 percent. "Tuberculosis," he wrote, "appears to be the greatest scourge among the natives of Alaska," apparently the first of many times that the disease was to be thus characterized.[31]

Dr. Milton H. Foster personally examined 1,364 individuals for evidence of disease during his five months visiting communities in Southeast Alaska and the Pacific Rim. He judged that possibly 30 percent of the Indians of Southeast Alaska at one time or another had suffered from pulmonary tuberculosis, and that perhaps 8 percent of the total were then in need of hospital treatment. In the towns of the Pacific Rim, however, he felt that only about 4 percent required early hospital treatment.[32]

Dr. Krulish also visited as many Native communities as possible, examining individual patients, talking with physicians and officials, and conducting sanitary surveys in the villages on the southern coast, Cook Inlet, the Bering coast, Yukon River, and the Arctic coast. He found tuberculosis to be the principal disease problem, predicting that if it was not eradicated in the near future it would exterminate the Alaska Native population in sixty or seventy years. Although he cited no figures, he discovered that the pulmonary form was most common among the Eskimos and that bone and joint tuberculosis was more prevalent among the people of the southern coast.

Overall, Krulish estimated that 15 percent of the Native population was infected with tuberculosis and in 7 percent the disease was in an active stage.[33] Later, when he examined everyone available in eighteen villages of Southeast Alaska—some 2,494 people out of an estimated population of 5,200—he found about 8 percent of the people had active tubercular infections, excluding those with "tubercular dispositions; those weakly constituted and susceptible to infection." Pulmonary tuberculosis was present in 5.4 percent of the population (a figure ranging as high as 13.9 percent in Haines), the remainder of the cases being diseases of the bones, glands, and joints. Although noting optimistically that the Indians' disease responded well to rest and open-air treatment, Krulish felt that untreated, pregnant women with the disease often progressed rapidly to death. "That tubercular girls should remain single," he concluded, "is therefore obvious."[34]

In the summer of 1913 Krulish accompanied the USRC *Bear* on its annual cruise north to Point Barrow. Once more he found tuberculosis "the most important and prevailing disease" among the northern Eskimos, estimating that 6 to 9 percent of the population had active disease.[35] The regular medical officer of the *Bear* that summer was Dr. J. A. Watkins, who rendered medical care to 281 persons during the cruise; of these, 13 percent of those seeking treatment had some type of tuberculosis.[36] Among 2,010 Eskimos whom Dr. Neuman examined in Nome during his extended practice there in the 1910s and 1920s, about 16 percent had some form of tuberculosis, nearly a third of them active. Of ninety deaths reported in 1929–30 by bureau doctors and nurses from twenty-two Eskimo villages, some forty-six (51 percent) were attributed to tuberculosis.[37]

Although none of the available statistics document the trend, several observers pointed out that active tuberculosis cases and deaths became more frequent following epidemics of influenza, measles,[38] and other respiratory diseases. Many individuals already weakened by tuberculosis received the coup de grâce from the new infections. Some cases of dormant tuberculosis were reactivated by new illness, and other individuals probably became infected with tuberculosis for the first time because of their weakened physical condition. These circumstances were particularly auspicious

for tuberculosis following the "Great Sickness" of measles and influenza in the summer of 1900, and again during the worldwide Spanish flu pandemic in 1918–19.[39]

Fighting Dirt, Spit, and Foul Air

The causative organism of tuberculosis had been known since Koch's discovery in
1882, but over the following generation controversy and confusion reigned about
the exact means of development, transmission, and prevention of the disease.
Nevertheless, physicians, nurses, and other health professionals expressed strong
convictions on how the spread of the disease could be interrupted.[40] A major handbook of the period summed it up thus: "The whole law and gospel of properly
trained tuberculous patients are contained in the expression 'Be ye clean.'"[41] This
quasireligious doctrine for the prevention of tuberculosis boiled down to four principles: 1) isolation of the infected individual; 2) maintenance of personal cleanliness and a sanitary environment; 3) control of spitting and the proper disposal of
sputum; and 4) sunshine and fresh air. The latter three items will be discussed in
this section; isolation will be discussed later in the chapter.

Scrupulous cleanliness of the individual and meticulous sanitation around
the home had been dogma in Western medicine since the Sanitary Movement in
England and America, which began in the mid-nineteenth century. As the result
of a number of seminal statistical studies, mortality rates and the incidence of
epidemic diseases, including tuberculosis, had been tied directly to poverty and
urban-slum living resulting from the Industrial Revolution. That bad water, poi-
soned air, crowded housing, and personal uncleanliness bred disease was an article
of faith, a concept that seemed to be validated by the work of Robert Koch, Louis
Pasteur, and Joseph Lister in the late nineteenth century on the role of bacteria in
the spread of disease.[42]

It was for some a short step from urban slums to the villages of Alaska, with
their crowded, dilapidated, and poorly ventilated homes. Many Alaskan doctors,
nurses, and teachers described in evocative detail the sanitary conditions inside and
outside the houses. These reports often had a sanctimonious tone, since most of
the observers were from middle-class urban or rural homes where water and soap
were plentiful and "cleanliness was next to Godliness." In a summary statement
in their 1913 *Medical Handbook for Teachers,* Drs. Krulish and Neuman set forth
the prevailing view: "The predisposing causes of tuberculosis are inherited weakness, frequent exposure to cold without sufficient protection of the body, wet feet,
overcrowded and poorly ventilated houses, general debility, the excessive use of
tobacco and alcohol, adenoids, and in fact any condition which tends to lower the
resisting power of the individual." Although the tubercle bacillus, they went on,
was the "active" cause of the disease, a "favorable soil" was necessary for its mul-
tiplication and activity. This was to be found in filth, dirt, moisture, and darkness,
while sunshine and dryness destroyed the organism.[43]

Dr. Krulish, following his first visit to arctic Alaska, had written of the Eskimos:

The home life of these natives is directly responsible for the majority of their ailments. Considering the long severe winters of continual darkness, during which
period these people live indoors in small, overcrowded, overheated, and unventilated
quarters,... it is remarkable that so many escape infection.... The all-night dances,
which are of weekly occurrence during the winter in every village, at which event 50
to 60 people crowd into an igloo having a floor space of about 16 feet square, under
the most insanitary conditions, where singing, dancing, smoking, coughing, and
expectorating prevail to a certain extent during the performance, are also important
factors in the dissemination of tuberculosis and other diseases.

He went on to incriminate common drinking cups, bowls, towels, and nursing
bottles, the premastication of food, and the children's habit of exchanging gum
and candy and placing pencils in their mouths.[44]

Dr. Joseph H. Romig, originally a Moravian missionary on the Kuskokwim,
summarized the threat of tuberculosis transmission when he wrote in 1908, after
a local survey of Native homes:

The ventilation of these houses was the poorest one could imagine, and the air was
laden with dust, germs, and foul odors. There were 141 people living in the 37 houses
visited, and of this number 22 had in the recent past suffered with pulmonary hemorrhage (tubercular); a larger number were subject to chronic cough...; promiscuous
expectoration was common on any part of the floor, and in the larger proportion of
houses the people as well as the houses were dirty and looked as if soap and water
were seldom used.[45]

Teachers, who lived year-round in the village and knew all the children and
their parents, had the responsibility after 1908 to visit—perhaps "inspect" is a better word—each home to ensure that hygienic rules were being followed. Special
responsibility fell to the so-called teachers of sanitation, nurses who, among other
duties, were "to visit the homes of the natives, instructing them in matters pertaining to health and endeavoring to introduce sanitary methods of living."[46] A
recruitment circular for this position noted that the duties were "somewhat similar
in character to the work of social settlement centers among the foreign population
in our large cities."[47] These teachers often found themselves overwhelmed by the
conditions they saw. A teacher at Barrow told of a family in which the older children had "running sores on the neck from ear to ear," of years' duration, presumably from scrofula, and constantly dripped pus and scales, yet they continued to use
common dishes and washbasins with other members of the family.[48]

A report by Ada J. Van Vranken, a nurse at Seldovia and one of the first of the teachers of sanitation, reflected the enormity of the task set before her, as she saw it:

> The sanitary conditions in the native villages are appalling. What we will call homes really are single rooms inhabited by several families, varying in number from 8 to 16 and used as kitchen, bedroom and living room.... The beds are wooden, holding vermin in their many cracks and crevices.... Filthy skins of all kinds, unused or cast off wearing apparel, and gunny sacks are used as bed covering.... The total ignorance of the source of infection and the unsanitary conditions of the native houses and their villages contribute largely to the spread of tuberculosis.

Van Vranken approached her task as a zealot:

> Visits were made each week day in order to become acquainted with the people, to ascertain the actual conditions, to teach mothers...the hidden dangers of promiscuous spitting, and the needs of cleanliness. Saturday was chosen as inspection day, and the natives soon learned that the nurse expected to see the results of her week's teaching. They soon began to understand that cleanliness meant the prevention of disease, and gradually they grasped the idea that their floors should be washed at least once a week, that the beds should be clean and made up neatly, and unnecessary rubbish thrown out.

In the school she worked in a more controlled environment:

> My principal rules were: Keep clean. Wash your face. Wash your hands. Wash your neck. Wash your ears. Wash your teeth every day. Bathe your whole body with soap and warm water at least once a week. After these rules were well understood any child who came to school with a dirty face was brought before the class for consideration. The usual verdict was "Scrub 'em good with soap and warm water." After the assistants were through with him the subject was usually a shining example of cleanliness.[49]

A nurse at St. Michael also pitched headlong into changing both environment and culture.

> I visited the native village and the houses, finding the former very insanitary and the latter dirty and poorly ventilated. All the houses are too small to accommodate the large families occupying them.... I soon started the natives cleaning their houses and their village, which required much time and patience. Not until this spring could

I begin to see much improvement in the village and in a few houses.... During the year there were six deaths, all from tuberculosis, and three births.[50]

The approach of Dr. Frank Lamb in Nulato was equally aggressive. After a massive general spring cleanup of the village, including such measures as sprinkling chloride of lime around the outsides of building and fumigating the interiors, he turned his attention specifically to tuberculosis. He gave talks on tuberculosis, care of the tuberculous and their families, and care of their homes. He took all infants away from tuberculous nursing mothers and started them on formula. He then "induced" the Natives not to spit on the floors of their homes, but instead to use a small receptacle containing an antiseptic.[51]

Another nurse at St. Michael was encouraged that several families asked that their houses be fumigated after the death of a family member with tuberculosis, and others asked for chloride of lime for disinfecting drains and holes. She felt she was making progress, since formerly the people had to be "forced" to comply.[52]

Some of these statements and actions might seem today like patronizing and blatant attempts to impose Western values. The nurses and doctors, however, were generally not racially motivated, but rather committed individuals who believed that they were improving the lives of the people. They would likely have approached their jobs in a similar manner among poor European immigrants in the Lower East Side of New York.

Despite some opposition to these prescribed changes of behavior, there is evidence that many villagers took the cleanliness campaign to heart. Repeatedly, teachers and health workers were able to report that people were scrubbing their floors, cleaning up refuse and trash, and washing themselves more often.[53] The superintendent for the Upper Yukon wrote in 1915 that "nearly all the cabins in our school villages are washed and scrubbed once a week, but it is a difficult matter to keep them clean, as so many unsuitable things are brought into the cabins.... The personal cleanliness of the younger generation of natives has much improved. In regard to the old natives, it is a hopeless task...." He felt, however, that the school-age generation would ultimately pass on their new "spirit of cleanliness" to the next generation.[54]

In spite of all of the earnest effort, this single-minded preoccupation with dirt and cleanliness was of little value in the control of tuberculosis, although attempts to improve ventilation and reduce crowding in the homes may have done some good.

Among the efforts of the teachers, nurses, and physicians, the control of spitting was probably the most helpful. Indiscriminate spitting in tuberculous homes evoked the greatest fear of contagion and also a certain measure of disgust among non-Natives in the villages. They correctly believed that sputum was the most important factor in the spread of tuberculosis, although it was really not the sputum itself but rather the act of coughing that was responsible for transmission.

In the first quarter of the twentieth century, it was assumed that sputum retained its infectiousness for long periods, especially when it dried and became airborne as dust. In their medical handbook for Alaska teachers, Drs. Krulish and Neuman wrote of the dangers of sputum:

> The tubercle bacillus occurs in the sputum of tuberculous persons, and is in the air almost everywhere. It is dangerous to live in a room with a consumptive. With every cough hundreds of these germs are expelled into the air, unless a handkerchief is held before the mouth during every coughing spell; this is known as "droplet infection." The sputum of such a person contains the seed of the disease in great numbers. If this sputum is not collected and destroyed properly, but is allowed to dry and be scattered by the wind, the disease may be widely disseminated.[55]

Pulmonary tuberculosis is indeed acquired by the inhalation of tiny droplet particles containing viable bacteria produced by the coughing, sneezing, singing, and even talking of an infected individual. The tubercle bacillus, however, is quite easily killed by drying and sunlight, and thus dried sputum mixed with dust or contaminating physical objects in the household is not now believed to be an important factor in the spread of tuberculosis.[56]

Dr. P. H. J. Lerrigo, a physician employed as a teacher on St. Lawrence Island, gave a graphic, if rather facetious, description of the conditions as he saw them in 1900:

> Inside the houses [in Gambell] the accumulated expectoration of germ-laden sputum has rendered the upper soil most unhealthful, and the germs and grease cleaving to the walls and supports form a happy hunting ground for any sportive bacterium which may feel inclined to propagate his species in undisturbed felicity.
>
> In the living rooms, which are curtained from the main dwelling by heavy reindeer hides, the conditions are even more favorable to the growth of microscopic fauna. The rooms are small, the dimensions being, in width, about 8 feet; in height, 5 feet, and varying from 10 to 15 feet in length.... Their beds are reindeer hides, upon which the sputum of a sick person will often fall and dry.[57]

A teacher at Eagle told with horror of a woman almost dead with tuberculosis who, though she had a bucket beside her bed, often spit on the floor. The Indians held three potlatches that year in the room where she lay sick, eating on the floor, as was customary at a feast. When another woman in the village had a major pulmonary hemorrhage, all the Indians gathered to visit and allowed their children to crawl over the bedding and floor.[58] A teacher in Bristol Bay described a woman in the last stages of tuberculosis using a cooking vessel as a sputum cup, and then merely rinsing it with cold water before cooking in it.[59] A public health nurse working in

Kodiak in 1923 reported that in the Russian Orthodox church services tubercular patients were carried up to kiss the cross held by the priest, and that others followed and kissed the same cross.[60]

Van Vranken countered the dangers of "promiscuous spitting," as she termed it, by encouraging the use of makeshift sputum cups:

> A tin can holding a cornucopia made from newspaper was improvised as a cheap sputum cup. They were taught that this cornucopia was to be burned and replaced with a new one twice a day and the tin can boiled once a day. The rule, "Do not spit on the floor, spit in a piece of paper and burn," was made and enforced. The results were most encouraging, for seldom is this unsightly mark of ignorance now seen about the homes, nor does a native ever spit on the floor in my presence.

This last phrase suggests that she recognized that her efforts had their limitations.[61]

Their faith in these methods is shown by the teachers in Sitka, who allowed a young girl "wasting away with tuberculosis" to attend school with what they thought was no danger of contagion, because their rooms were properly ventilated and it was a "hard and fast rule of this school" that sputum be properly disposed of in paper and burned in the stove.[62] Even disposal in the stove, however, could be a problem. One observer noted that some Eskimos spit in a coffee can, but then threw the contents outdoors because there was so much of it that it extinguished the fire.[63]

Dr. Otto George described the scene in Akiak in the 1930s when he was taken on rounds with Lulu Heron, a public health nurse stationed at Bethel: "Those ill with tuberculosis lay on beds or squatted on the floor, each with a coffee can or a paper cup handy by his side. The nurse pointed with pride to some progress; one used his sputum cup; another kept his dishes separate from the others."[64] A Native woman who grew up in Akiak in that period told of how a neighbor child had a bad habit of spitting on the floor and wiping it up with her boots. When the child left the house, her mother would get out the Clorox and scrub brush and clean the floor as well as all the dishes and cups that had been used. "We seemed to always use a lot of Clorox," she remembered.[65]

The widespread practice of premastication of an infant's food by the mother or someone else was singled out for special censure. A bureau physician in the Lower Yukon District noted that this was one of the most difficult local customs to break. Sometimes the baby was only a few days old when the food was chewed by a person with active tuberculosis.[66] Other modes of transmission were thought to include adults exchanging tobacco quids, families using common drinking cups and towels, mothers using unclean nursing bottles, two children using the same bottle nipple, and several people eating with their fingers from the same bowl.[67]

Some teachers agreed that the Natives were trying to follow the instructions on sputum disposal. The teacher at Chogiung wrote, "They do get more fresh air, and they are careful to expectorate in cans partially filled with grass that they burn."[68] A teacher of sanitation at Nome noted that the Eskimos there were careful about the proper use of sputum cups, adding resignedly that "about the only thing we can do is to give them sputum cups, and talk to them a great deal about the importance of using them and the serious results that come from not using them. All the deaths, except one, in the past year have been from tuberculosis. . . ."[69]

The third precept of tuberculosis prevention in that era was proper ventilation, and it remains today one of the basic principles for minimizing the spread of tuberculosis. Unlike the other measures, the persistent efforts of the teachers, nurses, and doctors in Alaska in the early twentieth century to improve ventilation probably did reduce transmission of the disease.

Summing up the case for ventilation in their *Handbook*, Krulish and Neuman wrote:

> Tuberculosis is practically a disease due to living under unhygienic conditions—oxygen starvation. . . . Ventilation is the necessity that is most neglected by the native, but still the most vital to his welfare. It is a matter of prime importance and should receive the immediate and most careful attention of teachers.

The secret of ideal ventilation was to supply the proper quantity of air without creating a draft in the room. At school they prescribed that the windows be left open about two inches from the top during class time, but during recess and lunch hour they were to be opened top and bottom until the students returned. At home, ventilation could be achieved in the summer simply by opening the windows and doors, although few did. The winter posed more problems, although at least some of the "foul air" could be exhausted by boring a few two-inch holes just below the eaves. People were told to sleep with their windows open, although they must remain warm and well covered, except for the head.[70]

Alaska Natives protected themselves against the rigors of the climate by making the windows and door frames of their homes as airtight as possible. Many traditional homes had little more than a smoke hole in the roof for ventilation. The teachers at Hooper Bay reported in 1916–17 that 220 people lived in 21 "igloos" and 4 log houses. The igloos, they wrote, presumably with some hyperbole,

> average about eight by ten feet, while the smallest, in which two families live, is five by six feet. The ceilings are very low and I have difficulty in standing upright in most of them. In summer, the ventilation is good, consisting of a large window in the roof . . . and the door through which one has to stoop to enter. . . . The conditions

during the winter, however, are deplorable, as the window is closed by a huge block of ice, while the door is sealed as tight as possible.[71]

In Southeast Alaska a visiting doctor noted the large Tlingit homes, which sometimes housed four to six families. In one he counted thirty-four people, several with active tuberculosis, living in a space thirty by thirty by eight feet. There were several windows in each house, but these were never opened in the winter.[72]

As for more "modern" homes, Dr. Hutton described the situation in Eagle in 1907:

A portion of them reside in fairly good, one-room frame houses with glass windows, which they never employ for ventilation. On the contrary, the ingress of all air is sacredly prevented by the thorough caulking of windows, doors and cracks, and the houses being without chimneys, air can not enter.[73]

Some Natives embraced the idea of ventilation. The teacher in Barrow reported that "every house, even trapping igloos, had at least one ventilator in the roof. The fresh air idea seems to have taken good root here and the ventilators in winter and the tents in summer help the general health in a very material way."[74] At Nome the parents of one girl with advanced tuberculosis cut a good-sized window in their cabin to allow her more air and sunlight.[75] Others also tried their best to please the teachers and nurses by opening the windows, at least during the summer months. A nurse at Nome wrote, "At the beginning of the term I gave an evening talk at the schoolhouse explaining the necessity of cleanliness and proper ventilation in the homes.... Holes for ventilation have been made in all the cabins that did not already have them."[76]

Recapitulating the principles they believed would reduce the spread of tuberculosis in Native villages, Drs. Krulish and Neuman wrote in their *Handbook*:

The consumptive should be isolated when possible, and it is especially important that he should sleep alone. He should be supplied with a proper receptacle for the sputum. The spit cup should at all times contain a solution of carbolic acid and be supplied with a cover to prevent flies from carrying the germs; the cup should be emptied and the sputum burned twice a day or oftener if necessary.... The patient should have his own dishes, and they should be sterilized by boiling after each meal. Caution the family against the danger of kissing, and give instructions regarding ventilation of the room and especially regarding the collection and disposal of the sputum.

After the death of the patient his clothes and bedclothing should be burned. His room should be sealed as tightly as possible and disinfected by burning sulphur, using 10 pounds of sulphur to every 1,000 cubic feet of space.

They further advocated weekly lectures in the schoolroom on tuberculosis prevention. Signs reading "Do not spit on the floor; to do so may spread consumption" should not only be posted conspicuously, but the text should be read aloud daily by the entire student body. Multiple sputum cups should be strategically located around the classroom for the use of students who cough during school. Each day a different student should have charge of proper disposal of the contents of the sputum cups, under the watchful eye of the teacher. Students were to be cautioned about putting pencils or marbles in their mouths and especially instructed not to exchange candy and chewing gum. All drinking cups were to be of disposable paper.[77]

Although some Natives cooperated and a few became believers, more commonly the best efforts of the teachers, nurses, and doctors on the issues of cleanliness, spitting, and ventilation were met with resistance. Many Natives must have viewed these rules with a mixture of contempt, indifference, and amusement. Despite the resistance, however, these efforts, wrought by committed and enthusiastic health workers, probably had some positive effect in slowing the spread of tuberculosis, although less than they might have believed.

Thus, in the first three decades of the twentieth century, the staff of the Bureau of Education mounted an intensive educational campaign against what was perceived as the greatest health threat to the Alaska Natives. The content of the message was in accordance with the precepts of the time: personal and village cleanliness, control of spitting, and ventilation. They pursued this effort sincerely and with almost religious fervor, because in the isolated villages it seemed the only course open to them. No evidence exists to show that the campaign was successful in its goal of reducing tuberculosis, which seemed to continue its inexorable advance.

Seeking Isolation: The Early Campaign for Sanatoriums

In the absence of effective treatment, isolation of the people with active disease was the mainstay of tuberculosis control in the first half of the twentieth century. Attention to cleanliness, indiscriminate spitting, and ventilation were each important and useful measures, but the essential task of keeping the sick away from the healthy in small, crowded Alaskan homes was effectively impossible, as it was in many of the tuberculosis-infested slums of the major cities of the United States and Europe. Thus, the only practical way to isolate those with active disease was to maintain separate facilities where the sick could rest, eat a healthy diet, and experience the benefits of fresh air and sunshine. Such a regimen, many thought, also offered the best hope of cure.

Many observers saw the need for tuberculosis hospitals for Alaska Natives. Governor Knapp, in his report for 1889, had first proposed that the government build hospitals for the treatment of "chronic and hereditary diseases among the natives," the current euphemisms for syphilis and tuberculosis.[78] Governor Brady took up the cause in 1901 and again in his final report in 1905, noting that consumption continued to make "sad inroads" on the Native people:

> They do not know how to combat it, and not knowing the nature of the disease, their habits are sure to spread it. This need can be met in an efficient and intelligent manner by the Government providing a central hospital, well provided in all its details. It would probably be well to put it under the direction of the Marine-Hospital Service.... The physician in charge should be instructed that he himself or one of his helpers should visit every community and give talks on consumption—what it is and how to avoid it—talks on contagion and cleanliness, and upon such visits he should look after the sick and disabled in every house, and provide necessary remedies.[79]

Perhaps picking up on these suggestions, the School Service in 1908 proposed a hospital for the isolation of tubercular patients, with a place both for those beyond hope of recovery and those likely to get well.[80]

In 1911 Dr. Milton Foster asserted that by far the most important health need in Alaska was the immediate establishment of a 200-bed tuberculosis sanatorium for the treatment of the 6,000 cases of tuberculosis he estimated were in the District of Alaska. He had no faith in home or village care for the tubercular, and was convinced that a "free, central sanitarium" was the only practical solution to the problem. In his personal view, Haines would be a good location for such a facility because of its climatic conditions and relative ease of access. He estimated the cost of constructing and equipping such a hospital to be about $180,000, with annual maintenance costs running an additional $75,000.[81] Dr. Krulish was also convinced that a tuberculosis facility was essential and agreed that the best location was the Chilkat Valley, between Haines and Klukwan. Krulish even suggested that such an institution could also be used as a "preventorium" for children of school age predisposed to the disease but not yet ill.[82]

A few in this era felt that a tuberculosis hospital should in fact be a detention hospital, where patients could be forced to undergo treatment. This was the view of a teacher at Eagle, who felt that a certain Native was infecting other persons because of running sores. "This native ...," he wrote, "should be treated like a leper, and removed from the village." Governor Riggs also hinted at such a radical solution in 1920.[83]

Governor Strong in FY1915 asked Congress for an appropriation of $125,000 annually for the Bureau of Education to establish and maintain Native hospitals, including a "tubercular sanitarium," and the new territorial legislature, in its second biennial session, passed a memorial in support. The following year the governor once again urged funds for "sanitariums."[84] The bureau asked for funds in

FY1917 for the erection and maintenance of a fifty-bed sanatorium in the Chilkat Valley. The governor added his strong support, bluntly stating, "Congress should either attend to the needs of the natives in a comprehensive and sufficient manner or else do nothing at all and allow the race to die out as quickly as possible."[85]

Since the budget pressures of wartime Washington did not realistically permit the construction of a new hospital that year, the commissioner of education, counting on at least a supplemental congressional appropriation, entered into discussions with the Women's Board of Home Missions of the Presbyterian Church for the lease of their hospital building in Haines for use as a sanatorium. This hospital was one of the few in the region that had opened its doors to Natives. In 1918 the bureau agreed to pay a "nominal rental" of $200 per month for the building for ten months and subsistence costs of approximately $2,450 for the patients who could not pay for their own care. The mission would be responsible for obtaining necessary medical consultation services.[86]

The Haines Sanitarium opened officially on October 1, 1918, and shortly thereafter the great epidemic of Spanish influenza struck Alaska, causing many deaths and great social disruption at Fort Seward and in the villages to the south. As a result, the hospital effectively served only Klukwan and Haines until after the middle of February 1919, when quarantine travel prohibitions were lifted.[87] Those with tuberculosis were reluctant to leave home when sick, or if they did, they got desperately homesick soon after arrival at the hospital.[88] The contract for the Haines Sanitarium was apparently not renewed the following fiscal year, for there is no further mention of it in official reports.

In the context of the inevitable increase in tuberculosis that occurred among the weakened survivors of the great flu epidemic of 1918–19, Governor Scott C. Bone in 1923 urgently recommended that at least three sanatoriums be established—in Southeast Alaska, in the Yukon Valley, and in northwestern Alaska. He wrote that it was "regrettable" that Congress could not realize the importance of such a project, since "the native inhabitants are of inestimable value to the Territory and their preservation is of great concern to the Territory and its white inhabitants." No hope of "uplift, education, and economic improvement" could be achieved among the Natives without adequate attention to their physical welfare. The price tag of $325,000, however, even for such lofty goals, was too much for Congress to stomach.[89]

Since the bureau had built several new hospitals for the Natives, with plans for more, the non-Native population also felt the need for their own medical care facilities. Such requests appeared from time to time during this period in the correspondence of the governor. In February 1924 Clara Goss of Unalaska sent Governor Bone a forty-line bit of doggerel, with a few lines devoted to tuberculosis, urging him to construct a hospital in her community:

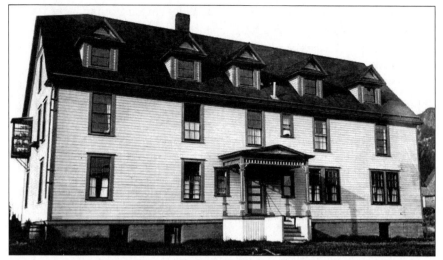

:: Haines Sanatorium, established 1919 by the Bureau of Education. ::
(Courtesy of the Sheldon Museum and Cultural Center, Haines, Alaska)

Sun rooms, and big wards for the dang'rous infection,

X-rays for our ails, and their rapid detection. . . .

A porch for T.B.'s, full of glass for the sun,

To enable the victims the asourge [scourge?] to o'ercome . . .

The governor's reply, if any, has not been preserved.[90]

Two years later, in 1925, Governor George A. Parks asked that an abandoned military hospital at Fort Gibbon near Tanana be turned over to the Bureau of Education to provide a place where the doctors and nurses from the bureau's Yukon medical boat *Martha Angeline* could work during the winter months.[91] Tanana was a particularly good location for such a facility because it was accessible by water from the Yukon River drainage throughout the warmer months, and during the wintertime was the crossroads of several trails. The cold, dry air of the winter months was believed to have a beneficial effect on tubercular cases.[92]

Governor Parks visited the new facility the following summer and reported that conditions there were "very satisfactory." The physician in charge, Dr. E. W. White, was using some rather unorthodox and "experimental" treatment methods, including sun therapy, but according to the governor some of the patients had been completely cured.[93] He regularly wrote to Governor Parks about his ambitious plans and his budgetary requests, seemingly in an attempt to circumvent bureau officials. His requests included various types of proprietary lamps for "general radiation," "concentrated and deeper treatment," and infrared treatment. He also tried to obtain an x-ray machine for the hospital.[94]

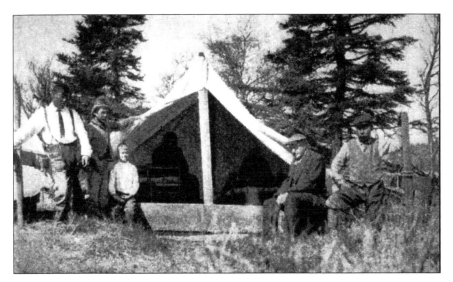

:: Tuberculosis patients cared for in tents at Kanakanak, circa 1916. ::
(Photo originally published in "Report on the Work of the Bureau of Education for the Natives of Alaska 1915–16," Bureau of Education Bulletin No. 32, 1917)

Tanana helped relieve the situation in the north, but tuberculosis beds were still urgently needed in the southeast. As early as April 1925, the territorial legislature had passed House Joint Memorial No. 14 stating that there was a "great, crying, human need for a detention ward, or temporary quarters of some kind" at the Juneau Native Hospital where tubercular cases could be cared for.[95]

Other small steps toward confronting the massive tuberculosis problem were being made by the missions. By 1925 the Episcopal Mission hospital at Fort Yukon had three or four beds set aside for tuberculosis, and a few more were available at the Methodist Hospital in Nome. By 1926 several mission boarding schools on the Yukon, including the Episcopal school at Anvik and Catholic schools at Akularak and Holy Cross, were making special provisions to "segregate" the tubercular children, though there was little they could offer by way of treatment.[96]

Separate and Ventilated: The Idea of Tuberculosis Camps

Despite the repeated pleas for tuberculosis hospitals, no funds were forthcoming. As a stopgap measure and relatively low-cost alternative, several officials suggested the construction of tuberculosis "camps," where patients with active disease could be isolated and treated apart from other patients. The idea behind such camps— either tents or small rude cabins for tuberculosis patients—was not entirely a matter of economics. Several observers had noted that Natives with tuberculosis tended to improve when they were away from the village hunting or at fish camp. As early as 1908 a doctor who had lived on the North Slope for a year remarked that the pulmonary tuberculosis cases improved markedly in the summer while people lived largely outdoors, only to relapse during the winter.[97] Foster had noted in 1911 that some cases subject to pulmonary hemorrhages every winter seemed to recover a fair degree of health during the summer while in their fishing camps and living out of doors. Likewise Krulish, in his manual for teachers, wrote that the effect of outdoor life on Natives could be plainly seen in the condition in which they returned to their villages after the summer camping season. He was convinced that many persons suffering from tuberculosis were still alive because of this yearly outing.[98]

In 1909 Dr. Henry De Vighne recommended "model sanitary camps" in the form of cabins or tents for the treatment of tuberculosis during the off-season from fishing in Southeast Alaska. These would be located near proposed Native hospitals, and the patients provided with water and fuel and a specially prepared diet provided by the government.[99] In response, the commissioner of education the following year asked for funding for a "sanitary camp" in Southeast Alaska where tuberculous Natives could be "segregated" and receive systematic treatment for their disease.[100]

The idea of tents for the tubercular patients, at least during the summer months, seems first to have come from the teacher at Chogiung, who wrote in 1912, "It seems to me that the tuberculosis patients could be helped if they could be put in tents during the summer, and in some clean, airy place during the severe months, and given wholesome, clean food." Within a couple of years, at least two bureau physicians, unable to obtain cabins for their tuberculosis patients, did indeed resort to tents. Dr. L. H. French may have been using tents at the Kanakanak Hospital as early as the summer of 1915, and by the summer of 1918 Dr. Lamb at Akiak also reported treating the tuberculous in tents.[101] As late as 1929, the physician at Kotzebue reported that his wife "had established a regular outside program for tuberculars in tents." Although the project was still in the experimental phase, the doctor thought that it promised a solution to the single largest medical problem in the district.[102]

The use of cabins seemed a more lasting solution than tents. Dr. J. W. Reed, the bureau physician at Bethel, suggested in 1914 that a series of cabins be constructed, plus a small hospital for surgical cases, in the "pines" above Bethel. These cabins would have to be heated, well lit by sunlight, and easily cleaned. The following year Reed, now assigned to Russian Mission on the Yukon, envisioned "several well-built cabins with glass on two sides, with plain furniture and inside finishing so that a hot solution of any antiseptic could be sprayed all over the room." These cabins would be large enough to accommodate one or two tuberculosis patients, and the nurse should have authority to make the "inmates" keep them in good order. Those in the early stages of the disease could put up enough fish in the summer to feed the doctor's dog team during the entire winter, as well as supply the hospital and tubercular patients with dried fish for their own use. Nearby the tuberculosis camp would be a village for the families of those in the tubercular camp and for "young men and women who are anxious to lead a civilized life."[103] His utopian concept remained just that, although the basic idea persisted in various forms.

In 1915 Dr. Lamb, then at Nulato, recommended construction of a large central hospital for tuberculosis, but failing that, he suggested that the bureau rent a suitable building in each village for the segregation of all advanced cases of tuberculosis, with one family to a building. There the local teacher or nurse could provide medical supervision of the patients under the orders of the nearest physician.[104] In fact, Dr. Neuman, the bureau physician at Nome, was able to put into practice just such an arrangement that year when the government purchased a "comfortable cottage" there for patients with active tuberculosis. The following year the superintendent of the Northwestern District pointed with pride to the bureau's cabin on the Sand Spit in which two tuberculosis patients had been housed for the past year, with the government furnishing food and fuel.[105]

Between 1917 and 1926, three different governors recommended that cabins be erected for tuberculous patients in conjunction with existing Native hospitals. Beginning in 1918, such camps were already being used at Akiak and Nulato, and by 1926 the bureau had constructed additional four-room isolation cottages at Akiak, Nulato, White Mountain, and Eklutna. In 1927 Governor Parks urged that more such cottages be built, as a low-cost alternative to more hospitals, but no further funding was forthcoming.[106]

In summary, the period between 1906 and 1931 saw the beginnings of a program to fight tuberculosis in the villages of Alaska. Education about the disease, attention to village and home sanitation, personal cleanliness, management of spitting, and the ventilation of living areas were methods that shared the virtue of costing little, but, except for ventilation, probably were generally ineffective. The need for isolation and treatment in hospitals was clearly recognized from the beginning, but the capital costs involved led to only a few tuberculosis beds being made available in hospitals, cabins, and even tents. Real disease control was still a distant hope.

Notes

1. Ruth M. Raup, *The Indian Health Program from 1800 to 1955*, DHEW, PHS, March 11, 1959.

2. Sheldon Jackson, "Education in Alaska. 1889–90," chapter 17 of *The Report of the Commissioner of Education for 1889–90*, US Department of the Interior, Bureau of Education, whole no. 191 (Washington, DC: GPO, 1893), 1290.

3. US Department of the Interior, "Report of the Commissioner of Education," in *Reports of the Department of the Interior for the Fiscal Year Ended June 30, 1907* (Washington, DC: GPO, 1908), 372–85.

4. US Department of the Interior, "Report of the Commissioner of Education" (1908), 391–92, 377.

5. A lively account of Dr. De Vighne's adventures may be found in his book *The Time of My Life* (Philadelphia: J. B. Lippincott, 1942).

6. US Department of the Interior, "Statement of the Commissioner of Education," in *Reports of the Department of the Interior for the Fiscal Year Ended June 30, 1908* (Washington, DC: GPO, 1909), 9–10, 1025–26, 1042.

7. US Department of the Interior, "Report on Education in Alaska," in *Report of the Commissioner of Education for 1909*, whole no. 437 (Washington, DC: GPO, 1910), 1298–99, 1311.

8. Walter E. Clark, *Report of the Governor of the District of Alaska to the Secretary of the Interior 1910* (Washington, DC: GPO, 1910), 19–20.

9. John F. A. Strong, *Report of the Governor of Alaska to the Secretary of the Interior 1917* (Washington, DC: GPO, 1917), 15, 21.

10. Dates preceded by "FY" refer to the fiscal year of the federal government, which at that time ran from July 1 through June 30 of the following calendar year.

11. US Department of the Interior, "Report on Education of the Natives of Alaska and the Reindeer Service," chapter 33 of the *Report of the Commissioner of Education for 1910*, whole no. 448 (Washington, DC: GPO, 1911), 1346, 1356.

12. Letter from C. H. Slightam to E. E. Brown, November 5, 1910, BIA Correspondence, roll 42; letter from W. T. Lopp to the Commissioner of Education, September 21, 1910, BIA Correspondence, roll 42: 924–26.

13. W. T. Lopp, December 31, 1911, in US Department of the Interior, Bureau of Education, Alaska School Service, *Report on Education of the Natives of Alaska and the Reindeer Service, 1910–11*, whole no. 484 (Washington, DC: GPO, 1912), 11.

14. Letter from L. H. French to the Commissioner of Education, July 1, 1912, BIA Correspondence, roll 19.

15. Lopp, *Report on Education of Natives, 1910–11*, 16.

16. Milton H. Foster, "Reports of Dr. Milton H. Foster," in *Report on Education of Natives, 1910–11*, 66–78.

17. Letter from Emil Krulish to the Surgeon General, USPHS, July 26, 1915 (Annual Report), personnel records, USPHS; Emil Krulish, "Report on Health Conditions among the Natives of Alaska," in US Department of the Interior, "Report on the Work of the Bureau of Education for the Natives of Alaska, 1911–12," *Bureau of Education Bulletin*, no. 36, whole no. 546 (1913): 31–33.

18. Emil Krulish and Daniel S. Neuman, *Medical Handbook*, US Department of the Interior, Bureau of Education, Alaska School Service (Washington, DC: GPO, 1913).

19. US Department of the Interior, "Report on the Work of the Bureau of Education for the Natives of Alaska, 1912–13," *Bureau of Education Bulletin*, no. 31, whole no. 605 (1914): 6–7, 11, 14.

20. US Department of the Interior, "Report on the Work of the Bureau of Education for the Natives of Alaska, 1913–14," *Bureau of Education Bulletin*, no. 48 (1915): 5–7, 9, 12.

21. John F. A. Strong, *Report of the Governor of Alaska to the Secretary of the Interior 1916* (Washington, DC: GPO, 1916), 52.

22. US Department of the Interior, "Work of the Bureau of Education for the Natives of Alaska, 1916–17," *Bureau of Education Bulletin*, no. 5 (1918): 7, 23, 9; Thomas Riggs, Jr., *Report of the Governor of Alaska to the Secretary of the Interior 1919* (Washington, DC: GPO, 1919), 58.

23. Thomas Riggs, Jr., *Report of the Governor of Alaska to the Secretary of the Interior 1919* (Washington, DC: GPO, 1919), 9–11, 15, 55–56, 58–59.

24. Thomas Riggs, Jr., *Report of the Governor of Alaska to the Secretary of the Interior 1920* (Washington, DC: GPO, 1920), 72.

25. US Department of the Interior, *Annual Report of the Secretary of the Interior for the Fiscal Year Ended June 30, 1923* (Washington, DC: GPO, 1923), 49–50; US Department of the Interior, *A Course of Study for United States Schools for Natives of Alaska*, Bureau of Education (Washington, DC: GPO, 1926), 10–13, 38.

26. George A. Parks, *Report of the Governor of Alaska to the Secretary of the Interior, 1926* (Washington, DC: GPO, 1926).

27. H. O. Schaleben, "Report of Dr. H. O. Schaleben, Superintendent of Schools in the Southwestern District," in US Department of the Interior, "Report on the Work of the Bureau of Education for the Natives of Alaska, 1914–15," *Bureau of Education Bulletin*, no. 47 (1916): 29.

28. George A. Parks, *Annual Report of the Governor of Alaska to the Secretary of the Interior 1930* (Washington, DC: GPO, 1930), 18–19, 88–90; William Hamilton, "Work of the Bureau of Education for the Natives of Alaska," chapter 3 of the *Biennial Survey of Education, 1928–1930*, US Department of the Interior, Bureau of Education, *Bureau of Education Bulletin*, no. 20 (Washington, DC: GPO, 1931), 587–88.

29. Paul C. Hutton, "Diseases and Sanitary Conditions among Alaskan Indians," *The Military Surgeon* 22 (June 1908): 449–54. Because of the known proclivity of the Tlingit to show hemoptysis without evidence of tuberculosis, his figures may have been inflated.

30. Henry C. De Vighne, "Annual Report of Henry C. De Vighne, MD," in "Report on Education in Alaska," *Report of the Commissioner, 1909*, 1311.

31. H. E. Hasseltine, "Report of Asst. Surg. H. E. Hasseltine," in "Sanitary Conditions in Alaska," *Public Health Reports* 26, no. 18 (May 5, 1911): 631–36.

32. Foster, "Reports," 72.

33. Krulish, "Report on Health Conditions," 31–33; see also Emil Krulish, "Sanitary Conditions in Alaska," *Public Health Reports* 28 (1913): 544–51.

34. Emil Krulish, "Report on Health Conditions in the Native Villages in Southeastern Alaska," in "Report on the Work of the Bureau of Education, 1912–13," 53–55; Emil Krulish, "Sanitary Conditions in Alaska. A Report upon the Diseases Found among the Indians of Southeastern Alaska," *Public Health Reports* 29 (1914): 1300–4.

35. Emil Krulish, "Report on Health Conditions in the Eskimo Villages on the Arctic Coast," in "Report on the Work of the Bureau of Education, 1912–13," 50–53; see also Emil Krulish, "Sanitary Conditions among the Eskimos. A Report on Conditions in Native Villages along the Arctic Coast of Alaska," *Public Health Reports*, suppl. no. 9 (December 12, 1913).

36. J. A. Watkins, "The Alaskan Eskimo. The Prevalence of Disease and the Sanitary Conditions of the Villages along the Arctic Coast," *American Journal of Public Health* 4 (August 1914): 643–48.

37. H. Dewey Anderson and W. C. Eells, "Present Health Status of the Eskimos," in *Alaska Natives: A Survey of Their Sociological and Educational Status* (Palo Alto: Stanford University Press, 1935), 140–41.

38. I. A. Gilman, "From Report of Mrs. I. A. Gilman, Teacher, Seldovia," in "Report on the Work of the Bureau of Education, 1913–14," *Bureau of Education Bulletin*, no. 48 (1915), 41; Mark Said, "Annual Report of the United States Public School at Hydaburg, in Southeastern Alaska," in *Work of the Bureau of Education, 1916–17*, 61.

39. For detailed accounts of these two epidemics, see Robert Fortuine, *Chills and Fever: Health and Disease in the Early History of Alaska* (Fairbanks: University of Alaska Press, 1989), 215–26; and Ronald L. Lautaret, "Alaska's Greatest Disaster: The 1918 Spanish Influenza Epidemic," *The Alaska Journal 1986*, vol. 16, ed. Terrence Cole (Anchorage: Northwest Publishing Company, 1986), 238–43.

40. For an extended treatment of general attitudes and practices of the period regarding the spread of infection, see Nancy Tomes, *The Gospel of Germs: Men, Women, and the Microbe in American Life* (Cambridge: Harvard University Press, 1998). For a detailed account of views on tuberculosis specifically, see Katherine Ott, *Fevered Lives: Tuberculosis in American Culture Since 1870* (Cambridge: Harvard University Press, 1996). Note especially chapter 7, "Mapping the Hygienic State."

41. Edward R. Baldwin, "Individual Prophylaxis," chapter 1 in Arnold C. Klebs, ed., *Tuberculosis: A Treatise by American Authors on its Etiology, Pathology, Frequency, Semeiology, Diagnosis, Prognosis, Prevention and Treatment* (New York: D. Appleton & Co., 1909), 393–409.

42. George Rosen, *A History of Public Health* (New York: MD Publications, Inc., 1958), chap. 6.

43. Krulish and Neuman, *Medical Handbook*, 141.

44. Krulish, "Sanitary Conditions among the Eskimos," 8.

45. Joseph H. Romig, "Report of Joseph H. Romig, M.D., Regarding Sanitary Conditions in the Vicinity of Nushagak, in Southwestern Alaska," in "Report on Education in Alaska" (1909), xxxiii.

46. "Report on Education of the Natives of Alaska, 1910," 1356.

47. Louise C. M'Connel, "Annual Report of Miss Louise C. M'Connel, Teacher of Sanitation in the Southeastern District," in "Report on Education of the Natives of Alaska, 1910," xx–xxix.

48. D. W. Cram, "Annual Report of D. W. Cram, Teacher, Barrow, to the Commissioner of Education, July 1, 1912," BIA Correspondence, roll 1.

49. Ada Van Vranken, quoted in US Department of the Interior, Bureau of Education, "Report on Education of the Natives of Alaska and the Reindeer Service," chapter 33 of the *Report of the Commissioner of Education for 1910*, whole no. 448 (Washington, DC: GPO, 1911), 1357–60.

50. Carrie W. Jordan, "Report of Mrs. Carrie W. Jordan, Nurse, St. Michael," in "Report on the Work of the Bureau of Education, 1913–14," *Bureau of Education Bulletin* , no. 48 (1915), 42.

51. Frank W. Lamb, "Report of Dr. Frank W. Lamb," in "Report on the Work of the Bureau of Education for the Natives of Alaska, 1914–15," 41. Dr. Lamb, incidentally, was later transferred to Akiak and was struck down by influenza on December 23, 1918, while on temporary duty in Old Hamilton. See May Wynne Lamb, *Life in Alaska. The Reminiscences of a Kansas Woman, 1916–1919* (Lincoln: University of Nebraska Press, 1988), 140.

52. L. G. Petrie, "Annual Report of Mrs. L. G. Petrie, Nurse at St. Michael, in Western Alaska," US Department of the Interior, "Work of the Bureau of Education for the Natives of Alaska, 1917–18," *Bureau of Education Bulletin*, no. 40 (1919), 33–34.

53. See, for example, George E. Boulter, "Report of George E. Boulter, Superintendent of Schools in the Upper Yukon District," in "Report on the Work of the Bureau of Education, 1913–14," 22.

54. George Boulter, "Report of George Boulter, Superintendent of Schools in the Upper Yukon District," in "Report on the Work of the Bureau of Education, 1914–15," 27.

55. Krulish and Neumann, *Medical Handbook*, 141–42.

56. Jack J. Adler and David N. Rose, "Transmission and Pathogenesis of Tuberculosis," in *Tuberculosis*, ed. William N. Rom and Stuart M. Garay (Boston: Little Brown and Company, 1996), 130–32.

57. P. H. J. Lerrigo, "Report from St. Lawrence Island," in Sheldon Jackson, *Introduction of Domestic Reindeer into Alaska. Tenth Annual Report, 1900* (Washington, DC: GPO, 1901), 102.

58. "Annual Report, 1912–13, of the Teacher at Eagle to the Bureau of Education, Seattle," BIA Correspondence, roll 6.

59. Thomas Vincent Calkins, *Educating the Alaska Natives* (PhD thesis, Yale University, 1931; Ann Arbor, MI: University Microfilms, 1970), 147.

60. Stella Louisa Fuller, in *With a Dauntless Spirit: Alaska Nursing in Dog-Team Days, Six Personal Accounts*, ed. Effie Graham, Jackie Pflaum, and Elfrida Nord (Fairbanks: University of Alaska Press, 2003), 136.

61. Van Vranken, "Report on Education of the Natives of Alaska," 1358.

62. Cassia Patton and Jeannette W. Wright, "Annual Report of the United States Public School at Sitka," in "Report on the Work of the Bureau of Education, 1912–13," 48.

63. Hasseltine, "Report."

64. Otto George, *Eskimo Medicine Man* (Portland: Oregon Historical Society, 1979), 95.

65. Sis Laraux [Rosanna L. Troseth], *Our Side of the River: Growing Up and Living on Our Side of the River in Old Akiak on the Kuskokwim* (Palmer, AK: Publication Consultants, 1994), 52–53.

66. Bruce H. Brown, "Report of Dr. Bruce H. Brown," in "Report on Education of the Natives of Alaska [1910]," 79–80.

67. Krulish, "Report on Health Conditions on the Arctic Coast," 50–53.

68. "Annual Report of the Teacher at Chogiung to the Commissioner of Education, June 30, 1912," BIA Correspondence, roll 3.

69. Harriet R. Kenly, "Annual Report of Harriet R. Kenly, Teacher of Sanitation at Nome, to the Commissioner of Education, July 1, 1914," BIA Correspondence, roll 18.

70. Krulish and Neuman, *Medical Handbook*, 165–69.

71. "Annual Report of the Sullivans, Teachers, Hooper Bay, to the Commissioner of Education, 1916–1917," BIA Correspondence, roll 9.

72. Hasseltine, "Report."

73. Hutton, "Diseases and Sanitary Conditions."

74. T. L. Richadson and Carrie L. Richardson, "Annual Report of T. L Richardson and Carrie L. Richardson, Teachers at Barrow, to the Commissioner of Education, June 30, 1915," BIA Correspondence, roll 1.

75. Kenly, "Annual Report, July 1, 1914."

76. Anna E. Carlson, "Nurse's Report of Work, Elim, Winter 1916–17," BIA Correspondence, roll 7.

77. Krulish and Neuman, *Medical Handbook*, 144–47.

78. Lyman E. Knapp, *Report of the Governor of Alaska for the Fiscal Year 1889* (Washington, DC: GPO, 1889), 28.

79. John G. Brady, *Report of the Governor of Alaska, 1901* (Washington, DC: GPO, 1901), 50; John G. Brady, *Report of the Governor of the District of Alaska to the Secretary of the Interior, 1905* (Washington, DC: GPO, 1905), 34.

80. US Department of the Interior, "Report on the Alaska School Service and on the Alaska Reindeer Service," chapter 26 of the *Report of the Commissioner of Education for 1908*, whole no. 402 (Washington, DC: GPO, 1909), 1042.

81. Foster, "Reports," 72–76.

82. Krulish, "Report on Health Conditions in Southeastern Alaska," 55.

83. Letter from George E. Boulter, teacher at Eagle, to the Commissioner of Education, May 1, 1911, BIA Correspondence, roll 6; Riggs, *Report of the Governor of Alaska, 1920, 62.*

84. Strong, *Report of the Governor of Alaska, 1915*, 29; Strong, *Report of the Governor of Alaska, 1916*, 52.

85. Strong, *Report of the Governor of Alaska, 1917*, 21.

86. Letter from R. P. Claxton, Commissioner of Education, to M. C. Allaben, Women's Board of Home Missions of the Presbyterian Church, September 20, 1918, BIA Correspondence, roll 8: 140; Thomas Riggs, Jr., *Report of the Governor of Alaska to the Secretary of the Interior 1918* (Washington, DC: GPO, 1919), 14–15.

87. Letter from Charles W. Hawkesworth, Superintendent, Southeast District, Bureau of Education, to the Commissioner of Education, June 30, 1919, BIA Correspondence, roll 44: 337.

88. Riggs, *Report of the Governor of Alaska, 1919*, 58–59; W. T. Lopp, Chief, Alaska Division, Bureau of Education, to M. C. Alleben, January 18, 1919, BIA Correspondence, roll 8.

89. Scott C. Bone, *Report of the Governor of Alaska to the Secretary of the Interior, 1923* (Washington, DC: GPO, 1923.)

90. Letter from Clara Goss to Scott C. Bone, February 20, 1924, Governor Correspondence, roll 111: 23.3.

91. George A. Parks, *Report of the Governor of Alaska to the Secretary of the Interior, 1925* (Washington, DC: GPO, 1925), 4, 6; George A. Parks, *Report of the Governor of Alaska to the Secretary of the Interior, 1926* (Washington, DC: GPO, 1926).

92. George A. Parks, *Report of the Governor of Alaska to the Secretary of the Interior, 1927* (Washington, DC: GPO, 1927), 6, 8, 66–67; George A. Parks, *Annual Report of the Governor of Alaska to the Secretary of the Interior 1930* (Washington, DC: GPO, 1930), 19.

93. Letter from Eben W. White to Governor Parks, October 25, 1928, Governor Correspondence, roll 155: 23.3. There is evidence that Dr. White, who in 1929 was transferred to Kotzebue against his will, was very unpopular among the Indians around Tanana because of the supposed poor quality of his care. See the report of a meeting at Tanana, June 23, 1929, from E. W. Sawyer to Governor Parks, Governor Correspondence, roll 177.

94. Letter from E. W. White to George A. Parks, September 12, 1928, Governor Correspondence, roll 155: 23.3; Letter from E. W. White to George A. Parks, November 3, 1928, Governor Correspondence, roll 155: 23.3.

95. Legislature of the Territory of Alaska, House Joint Memorial No. 14, *Laws of Alaska, 1925* (Juneau, Alaska, 1925), 181; Legislature of the Territory of Alaska, Senate Joint Memorial No. 8, April 19, 1927.

96. Letter from Marie Falldive (?), Red Cross Nurse, to Governor George A. Parks, August 22, 1925, Governor Correspondence, roll 134: 23.3; Letter from Governor Parks to the Commissioner of Education, August 17, 1926, Governor Correspondence, roll 133: 23.3.

97. G. P. Howe, "Medical Notes on Northern Alaska," *Boston Medical and Surgical Journal,* 158 (May 21, 1908): 794–97.

98. Krulish, "Sanitary Conditions in Alaska," 544–51.

99. De Vighne, "Annual Report," 1318.

100. "Report on Education in Alaska" (FY1910), 1363.

101. "Annual Report of the Teacher at Chogiung, June 30, 1912"; "Report on the Work of the Bureau of Education, 1915–16," photo following p. 40; Lamb, "Annual Report," 31.

102. Earl M. Forrest, "Annual Report of the United States Public School at Wainwright, in Arctic Alaska, in "Work of the Bureau of Education, 1917–18," 36.

103. J. W. Reed, in "Report on the Work of the Bureau of Education, 1913–14," 39–40; J. W. Reed, "Report of Dr. J. W. Reed, Russian Mission," in "Report on the Work of the Bureau of Education, 1914–15," 39–40.

104. Lamb, "Report of Dr. Frank W. Lamb, 1914–15," 42; Frank W. Lamb, "Report of Dr. Frank W. Lamb, in Nulato," in "Work of the Bureau of Education, 1916–17," 37.

105. D. S. Neuman, "Report of Dr. D. S. Neuman, Nome," in "Report on the Work of the Bureau of Education, 1915–16," 43–44; Walter C. Shields, "Report of Walter C. Shields, Superintendent of the Northwestern District," in "Report on the Work of the Bureau of Education, 1915–16," 22.

106. Strong, *Report of the Governor of Alaska, 1917,* 15, 20–21; Walter H. Johnson, "Report of Walter H. Johnson, Superintendent of the Western District," in "Work of the Bureau of Education, 1917–18," 20. Bone, *Report of the Governor of Alaska, 1923*; Parks, *Report of the Governor of Alaska, 1926*; Parks, *Report of the Governor of Alaska, 1927,* 6, 8.

: 3 : Arming for the Coming Conflict

The First Skirmishes

The Dimensions of the Disease

The first systematic study of tuberculosis mortality rates in Alaska was carried out by Frank S. Fellows, a Public Health Service officer appointed in 1931 as the medical director of the Office of Indian Affairs in Alaska. His study, published in 1934, was a detailed epidemiological analysis of Alaskan death certificates from the period 1926 to 1930, plus some incomplete data from 1931 and 1932. Fellows clearly recognized that the records on which his study was based had many short-comings. Death certificates at the time were filled out by "an interested person" in the community in which the death occurred. In the larger towns or in Native communities with a hospital or clinic, the task fell to the local physician or nurse, but elsewhere the task devolved by default to the teacher, magistrate, missionary, trader, or even the parents or other relative of the deceased. Some deaths were not reported to the authorities at all. In Alaska as a whole during this period, some 40 percent of death certificates were completed by a nonmedical person, with the figure much higher in the northern and western regions. Most wasting diseases, whatever the cause, were called tuberculosis; at the same time cases of tuberculous meningitis, miliary tuberculosis, scrofula, pericarditis, and pleurisy were usually not recognized as tuberculous at all. Moreover, some 9 percent of Native deaths in the territory in the period 1926 to 1930 were listed as "cause unknown."

Fellows felt that since three-quarters of deaths in Southeast Alaska were certi-fied by physicians and many of the remainder by nurses, the mortality figures for this area were much more accurate than those from other parts of the territory, even though he suspected that the tuberculosis problem was less severe on the Panhandle.

Of the 1,062 deaths attributed to tuberculosis from 1926 to 1930, 92.5 percent were in Natives, with tuberculosis causing 35.5 percent of Native deaths. The tuberculosis death rate for all Natives was estimated to be 655 per 100,000, com-pared to 56 per 100,000 for whites, a ratio of 11.7 to 1. In Southeast Alaska alone, however, where socioeconomic conditions were better than in the bush, the death rate among Natives was 888 per 100,000, compared with 42 per 100,000 for whites, a stunning ratio of 21.1 to 1. One particularly ominous finding was that during the period 1927 to 1932, the annual tuberculosis mortality rate in Southeast Alaska steadily rose from 818 per 100,000 to 1,302 per 100,000, although this increase might have been the result of more complete reporting.

When the figures were examined by age and sex, Fellows found that those under one year and those from twenty to twenty-nine years old were most at risk. Females aged twenty to twenty-nine (the prime childbearing years) had the horrific mortality rate of 1,704 per 100,000—that is to say, one out of every fifty-nine people in that cohort died each year from tuberculosis. The figures in the more remote areas could have been much higher.[1]

The territorial epidemiologist J. A. Carswell reported on tuberculosis in Alaska for the seven-year period 1930 to 1936. He found the average annual tuberculosis mortality for the period to be 810 per 100,000 for those he called "Indians" (all Alaska Natives) and 52 per 100,000 for whites, a ratio of 15.6 to 1. Carswell, like Fellows, had little confidence in his data, particularly since he felt that nonmedical personnel tended to overstate tuberculosis as a cause of death.

He also reported on some preliminary morbidity data based on his two-year experience with tuberculosis clinics, mainly in the larger communities of Alaska. At these clinics doctors tried to examine all Natives in the vicinity, while whites were self-selected, usually because of symptoms. Among the 1,830 Natives examined from December 1936 to April 1938, 30.3 percent were thought to have x-ray evidence of present or past tuberculosis. Of these, 13.1 percent had signs of active tuberculosis and another 3.4 percent were suspicious for activity.[2]

Other reasonably reliable figures came from the BCG vaccine[3] studies undertaken by Dr. Joseph D. Aronson in Southeast Alaska. In 1935 Aronson and his colleagues from the Henry Phipps Institute of the University of Pennsylvania undertook a long-term study of BCG vaccination among American Indians. With the support of the Office of Indian Affairs and the US Public Health Service, they began their work in 1936 in several Plains and western reservations, and in the winter of 1937–38 extended it to the Indians of Southeast Alaska. There, children under the age of nineteen were x-rayed, then tuberculin tested. Half of those who failed to react then received an intradermal injection of BCG vaccine prepared in the field under Aronson's supervision. In their initial studies, they found that 25 percent of 2,990 Indians examined showed radiographic evidence of tuberculosis and that 6.3 percent of the total manifested probably active disease.[4]

Summing up the experience of the first few survey years, Governor Ernest Gruening reported that between December 1936 and January 1941, 7,523 persons had chest x-rays in these clinics and that 2,838 Natives, or 9.46 percent, and 848 whites, or 2.96 percent, had active pulmonary tuberculosis. The department recognized that these figures were skewed by the fact that surveys in predominantly Native villages usually involved the entire population, while those in largely white communities were limited to those who volunteered to be tested, usually because of symptoms.[5]

Thus, by the beginning of World War II the true extent of the massive tuberculosis epidemic in Alaska was beginning to take shape. Far from the anecdotal reports of teachers in the early years of the century, it was becoming clear that tuberculosis was the principal health problem of the territory, especially among Alaska Natives, and that it was out of control. It was also evident that public health resources to combat this scourge were totally inadequate. The mortality and morbidity figures from this era may have been unreliable, but they eloquently described tuberculosis as it was perceived by both health officials and the public at large.

The Alaska Native Service Medical Program

On March 16, 1931, all activities of the Bureau of Education in Alaska, including the medical program, were transferred to the Office of Indian Affairs (OIA), thus bringing the federal educational and medical services for Alaska Natives in line with those for the rest of Native Americans. The Bureau of Education's Alaska program, its only field operation, ceased to exist. The new OIA Area Office, based in Juneau, became known as the Alaska Native Service (ANS).

Under the new agency, the medical budget for FY1931 rocketed to $268,760, an increase of more than 56 percent in a single year. Two new sixteen-bed hospitals of similar design were constructed that year in Kotzebue and Mountain Village, with the Kotzebue facility having special provisions for the treatment of patients with tuberculosis. Other Native hospitals in operation at the time of transfer were those at Juneau, Akiak, Noorvik, Kanakanak, and Tanana, and the Yukon River health boat *Martha Angeline* continued its operation.[6]

On September 4, 1931, Dr. Frank S. Fellows, a career officer in the US Public Health Service, was named medical director of the Alaska Medical Service, and promptly set out by steamship, Coast Guard vessel, and airplane to visit remote schools and hospitals, where he assessed the health situation and provided training for teachers. In a survey of the health of Natives in villages with OIA schools, he found 411 tubercular adults, 207 tubercular children, and 28 orthopedic hospital cases, most probably due to tuberculosis, in a population of 14,895.[7]

The Tanana Hospital, with its favorable location at the junction of two great rivers, continued to expand its program in tuberculosis, and the governor reported that Natives "with certain phases of tuberculosis" appeared to make excellent recoveries in that climate. As early as 1927 the governor had recommended adding a tuberculosis annex to the existing Juneau Native Hospital, a proposal supported by the Alaska senate in its Joint Memorial No. 8 that year. By the summer of 1931, this hope had finally come to fruition and a twenty-six-bed annex for the care of tuberculosis had been constructed behind the Juneau Hospital, effectively doubling the bed capacity. The hospital also added a laboratory technician to the staff and installed a new x-ray machine in support of the tuberculosis program.[8] In 1932 the

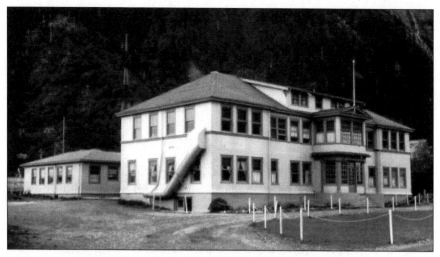

:: Juneau Native Hospital, built in 1916 by the Bureau of Education and later operated by ::
BIA and PHS. Building in the background is the tuberculosis wing.
(Courtesy of Margery Albrecht)

average census of tuberculosis cases at the new tuberculosis annex at Juneau was
more than twenty-two.[9]

As the result of new construction and hospital closures, the bed capacity of
the Native hospitals as of June 30, 1933, was 135, distributed among Juneau,
Kanakanak, Kotzebue, Mountain Village, Tanana, and Unalaska. The only beds
exclusively for tuberculosis were thirty at the Juneau annex, since the small general hospitals had neither the space nor the isolation facilities for the treatment of
the disease.[10] Thus, although tuberculosis was recognized as the most significant
health problem among Alaska Natives, only a small percentage of cases could be
hospitalized. Each year the medical director had sought the necessary funds for an
expanded tuberculosis campaign, but with the economic woes of the Depression
he had to be satisfied with an increased emphasis on tuberculosis education by the
public health nurses in the villages.[11]

As prosperity began to return to the nation, the ANS health appropriations
increased from $440,000 in FY1940 to nearly $520,000 in FY1942, despite the gathering clouds of war. The new forty-three-bed Bethel Hospital opened several months
ahead of schedule in January 1940, briefly bringing the number of Native hospitals
to eight, the most ever. In FY1941 two replacement thirty-two-bed hospitals of
similar design were completed at Kanakanak and Tanana.[12]

As Alaska mobilized for war, it became more and more difficult to recruit and
retain professional staff, despite the increasing appropriations. Many physicians
were either drafted or called to active duty as reserve officers, especially after the
attack on Pearl Harbor. Nurses also volunteered in numbers for military service,

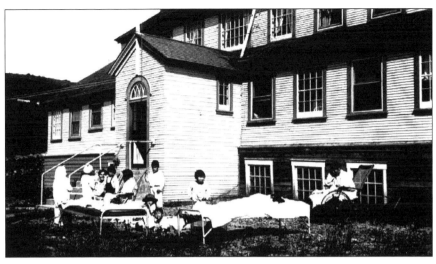

:: Tuberculosis patients getting fresh-air treatment at Mt. Village ANS Hospital during the 1930s. ::
(Photo by Mae Alexie, author's collection)

leaving some Native villages without a resident health professional. Transportation became more difficult, since most available civilian aircraft and ships were commandeered in support of the war effort. Many Natives volunteered for military service and served with distinction, though many more were rejected for medical reasons. As late as 1954, about 40 percent of the 1,300 Eskimos who applied for the Eskimo Scouts National Guard unit were rejected outright as physically unfit, and after additional screening 120 more were disqualified, most because of tuberculosis. According to Lt. Col. C. Earl Albrecht, who commanded the medical unit at Fort Richardson during the war, the Eskimos were superior soldiers, "but their health was so poor, and they were so riddled with tuberculosis, that they could not demonstrate their real ability."[13]

On June 3, 1942, a Japanese task force attacked Dutch Harbor in the Aleutians, bombing Fort Mears with carrier-based planes. The following day a second air attack occurred, this time spilling over into the nearby Aleut community of Unalaska, where the BIA hospital was totally destroyed. Fortunately, all patients had been previously evacuated as a safeguard, and no one was hurt.

Following this attack and the subsequent Japanese invasion of Attu and Kiska, all Aleuts were forcibly relocated from their homes in the Aleutian and Pribilof islands. With sometimes only hours of advance notice, about 880 Aleuts were forced to abandon their homes and board ships, which took them to four sites in Southeast Alaska, the largest of which was an abandoned cannery at Funter Bay, nineteen miles southwest of Juneau. There, ostensibly for their own safety, the Aleuts spent the remainder of the war under primitive conditions in cold, drafty, damp, barracks-style buildings, most with no plumbing or electricity, and with little privacy. At Funter Bay, whole families lived in ten-by-ten-foot cubicles separated only by a hanging blanket. Sanitation was primitive and the water supply unsafe. The health of the people, already precarious before the relocation, suffered as the war continued. Some idea of the prevalence of tuberculosis in the group is revealed in a 1945 medical report on a group of seventy-one returning Aleuts who had spent the war years at Killisnoo, another evacuation site. In the group there were twenty-nine individuals (41 percent) with tuberculosis, including two pregnant women and three with far advanced disease.[14] Overall, about 10 percent of the relocatees died during the two years of their confinement, and many more died in the years that followed of tuberculosis and other diseases they contracted during their bitter sojourn in Southeast Alaska.[15]

Some effort was made to carry on the struggle against tuberculosis during the war years. Native children continued to receive care for bone and joint tuberculosis at the Seattle Children's Orthopedic Hospital and the Tacoma Indian Hospital, the territorial Department of Health continued tuberculosis case finding, and Aronson's BCG program in Southeast Alaska went forward.[16] Staff shortages continued, however; in FY1944 the OIA in Alaska employed only four physicians, the fewest since the medical program began under the Bureau of Education some thirty-five years before. Six hospitals—at Juneau, Kanakanak, Bethel, Tanana, Kotzebue, and Barrow—continued to operate, with a total bed capacity of 174, nearly 40 percent of them set aside for the care of tuberculosis.[17] At the end of the war, sixty-nine tuberculosis beds were available in ANS facilities.[18]

The Birth of the Alaska Tuberculosis Association

The National Association for the Study and Prevention of Tuberculosis—after 1918 the National Tuberculosis Association (NTA)—was founded in 1904, with some of the greatest names in American medicine among its board members, including its first president, Dr. Edward L. Trudeau. Over the next half century it was in the vanguard of tuberculosis education, prevention, and control efforts in the United States. In 1910, the NTA borrowed from Denmark the idea of selling special stamps at Christmastime as a method of fund-raising to support its educational efforts. These so-called Christmas Seals, with their distinctive Cross of Lorraine, became a fixture on the envelope of nearly every Christmas card sent in the United States up until mid-century.[19]

In 1934, the NTA office in New York contacted a number of prominent Alaskans and asked if their names might be used as sponsors for the sale of Christmas Seals in Alaska. The list ultimately included Governor John Troy as chairman, together with several well-known Alaskan physicians, the territorial commissioner of health, officials from the Alaska Native Service, and businessmen from around the territory. Frances Paul of Juneau, the wife of prominent Tlingit political leader William L. Paul, was also on the list. The first appeal of the Alaska Tuberculosis

Committee went out to approximately 13,500 people on November 15, 1934, and brought in $3,375.[20]

An early goal of the NTA was to try to determine the true extent of tuberculosis in Alaska. Here opinions diverged widely, with officials of ANS and the health department recognizing the peril all too clearly, while some in the private sector seemed unable to sense the danger. One prominent Anchorage attorney complained to the governor that his town was being flooded with some kind of stamps in a money-raising scheme that ought to be stopped. The goal was purported to be for tuberculosis control, but everyone knew, he asserted, that the Alaska Native Service took care of all the Indians and Eskimos and that white people didn't get the disease.[21]

On March 16, 1936, Dr. W. W. Council, the part-time territorial commissioner of health, called a meeting of the Alaska Tuberculosis Committee to announce a general tuberculosis survey of Alaska using territorial funds matched with federal funds available under the new Social Security Act. During this meeting the committee was formally organized as the Alaska Tuberculosis Association (ATA), with Dr. Council as president.[22]

By April 15, the epidemiologist Dr. Carswell was able to report that the tuberculosis survey had already reached twenty communities. The survey staff had applied 3,556 tuberculin tests, taken 1,277 x-rays, performed 1,041 physical examinations, and presented 46 public lectures and talks before 3,062 people. The survey had turned up 102 active cases of tuberculosis in adults and another 132 in children. Ten percent of the children at the Bureau of Indian Affairs' Wrangell Institute were found to have active disease. These impressive figures stirred up the controversy again on how the ATA should be spending its limited resources. Most members of the board felt that funds should be used for care of the sick thus found, or for the erection of a hospital, rather than in further support of the survey. Everyone agreed that the organization had to make greater efforts to raise public consciousness about tuberculosis.[23]

The year 1938 was the last in which the organization was run completely by volunteers. The board organized itself into specialized committees, including Christmas Seals sale, publicity, health education, school hygiene, and health movies.[24] Carswell again stressed the importance of obtaining accurate information for presentation to the legislature to bolster their case for a tuberculosis sanatorium.[25]

The x-ray survey begun in FY1937 continued and expanded in 1938 and 1939. The teams were mainly reaching communities with a predominantly white population, however, even though everyone was well aware that most of the tuberculosis was in the more remote Native communities.[26]

Despite this good work, however, ATA was only helping to define the problem, not address it. Active tuberculosis was being found, but little could be done without a sanatorium where the patients could be treated. The association received numerous letters—some pathetic, some angry—from patients pleading for help, and it did what it could to publicize the urgent need for a tuberculosis hospital by writing letters, buttonholing visiting dignitaries, and educating the public. Finally, in FY1942 Congress crowned ATA's efforts by appropriating funds for the construction of a large sanatorium at Saxman, near Ketchikan, but the outbreak of war put the plans on the back burner.[27]

The early war years brought an initial decrease in the association's activities, but in August 1943 the ATA turned a major corner by hiring Bess Winn as its full-time executive secretary. In a single year, receipts from Christmas Seal sales jumped from $2,700 to $14,146. Winn was a woman with a mission, and plunged into her work with enthusiasm. In one of the earliest issues of the new territorial publication *Alaska's Health*, she set forth her stand in an article titled, appropriately, "What We Hope to Do." She described the value of the sale of Christmas Seals in two ways: they gave many people a chance to have a part in a worthy cause, and at the same time they aroused the curiosity of the public about a serious problem. The association, she wrote, would continue its educational efforts and work especially toward the establishment of tuberculosis hospitals in the territory. She concluded with an appeal:

> Perhaps new institutions will be possible in the not too distant future. Perhaps after the war the Government might be persuaded to leave us some of its well equipped military hospitals.... Will we, the people of Alaska, buy more seals during the forthcoming Christmas season and thus help provide wider education, earlier diagnosis, better treatment, and more hospitals?[28]

That same year Representative Bill Egan of Valdez introduced a bill in the legislature asking for $240,000 to contract with hospitals for the care of tuberculosis patients. That august body was not yet ready for such largesse, although it did appropriate $25,000 for the purpose, plus another $3,000 for tuberculosis control.[29]

In 1944 Winn set forth ATA's program philosophy more clearly. An important guiding principle was that its limited funds must not be dissipated on a few cases, but rather divided in a manner that would benefit all. She then outlined four priorities that the organization had established: 1) tuberculosis education of the general public and in the public schools; 2) continuing support for the territorial x-ray survey, with emphasis on expectant mothers [!], crippled children, indigents, and high school students; 3) teaching home care of tuberculosis through pamphlets and other publications; and 4) rehabilitation of Alaskan patients in sanatoriums in the Seattle area.[30]

ATA was becoming a major force in the fight against tuberculosis in Alaska. The organization, enthusiastically led by Winn and composed of dedicated volunteers throughout the territory, was the first to take the initiative for tuberculosis control in Alaska. ATA remained in the thick of the battle against tuberculosis, raising and strategically allocating funds to meet pressing needs, expanding the vision of the health department, and keeping the attention of politicians and the general public clearly focused on the danger that tuberculosis posed to the people of Alaska.

Beginnings of the Territorial Health Department

The Second Organic Act, rather grudgingly passed by Congress on August 24, 1912, finally provided for a bicameral Alaskan legislature, although its powers were severely restricted. When the new legislative body convened for the first time the following March, it passed a law designed to restrict the spread of communicable disease in the territory. First, however, it was necessary to develop an administrative infrastructure to enforce it. The law designated the governor, then an official appointed by the president, as the ex officio commissioner of health. He in turn was authorized to appoint four licensed physicians to serve as assistant commissioners, one in each of the four judicial divisions (later called districts) into which the territory had been divided for administrative purposes. The act delegated to the commissioner the responsibility for supervising "the interests of the health and life of the citizens of the Territory," including the authority to make and enforce quarantine regulations, collect communicable disease reports, isolate any person to prevent the spread of contagious diseases, and carry out a host of specific powers to improve community sanitation.

The new law was prompted by many frightening infectious diseases, including smallpox, influenza, measles, typhoid, scarlet fever, diphtheria, "infantile paralysis" (poliomyelitis), whooping cough, and mumps, all prevalent in Alaska in those years. As for tuberculosis, the law went on, "All cases of tuberculosis..., where the usual precautions to prevent the spread of the disease to others are wilfully neglected and where other persons are liable to become infected on account of this negligence, shall also be considered as capable of conveying contagious or infectious disease," and were therefore subject to the provisions of the law. Any such disease had to be reported to the local board of health, which was empowered to investigate and quarantine if necessary. Following the death, recovery, or removal of a patient with communicable disease, including tuberculosis, the sick room was to be "cleansed and disinfected" under the supervision of the board of health.[31]

The great Spanish influenza epidemic struck Alaska in the fall of 1918, beginning in Norton Sound and later appearing in many of the coastal towns of the Pacific Rim. The following spring the epidemic stalked the fishing villages of the Aleutians and Bristol Bay, leaving a swath of suffering and death. Governor Thomas Riggs, Jr., acting with commendable dispatch and no little administrative courage, arranged for medical support, relief of destitution, and support for the many new orphans resulting from the epidemic. When the legislature met in March 1919, it declared an emergency and reaffirmed the powers of the commissioner, assistant commissioners, and local boards of health to deal with the threat of infectious disease, specifically the current epidemic. No longer did the commissioner simply have the "power," but the law now provided that "it shall be his duty" to make and enforce quarantine regulations, with such rules and regulations having the "force and effect of law."

Later in the session the legislature passed senate Bill 53, which repealed the 1913 law and reorganized the health authority of the territory. Under its provisions the governor could appoint a US Public Health Service officer as commissioner of health of the territory of Alaska, or designate any qualified licensed physician and "competent sanitarian" as commissioner. The statute delegated broad powers to the commissioner, particularly with respect to communicable diseases. Tuberculosis is mentioned as only one of twenty-three diseases to be reported and quarantined, with language nearly identical to that of the 1913 law. No individual suffering from a communicable disease, or a member of his or her household, was permitted, without the express permission of the health officer, to attend any public gathering.[32]

By 1922 the commissioner had promulgated rules and regulations governing the quarantine and isolation of contagious diseases to all physicians, health officers, and teachers.[33] Beginning in about 1925, teachers, priests, and other officials were expected to report deaths and forward death certificates, including a best estimate of the cause, to the secretary of the territory and, after 1927, the territorial auditor. These reports, although a beginning, were not only incomplete, they suffered from many deficiencies of fact, as we have seen above.[34]

The 1931 legislature passed house Joint Memorial No. 4 asking the president, secretary of the interior, and Congress to increase appropriations for the care of Alaskan "Indians," citing recent statistics showing that 36.5 percent of deaths in the past fifteen years among Alaskan Indians and those of mixed blood were caused by tuberculosis, compared with only 1.7 percent in the United States proper.[35] The 1935 legislative session produced house Joint Memorial No. 28, this time addressed to the president, Congress, and commissioner of Indian affairs, to deal with the tuberculosis problem. After pointing out that three times as many Alaskans die of tuberculosis than of any other cause, and that "practically all of the victims of the White Plague are Natives," the resolution went on:

WHEREAS, the only facilities for handling this dreaded disease among the natives...consist of an annex to the Native Hospital in Juneau, Alaska; that this institution is not nearly large enough to care for the patients in this immediate vicinity, and that frequently it has been necessary to refuse admittance to many needy cases which necessitates returning these patients to their families and further exposing others and spreading the disease; that this single institution has demonstrated the wisdom of maintaining such institutions in every Division of the Territory and the need for such places is urgent;

NOW, THEREFORE, your Memorialists petition the Congress . . . to appropriate sufficient funds . . . to construct and operate such institutions in each of the four
Judicial Divisions of the Territory.[36]

While one would like to believe that the members of the legislature were genuinely concerned about the terrible tuberculosis epidemic then raging among the
Natives, the context suggests that the good people of Juneau and elsewhere were
more concerned that there were Natives with active tuberculosis walking the
streets and possibly exposing them to the dread disease.

In February 1936, following the passage of the Social Security Act the previous
year, for the first time outside funds became available for public health development in Alaska. In that year an expanded jury-rigged territorial Department of
Health (TDH) established a public health laboratory and hired five public health
nurses and two physicians.[37]

A provision of senate Bill 73, passed during the 1937 session, established a Division of Crippled Children's Services within TDH to prescribe and carry out a general plan for the care of "crippled and otherwise deformed children;" a requirement
necessary for the territory to participate in the programs available for crippled
children under the US Children's Bureau. Children under the age of fourteen who
were eligible for hospital care were treated at the Children's Orthopedic Hospital
in Seattle, while those aged fourteen to twenty-one were sent to Swedish Hospital
in the same city. By 1941, some 264 children had been identified as needing care, of
whom 63 percent, almost all of them Natives, were suffering from tuberculosis of
the bones or joints. Some concept of the size of the problem may be gained by the
fact that Alaska had 150 known cases of bone and joint tuberculosis in a population
of roughly 70,000 people, while the state of Washington, with a population of 1.7
million, had only 135.[38]

Among the first divisions to be created in the expanded health department in
1936 was that of Communicable Disease Control, which included responsibility for
the tuberculosis problem. The division's priority was a territory-wide tuberculosis
survey to try to learn the true extent of the disease in Alaska, working in close
cooperation with ATA and Aronson's study of the anti-tuberculosis vaccine BCG
in Native villages in Southeast Alaska. The tuberculin testing and x-ray surveys
continued over the next few years.[39]

At least some of those needing hospitalization for tuberculosis were able to
receive care. Non-Natives were all sent outside Alaska, where they either received
care at their own expense or were treated under some government program. The
Alaska Department of Public Welfare also gave partial or complete support to
some fifty-five tuberculosis patients in two Seattle hospitals during the two-year
period 1939–40, but unfortunately it was unable to underwrite the care of every
needy person with tuberculosis. Normally it accepted only those with a significant

hope of recovery, although rarely also patients with advanced disease in order to isolate them from others in the household.[40] Fishermen received care at the PHS Marine Hospital in Seattle.

The Division of Communicable Disease Control, supported in part by funds from the US Public Health Service, continued and even expanded its efforts in the early 1940s. By this time the division had two physicians, one of whom was designated "tuberculosis clinician," plus eleven public health nurses who spent a substantial portion of their time on tuberculosis. In addition, the doctors and public health nurses of ANS were supportive of the program, as were local health officers, where they existed. A rudimentary tuberculosis register was kept in Juneau, consisting of x-ray and tuberculin test reports.

The second priority, after identification of tuberculosis patients, was the isolation of active cases from the uninfected. The third goal was to investigate all contacts of active cases, in order to find other active cases needing treatment and isolation. The tuberculosis clinician spent the bulk of his time in this latter endeavor, x-raying and examining those with positive tuberculin tests, those in close contact with other active cases, and individuals referred for consultation. The staff participated in efforts to educate the public about tuberculosis, how it spread, and how it could be treated when hospitalization was not possible.[41]

By the end of FY1940, TDH estimated that less than one-third of the population had been reached by x-ray surveys, but they were beginning to reach such out-of-the-way places as Chitina, English Bay, Golovin, and Ruby.[42] In 1941 Dr. Palmer Congdon, the tuberculosis clinician, reported that the survey team had x-rayed 7,500 persons in forty-four communities from Ketchikan to Barrow.

By the outbreak of World War II, it was estimated by several techniques that about 2,500 Alaska Natives and perhaps another 200 whites had active tuberculosis in need of hospital treatment.[43] All agreed, however, that little more could be done to hold back the rising tide of tuberculosis without sanatorium beds for treatment.

During the war years, the territorial health department understandably turned much of its attention to the health consequences of the large numbers of military personnel and civilians who poured into Alaska. The US Public Health Service established a special District No. 11 for Alaska, under the direction of Dr. Earl W. Norris, who also served as the director of ANS medical services. Dr. George A. Hays, another PHS officer, was assigned to the health department as its executive officer. A major function of these officials was to coordinate public health activities among TDH, ANS, PHS, and the military services. Near the top of their list of priorities was sexually transmitted diseases—always a problem in a war zone. As for tuberculosis control, the emphasis shifted from case finding in the remote areas to protecting the troops and civilian contract workers from tuberculosis in and around the military bases.[44]

Preparing for the Postwar War

As Alaska emerged from the war zone in 1943, the Territorial Department of Health began planning for the postwar assault on tuberculosis and other health problems. The department initiated a new monthly publication in June 1943 called *Alaska's Health*, which reported to the public on the health needs of Alaska and the programs of the territorial government, particularly with an eye to the coming postwar period. In the very first issue was a detailed policy paper titled "Public Health Needs in Alaska," originally written in 1940 by Dr. Carl E. Buck and later revised by Dr. Hays. This paper set forth four principal recommendations for improving the health situation in Alaska, particularly with regard to tuberculosis. This report is worth a closer look because it sums up how tuberculosis in Alaska was viewed at the end of an era.

"The most important public health problem in Alaska is unquestionably tuberculosis," the relevant section began. Two problems stood in the way of progress: first, the totally inadequate hospital facilities for treatment and isolation; and second, the lack of understanding on the part of the white population that they also suffered from the disease and "that tuberculosis among the Natives for this reason, if not for humanitarian reasons, should be of real concern." Again, tuberculosis control was being couched in terms of protecting the whites from the sick Natives.

The main problem was clearly the lack of beds. No tuberculosis beds at all were available for white patients in Alaska, although the territorial Department of Public Welfare was paying for the care of approximately twenty-four patients in sanatoriums outside the territory. ANS at that time provided only seventy tuberculosis beds itself, and contracted for another twenty-five or so in private hospitals within Alaska. Even when patients were hospitalized, conditions were unsatisfactory. Many facilities had no trained nurses, and tuberculosis patients often roomed in close contact with other patients. In some hospitals Native patients were assigned bed linens just previously used by white patients. Those who complained about conditions in the hospitals were often discharged before they had received the maximal benefits—such as they were—of hospital care.

The report asserted that some 900 tuberculosis beds would be necessary for adequate care of the more than 2,000 active cases estimated to be at large in the territory. Although there would be advantages of scale to building a single large institution, it was thought to be more practical to plan for three—one in the "Eskimo area," one in central Alaska, and one in Southeast Alaska. The original idea was that whites and Natives would be served in each hospital, but in separate pavilions. For the central Alaskan hospital, the report expressed the hope that the 500-bed hospital at Fort Richardson might become available after the war, especially since the facility was well built and, conveniently, already divided into pavilions.

The new hospitals would be best suited for "hopeful cases," while the older military facilities might provide "custodial care" for the "older, less hopeful, cases." All the hospitals would utilize funds from multiple sources, including individual patients, ANS, PHS Marine Hospitals, the Veterans Administration, and the territorial Department of Welfare, not to mention those individuals who were "charitably inclined."[45]

In September 1943, Dr. R. R. Hendrickson, the TDH tuberculosis consultant, wrote an article for *Alaska's Health* in which he summarized for the public the status of tuberculosis treatment at the time. Noting that "no specific drugs, serums or vaccines have been found to prevent or combat tuberculous infection," he asserted that the disease could still be "eliminated entirely" if current knowledge were put to good use. The crux of the program was hospital treatment, both to benefit the individual patient and to prevent exposure of others to the disease. The three foundation stones of hospital therapy were explained to be bed rest, good diet, and surgical collapse of the lung. Bed rest should be absolute at first, but as treatment progressed, the patient could take limited exercise under supervision. A well-balanced diet was necessary to fuel the system and reinforce the body's own natural defenses, while surgical collapse served to put the diseased portion of the lung at rest to permit more rapid healing. The sanatorium also provided, at least in principle, the "mental rest and peace of mind" that was essential for recovery. A program of occupational therapy kept the hands and mind occupied and, if possible, helped the patient gain a marketable skill in keeping with his or her physical limitations after discharge.[46]

Even before the outbreak of the war, the TDH had tried to establish the agency on a firmer legal footing, so that it would be in a position to take full advantage of funding from various federal agencies. In late 1944, the staff drew up a proposed Health Bill for the consideration of the seventeenth territorial legislature and circulated it for comment to the regional health councils and various voluntary health organizations, including the Alaska Tuberculosis Association. The response was very positive and indicated that there was widespread support for the concept.[47] Governor Gruening, originally trained as a physician, also placed the bill high on his list of legislative priorities for the postwar period.

The idea of obtaining surplus military property after the war for use in the health program may have originated with Dr. Hays. Certainly he enthusiastically supported the idea of taking over not only former military hospitals but also equipment, supplies, vehicles, and even ships. Most of these assets he hoped to see used in the battle against tuberculosis.

In December 1943, when the military threat to Alaska was largely over, Governor Gruening suggested to Secretary of the Interior Harold Ickes that if some of the surplus hospitals and medical equipment no longer needed by the military were turned over to the territory, it would "go far to solve our long standing and really grave tuberculosis problem." Recognizing that the War Department might be reluctant to give up such properties, especially before the formal end of the hostilities, he asked the secretary to bring up the subject with the president in a cabinet meeting. Ickes in turn suggested that Gruening take up the matter first with PHS Surgeon General Thomas Parran and with the Army Medical Corps, after which he would consider asking for a cabinet-level meeting.[48]

Only a few days later, Lt. Col. C. Earl Albrecht, commander of the Fort Richardson Army Hospital, met with representatives of TDH, PHS, and the governor's office, following which he announced unofficially that he and other high-ranking army medical officers were also eager to see surplus hospitals turned over to the civilian authorities for use as tuberculosis hospitals.[49] A few weeks later, however, it became clear that the War Department was not ready to accede to the plan, even though Parran had personally put in a word with the military authorities.[50]

The first positive result of these and other negotiations in Washington was that in June 1944 Congress passed a bill authorizing the secretary of war to transfer outright to the Bureau of Indian Affairs the "hospital building and land valued at approximately $1,100,000, and the military stores, supplies, and equipment of every character in said hospital, . . . located at Skagway, Alaska." Congress then added an additional $200,000 over the regular appropriation for medical relief in Alaska for FY1945 in order to renovate and operate the hospital.[51] Although the governor had worked hard to effect this transfer to the Alaska Native Service, he hoped that the hospital would ultimately serve people of all races.[52]

Another facility the governor had had his eye on since at least 1943 was the army hospital at Fort Raymond, a few miles from Seward. This he hoped would serve as a temporary territorial sanatorium until plans for a permanent hospital in south-central Alaska could be realized. On September 15, 1944, Governor Gruening made a formal request for transfer of the hospital and its equipment to the territory, an appeal that ultimately resulted in the establishment in 1946 of the Seward Sanatorium (see chapter 5).[53]

Hays had also foreseen the value of floating public health clinics in Alaska and sought to effect the transfer of surplus military vessels to the health department. In late 1944, Dr. C. C. Carter, who had replaced Dr. Council the previous year as territorial commissioner of health, announced that within a few months a new marine mobile health unit would become available to serve the island communities of Southeast Alaska. This unit was a sixty-five-foot motor vessel, known as the *C-118,* or *Gene,* that the department had purchased from the War Shipping Administration for $9,500. It was to be manned by a crew of four, plus a physician, nurse-technician, public health nurse, clerk, and occasionally a sanitation officer. The vessel would be equipped with an x-ray unit, a laboratory for developing films, and a bacteriological laboratory, with the emphasis on diagnostic services.[54] The following spring, the first Alaska marine unit was put into service (see chapter 4).

Hays could assess the tuberculosis situation more hopefully in his 1944 report on public health in Alaska, as the war was finally winding down:

The most serious and costly problem [of public health] is that of tuberculosis. Health authorities estimate that more than 3000, and possibly 4500, Alaskans are suffering from active and contagious tuberculosis.... Our meager hospital facilities, (70 beds for tuberculosis), have been totally inadequate. However, this situation is not now as hopeless as it has been. It can be vastly improved and at the very minimum of expense.... [W]e are extremely fortunate because we can provide care without any appreciable capital investment for buildings and equipment, which, to the value of millions of dollars, can be had practically for the asking....

Within the past year, and after much promotion and negotiation on the part of several officials and agencies, nearly 300 new hospital beds have been obtained for the benefit of tuberculous Alaskans. The Skagway army hospital, completely equipped, was transferred from the War Department to the Alaska Indian Service and a Congressional appropriation of $200,000 was made for its operation for one year. The Seward army hospital, with most of its equipment, is, by agreement with the War Department, being held for the use of the Department of Health. We have only to obtain and furnish the money to put our suffering citizens in the beds to cure them or to prevent them from infecting others. There is every indication the Congress will make new and large appropriations for the control of tuberculosis. Some of this money will be rightfully Alaska's. But most of what may be allocated to Alaska will be forthcoming only when it can be honestly shown that Alaska is doing all she can for herself.

He went on to note that although the proposed surplus hospitals were of temporary construction, they would serve well for many years, at least until permanent ones—even then being contemplated by Congress—could be constructed. A recent meeting of the Federal Board of Hospitalization had in fact proposed two large general hospitals for Alaska, one with 350 beds in the Interior and another with 250 beds in Southeast Alaska.[55]

The decade of the 1930s, followed by the war years, saw both forward movement and setbacks in the battle against tuberculosis. The transfer of Native health services from the Bureau of Education to the Office of Indian Affairs was a positive step, although the greater resources initially allocated to health soon had to be scaled back because of the Great Depression and the new priorities of wartime. In the 1930s, for the first time, both the federal and territorial governments gained more reliable data on the extent of the tuberculosis epidemic. A major advance in these years was the establishment in 1936 of an ad hoc Territorial Department of Health to receive federal health funds dispensed under the Social Security Administration and the Children's Bureau. The new department undertook major new initiatives, including large-scale x-ray surveys, tuberculin surveys, and chest clinics in the major population centers. The 1930s also saw the founding of the Alaska Tuberculosis Association, a vigorous grassroots partner in the struggle against tuberculosis. The war years retarded all civilian health programs, yet planning for the postwar period continued throughout the war. The outlook for tuberculosis control in Alaska was at last beginning to brighten.

Notes

1. F. S. Fellows, "Mortality in the Native Races of the Territory of Alaska, with Special Reference to Tuberculosis," *Public Health Reports* 49 (1934): 289–98.

2. J. A. Carswell, "Poverty and Tuberculosis with Particular Reference to the Economic and Social Significance of High Death Rates among Alaskans," *Journal of the National Tuberculosis Association* 34 (1938): 233–46. Mortality figures by year from both Fellows and Carswell can be found in appendix A. Carswell also extrapolated the number of active cases by a standard measure of the time that the number of tuberculosis deaths times eighteen gives the total number of cases of tuberculosis in the population. He thus estimated 4,559 cases of tuberculosis among the Alaska Natives, or 15.2 percent of the population, a figure not unlike the estimates from a couple of decades earlier.

3. BCG (Bacille Calmette-Guérin) was a live tuberculosis vaccine developed by French researchers Albert Calmette and Camille Guérin between 1906 and 1921. The original strain was developed from *M. bovis* attenuated over many generations by growth in bile. Although widely tested in Canada and Europe, the vaccine, intended primarily for infants, was never popular in the United States, mainly because of concerns for its safety and the fact that vaccination caused a conversion of the tuberculin test, thus destroying its value for case finding. Where tuberculosis rates were especially high, however, Aronson and others thought it had a place. See Georgina D. Feldberg, *Disease and Class: Tuberculosis and the Shaping of Modern North American Society* (New Brunswick, NJ: Rutgers University Press, 1995), 125–37, 168–74.

4. Joseph D. Aronson and Carroll E. Palmer, "Experience with BCG Vaccine in the Control of Tuberculosis among North American Indians," *Public Health Reports* 61, no. 23 (June 7, 1946): 802–20; John W. Troy, *Annual Report of the Governor of Alaska to the Secretary of the Interior for the Fiscal Year Ended June 30, 1938* (Washington, DC: GPO, 1938), 47.

5. Ernest Gruening, *Annual Report of the Governor of Alaska to the Secretary of the Interior. Fiscal Year ended June 30, 1941* (Washington, DC: GPO, 1941), 52–53.

6. George A. Parks, *Annual Report of the Governor of Alaska to the Secretary of the Interior 1931* (Washington, DC: GPO, 1931), 101–3.

7. Parks, *Report, 1931*, 101–2; US Department of the Interior, *Annual Report of the Commissioner of Indian Affairs to the Secretary of the Interior for the Fiscal Year Ended June 30, 1932* (Washington, DC: GPO, 1932), 12.

8. Parks, *Report of the Governor of Alaska, 1927*, 6; Legislature of the Territory of Alaska, House Joint Memorial No. 14, *Laws of Alaska, 1925* (Juneau, Alaska, 1925), 181; Legislature of the Territory of Alaska, Senate Joint Memorial No. 8, April 19, 1927, Governor Correspondence, roll 144: 23.3; a rough drawing of new facility may be found in Governor Correspondence, roll 144: 23.3; Parks, *Annual Report of the Governor of Alaska, 1931*, 101–2.

9. George A. Parks, *Annual Report of the Governor of Alaska to the Secretary of the Interior 1932 for the Fiscal Year Ended June 30, 1932* (Washington, DC: GPO, 1932), 21–23, 95, 99–100.

10. George A. Parks, *Annual Report of the Governor of Alaska to the Secretary of the Interior 1932 for the Fiscal Year Ended June 30, 1933* (Washington, DC: GPO, 1933), 27–28; US Department of the

Interior, *Annual Report of the Secretary of the Interior for the Fiscal Year Ended June 30, 1933* (Washington, DC: GPO, 1933), 85–87.

11. John W. Troy, *Annual Report of the Governor of Alaska to the Secretary of the Interior for the Fiscal Year Ended June 30, 1934* (Washington, DC: GPO, 1934), 33–35; US Department of the Interior, *Annual Report of the Secretary of the Interior for the Fiscal Year Ended June 30, 1934* (Washington, DC: GPO, 1934), 95–96.

12. Edward F. Vollert, "Indian Service hospitals in Alaska," typescript, in Papers Presented at Public Health Nurses' Institutes held at Juneau, Alaska, Territorial Department of Health, March and April 1941.

13. Diamond Jenness, *Eskimo Administration: I. Alaska,* Arctic Institute of North America Technical Paper no. 10 (Montreal: Arctic Institute of North America, 1962), 49, 49fn.

14. Letter from Wallace C. Philoon to Don G. Foster, May 31, 1945, Governor Correspondence, roll 273. "Far advanced" tuberculosis was defined by x-ray appearance by the National Tuberculosis Association as disease in both lungs and more extensive than "moderately advanced." See the definitions of "minimal," "moderately advanced," and "far advanced" in the glossary.

15. John Tetpon, "Aleut Recalls Trauma of World War II Relocation," *ADN,* October 1, 1987; Linda Billington, "Aleut Recalls Horror of Internment Camps," *ADN,* November 3, 1995; "Aleuts Visit Southeast to Learn about Relatives Lost During WWII," Associated Press State and Local Wire, October 3, 1999; Stephen Haycox, *Alaska: An American Colony* (Seattle: University of Washington Press, 2002), 260–61.

16. Ernest Gruening, *Annual Report of the Governor of Alaska to the Secretary of the Interior for the Fiscal Year Ended June 30, 1940* (Washington, DC: GPO, 1940), 47–48; Ernest Gruening, *Annual Report of the Governor of Alaska to the Secretary of the Interior, Fiscal Year Ended June 30, 1941* (Washington, DC: GPO, 1941), 50–51; Ernest Gruening, *Annual Report of the Governor of Alaska to the Secretary of the Interior, Fiscal Year Ended June 30, 1942* (Washington, DC: GPO, 1942), 23–24; US Department of the Interior, *Annual Report of the Secretary of the Interior for the Fiscal Year Ended June 30, 1941* (Washington, DC: GPO, 1941), 443–44; US Department of the Interior, *Annual Report of the Secretary of the Interior for the Fiscal Year Ended June 30, 1942* (Washington, DC: GPO, 1942), 236, 255–56.

17. Ernest Gruening, *Annual Report of the Governor of Alaska to the Secretary of the Interior for the Fiscal Year Ended June 30, 1943* (Washington, DC: GPO, 1943), 23; Ernest Gruening, *Annual Report of the Governor of Alaska to the Secretary of the Interior for the Fiscal Year Ended June 30, 1944* (Washington, DC: GPO, 1944), 21.

18. Gruening, *Annual Report, 1942,* 19, 24.

19. George Rosen, *A History of Public Health* (New York: MD Publications, 1958), 389–90.

20. Form letter addressed "Hello Alaska!" signed by John W. Troy, November 15, 1934, ATA Collection.

21. Frances L. Paul, "The Beginnings of Tuberculosis Control in Alaska," typescript (April 1956), ATA Collection, 4.

22. Alaska Tuberculosis Committee, Minutes, March 16, 1936; ATA, Minutes, March 23, 1936; ATA, Minutes, May 29, 1936, ATA Collection.

23. ATA, Minutes, April 15, 1937, ATA Collection.

24. ATA, Minutes, July 6 and July 8, 1938, ATA Collection.

25. ATA, Minutes, September 14, 1938, ATA Collection.

26. Troy, *Annual Report, 1938,* 48; Troy, *Annual Report, 1939,* 55.

27. Gruening, *Annual Report, 1942,* 24.

28. Bess Winn, "What We Hope to Do," *AH* 1, no. 4 (September 1943).

29. Territory of Alaska, *Session Laws, Resolutions and Memorials, 1943* (Juneau: 1943), 136–37.

30. Bess Winn, "Tuberculosis in Alaska," *Alaska Life* (Dec. 1944), 36–41.

31. Territory of Alaska, *Session Laws, Resolutions and Memorials 1913* (Juneau: 1913), 69–74.

32. Thomas Riggs, Jr., *Report of the Governor of Alaska to the Secretary of the Interior, 1919* (Washington, DC: GPO, 1919), 9–11; Territory of Alaska, *Session Laws, Resolutions and Memorials 1919* (Juneau: 1919), 4–6, 99–107.

33. Scott C. Bone, *Report of the Governor of Alaska to the Secretary of the Interior, 1922* (Washington, DC: GPO, 1923), 67.

34. Fellows, "Mortality in the Native Races."

35. Territory of Alaska, *Session Laws, 1925,* 272.

36. Territory of Alaska, *Session Laws, Resolutions and Memorials, 1935* (Juneau: 1935), 219–20.

37. Courtney Smith, "History of Public Health Development in Alaska," typescript, in Papers Presented at Public Health Nurses' Institutes held at Juneau, Alaska, Territorial Department of Health, March and April 1941, 5.

38. Wayne S. Ramsey, "Crippled Children in Alaska," typescript, in Papers Presented at Public Health Nurses' Institutes held at Juneau, Alaska, Territorial Department of Health, March and April 1941, 2.

39. Troy, *Report, 1937,* 41, 43.

40. Deborah B. Pentz, "Social Implications of Illness," typescript, in Papers Presented at Public Health Nurses' Institutes held at Juneau, Alaska, Territorial Department of Health, March and April 1941, 4.

41. A. Holmes Johnson, "A General View of Tuberculosis in Alaska," *Diseases of the Chest* (September 1940): 266–69.

42. W. W. Council, *Territory of Alaska. Biennial Report of the Office of the Commissioner of Health, for the Period July 1, 1938 to June 30, 1940, Inclusive* (n.d.), 22–23.

43. Palmer Congdon, "Some Tuberculosis Problems in Alaska," typescript, in Papers Presented at Public Health Nurses' Institutes held at Juneau, Alaska, Territorial Department of Health, March and April 1941.

44. Courtney Smith, "Wartime Public Health in Alaska," *American Journal of Public Health* 32, no. 9 (1942): 965–70.

45. "Public Health Needs in Alaska," *AH* 1, no. 1 (1943): 6–9.

46. R. R. Hendrickson, "Why Tuberculosis Hospitals?," *AH* 1, no. 4 (September 1943).

47. "Alaska's Health Bill," *AH* 3, no. 8 (August 1945).

48. Letter from Ernest Gruening to Harold Ickes, December 9, 1943, Governor Correspondence, roll 248; Memorandum from Harold L. Ickes to Ernest Gruening, December 17, 1943, Governor Correspondence, roll 248.

49. Letter from E. L. Bartlett to Ernest Gruening, December 24, 1943, Governor Correspondence, roll 248.

50. Memorandum from Ernest Gruening to Mr. Thoron, January 5, 1944, Governor Correspondence, roll 248.

51. 58 United States Statutes, ch. 304: 607; 78th Cong., 2d. Sess.

52. Letter from Ernest Gruening to Anthony J. Dimond, September 28, 1944. Alaska, Territorial Government. Governor, General Correspondence, 1909–1958, RG 80-14, roll 248.

53. Letter from Ernest Gruening to Anthony J. Dimond, September 28, 1944, Governor Correspondence, roll 248.

54. "A Dream Becomes Reality," *AH* 2, no. 11 (November 1944); letter from B. W. Thoren to J. W. VonHerbulis, December 30, 1944, Governor Correspondence, roll 247.

55. George Hays, "Public Health Administration," in *Biennial Report of the Office of the Commissioner of Health, for the Period July 1, 1942 to June 30, 1944* (Juneau: 1944).

:4: By Land, Sea, and Air

The Public Health Campaign

The Territorial Government Takes Command

World War II forever changed the face of Alaska. The great influx of military personnel, the construction of new roads, airfields, harbors, and housing units, and the improvements in transportation and communication capabilities all portended a new era of prosperity. Although the war boom was greater than any of the gold rushes, there were also some disturbing trends. After 1943, Alaska became a backwater of the war, the military population decreasing from a peak of 152,000 in 1943 to a mere 19,000 in 1946. On the other hand, the civilian population of the territory had climbed from 74,000 in 1940 to 112,000 a decade later, as many who had come north to work in the war effort decided to cast their lot with the last frontier.[1] Many activities supporting the infrastructure of civilian life, including health services, had been suspended, or at least scaled back, during the war years. Much rebuilding and expansion were needed, especially in the public health sector.

The legislature convened in Juneau on January 22, 1945, its members eager to face some of these pressing problems of the coming peace. The Health Bill (senate and house Bill 52) set forth the legal authority for an Alaska Department of Health (ADH) for the first time. The agency was, among other things, "charged with the duty of administering laws and regulations relating to the promotion and protection of the public health, control of communicable diseases,... care of crippled children, [and] hospitalization of the tuberculous...." As previously noted, the legislation also created a board of health consisting of the governor and four members with staggered four-year terms, one from each of the four judicial divisions of the territory. The members, only one of whom had to be a physician, were nominated by the governor and subject to the approval of a majority of both houses. Among its other functions, the board was empowered to advise the commissioner to make and promulgate rules and regulations, notably with regard to the control of communicable diseases, including "the isolation of any person affected with and prevention of the spread of any contagious or infectious disease."

The bill became law on March 21, 1945. Of a total biennial appropriation of $133,880 for health and sanitation, the legislature appropriated $20,000 for communicable disease control (including tuberculosis), $25,000 for maternal and child health and the care of crippled children (90 percent of whom had tuberculosis of

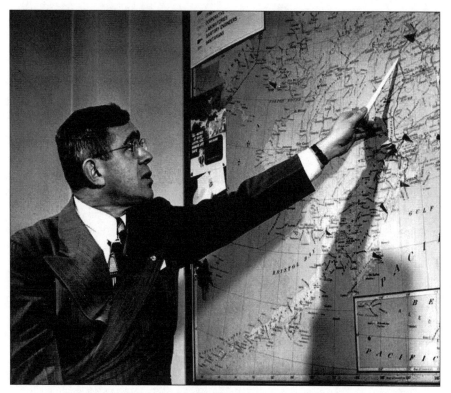

:: Dr. C. Earl Albrecht, first full-time Commissioner of Health for Alaska. ::
(Courtesy of Margery Albrecht)

the bones and joints), and $60,000 for the hospitalization of individuals with tuberculosis.[2] The law also authorized the board of health to appoint a commissioner of health who would serve a five-year term as the chief executive of the department. Significantly, the commissioner was required to be a "reputable physician" with training in public health administration. No more would public health be a sideline of a busy local practitioner.

Governor Gruening, however, wished to appoint his own commissioner and had his eye on Dr. C. Earl Albrecht for the post. Albrecht had come to Alaska in 1935 intending to serve as a Moravian medical missionary in Bethel, but instead found himself sent to Palmer as the physician for the Matanuska Agricultural Colony. From his military travel throughout Alaska during the war years as post surgeon at Fort Richardson, he had begun to appreciate the magnitude of public health problems facing the civilian population of the territory. The governor offered him the post soon after the bill passed.[3] Albrecht was initially reluctant but finally accepted the assignment in the spirit of his training as a medical missionary—to go where his faith directed him and where he could be most useful.[4]

In his first statement to his staff and the people of Alaska in 1945, Albrecht declared that the task of protecting the public health would not be easy in the immediate postwar era because of the shortage of trained personnel, the non-availability of supplies, and limitations resulting from inadequate appropriations. He also published the new health law in full in *Alaska's Health*.[5]

The board appointed by Governor Gruening[6] met for the first time during the first week of September 1945 and devoted its attention primarily to the problem of tuberculosis. In a strongly worded resolution, which it sent to every newspaper and radio station in the territory, the board declared that "tuberculosis has developed into the most critical health problem facing the people of Alaska at this time," with only 289 beds available for tuberculosis care (including those in the States) despite an estimated 4,000 active cases in the territory. Noting that the federal government was prepared to match federal dollar for territorial dollar for the care of tuberculosis patients, the board developed and presented what it felt was a realistic budget of $522,755 to "carry out an adequate hospitalization program" for tuberculosis for FY1947. Surplus army and navy hospitals, equipment, and supplies were currently available for transfer to the territorial government at little cost if sufficient funds could be mobilized. Since the next regular session of the legislature would convene only in January 1947 and by then this fleeting opportunity might be lost, the board urged the governor to call an extraordinary session of the legislature in March 1946.[7] After heated debate in the press about the advisability of calling the session, Governor Gruening finally announced on November 16 his intention to convene the special session in March 1946. Interestingly, in the long public statement announcing his decision, Gruening did not once refer to tuberculosis.[8]

By November Albrecht had distributed a detailed territorial plan for tuberculosis control procedures to all health department employees, physicians, hospitals, and other interested agencies throughout Alaska. In a New Year's message, Albrecht's optimism about the future of tuberculosis control in Alaska was reflected in his listing of five promising trends in public health in Alaska, four of them dealing with tuberculosis. He was particularly pleased by the recent founding of the Alaska Crippled Children's Association (ACCA), which agreed to sponsor a much-needed program to help the many children crippled by bone and joint tuberculosis.[9]

In February 1946 Albrecht established a Division of Tuberculosis Control in the department. On an earlier fund-raising trip to Washington, he had asked the National Tuberculosis Association for financial support for the Alaska tuberculosis program. The agency, however, had a strict policy against direct payments to states (or territories), although it offered to loan a tuberculosis educator to the department. In mid-February, Lois M. Jund, MPH, became the first professional staff member in the new Division of Tuberculosis Control. She plunged into the task at hand with enthusiasm, spending much of her first few months in Alaska writing tuberculosis teaching guides for use in the schools, developing exhibits, and meeting with community groups.[10]

In March, Dr. Leo J. Gehrig, a young PHS tuberculosis consultant, arrived in Juneau to take over the management of the division.[11] His special priorities were case finding and the development of new facilities for the isolation and treatment of the disease. Within a short time he had mapped out a nine-month plan for a massive x-ray survey throughout the territory. He also took the first steps toward the establishment of a central tuberculosis registry, although it did not become fully functional until January 1947.[12] Dr. Gehrig remained until 1948, when he was succeeded as chief of the ADH Tuberculosis Control Division by Dr. Duncan M. Chalmers.

Albrecht was particularly gratified by the mounting enthusiasm for building sanatoriums. OIA had requested funds for a 200- to 300-bed facility in Southeast Alaska to replace the temporary Skagway facility. The commissioner expanded the vision by vigorously supporting the idea of a 500-bed medical center in Anchorage and a 200-bed hospital in the northern region, perhaps at Fairbanks, each of them admitting both Native and non-Native patients. The plans for the two latter hospitals ultimately had to be pared down in the cold light of budget realities, but the hospital for Southeast Alaska seemed to be on track, supported by a flood of letters from communities and individuals in the region. Albrecht himself greatly encouraged such "spontaneous" outpourings, and undertook a number of public appearances to explain the needs.[13] In January 1946, he urged every community in Southeast Alaska to write hundreds of "convincing" letters to federal and territorial officials in support of the proposed OIA hospital construction plan for that region, assuring them, incidentally, that any hospital would also be open to whites. He tried to appeal to their better instincts by asking them to endorse the plan as a whole and not simply promote their own communities as a site. The response was gratifying, although a few did indeed promote the interests of their own community.[14]

The long-awaited special session of the legislature opened for a thirty-day period on March 4, 1946, with a limited agenda that included the tuberculosis problem. The governor's strategy was certainly to see the special session pass the tuberculosis legislation, but it was also essential for him to secure an appropriation in time to obtain the Fort Raymond Army Hospital and thus set the overall plan in motion. Commissioner Albrecht testified three times in support of the bill. The tuberculosis bill was taken up first, not only because of its importance, but probably also because it was the least controversial. The legislature did not fail them. The senate passed senate Bill No. 8 unanimously on March 9, 1946, and three days later the house followed suit, also unanimously. The governor signed the bill into law on March 15.[15] It carried an appropriation of $250,000 for the tuberculosis program— a figure that seems small today but in its time came to approximately one-tenth of the entire territorial budget.[16] In addition, the special session passed senate Bill 22, which set up a Health Surplus Property Fund with an initial appropriation of

$30,000, so that the health department could take advantage of any federal health property that might become available.[17]

The 1946 law authorized ADH to establish a comprehensive program for the control of tuberculosis. Among the primary provisions were the following:

- Arrange means by which all persons in Alaska may be x-rayed to determine the presence of tuberculosis
- Establish outpatient clinics and sanatoriums for tuberculosis
- Contract with private facilities for tuberculosis care
- Obtain surplus federal property that could be used for tuberculosis control
- Establish standards for the treatment of the tuberculous
- Gather tuberculosis statistics in cooperation with other territorial and federal agencies[18]

On May 10 Albrecht was pleased to announce that the War Assets Administration had transferred its hospital at Fort Raymond, near Seward, to ADH for lease to the Methodist Mission Board as a 150-bed tuberculosis sanatorium (for a fuller discussion, see chapter 5). Later in the spring Albrecht went to Washington and was able to parlay most effectively the fact that the territory was willing to spend one-tenth of its operating budget on tuberculosis control. He met with PHS Surgeon General Thomas Parran and other health officials, and testified before the House Sub-Committee on Appropriations. "I believe they were influenced, not unfavorably, in taking an active part in the proposed program," was his understated way of reporting on his mission.[19]

By January 1947 Albrecht could point with pride to the opening of the Seward Sanatorium and the continued operation of the Skagway Sanatorium. He was also pleased to report that Congress had appropriated $1.24 million for the construction of a new permanent sanatorium on Japonski Island, near Sitka. A tuberculosis education program was now in full swing and various mobile health units were already in active service, as will be discussed below.[20]

Albrecht returned to Washington in January 1948. A new development there was the so-called Alaska Program, directed by an interagency committee that included representatives of the departments of the Interior, Agriculture, and Commerce, as well as the Army, Navy, Federal Works Administration, and Federal Security Agency (which included the US Public Health Service). This group had a health subcommittee that made recommendations on many issues, including tuberculosis control. Albrecht was confident that this group would lead to larger health grants for Alaska, and his confidence was not misplaced.[21] That spring Congress appropriated $1.15 million for the new Alaska Health Program, which covered all aspects of public health and mandated cooperation between ADH and PHS. Activities in tuberculosis control made possible by the grant

included an expanded use of mobile x-ray units, the initiation of a BCG program, increased public health nursing coverage, and the establishment of an
arctic health research institute.[22]

Governor Gruening gave his special support to the tuberculosis control program whenever possible. In February 1948 his ire was aroused by a report that
the United States had spent $35 million to eradicate hoof-and-mouth disease in
Mexico—"a neighborly and useful act," he called it. "Yet it seems not unreason-
able," he wrote in a press release,

> to contrast this generous action and appropriation in behalf of a neighbor country's
> cattle, with the pitifully inadequate federal appropriations to stamp out a disease fatal
> to human beings, our American fellow citizens. Apart from the humanitarian aspects
> self-interest is no less involved, since tuberculosis, long unchecked, is extending its
> ravages to more and more of our citizens. Thirty-five million dollars would more
> than build and equip all the tuberculosis hospitals needed and leave a substantial
> balance for maintenance. It would also be a tiny fraction of the aid Uncle Sam is
> generously extending elsewhere in the world.[23]

In his *Biennial Report* for FY1948–50 Albrecht underscored that tuberculosis
remained the largest single health problem in Alaska, with 5,509 cases listed in the
case registry, 3,300 of which had been added in 1949 alone as a result of carrying
x-ray surveys into the more remote parts of the territory. That year a special study
had shown that the x-rays of 4,237 individuals were diagnosed as "active" or "questionably active," including 3,184 who were not hospitalized. Unfortunately, the
interpretation of the films lagged behind, especially in 1949, because of shortage
of personnel. In spite of these delays, some 21,487 films had been interpreted, plus
thousands more by the staffs of the highway and marine units.

By the early 1950s, ADH's aggressive tuberculosis control program was paying
real dividends. In both 1951 and 1952 accidents led the causes of death in Alaska,
and in the latter year tuberculosis actually dropped to third place, behind heart
disease.[24] By June 30, 1950, there were 439 tuberculosis beds in the territory,
mainly at Mt. Edgecumbe and Seward, with additional beds at the various ANS
field hospitals and at the mission hospitals in Nome and Fort Yukon. On April
15, 1950, the Division of Tuberculosis Control, Unit of Venereal Disease Control, and Unit of Acute and Chronic Disease Control were all administratively
joined into the Section of Communicable and Preventive Diseases.[25] This move
perhaps suggested a note of confidence on the part of ADH that tuberculosis
was beginning to decline, but it also was a disturbing trend in that it seemed to
downplay the significance of the disease, which still held many terrors for the
people of Alaska.

The Waning Years of the ANS Medical Program

At the end of World War II, the medical program of the Alaska Native Service was in shambles. Many of the physicians and nurses working in Native hospitals at the outset of the war had joined the military services, and most had not returned to Alaska after the war. Rising prewar health budgets were considerably cut back during the hostilities, and construction projects were put on indefinite hold. Six Native hospitals remained in 1945, at Juneau, Kotzebue, Barrow, Kanakanak, Bethel, and Tanana, the latter three having opened not long before the attack on Pearl Harbor. That year, all 82 available tuberculosis beds in ANS general hospitals were filled, not to mention 55 Native patients treated in Alaska under contract and 111 at the Indian Sanatorium in Tacoma, Washington.[26] In April the ANS Skagway Sanatorium opened in a surplus army station hospital.[27] By the end of the following fiscal year, the ANS program had begun to rebuild. All hospitals were filled to capacity, and the full-time staff rose 8 percent, from 150 to 162.

One interesting by-product of the war years was the great expansion of the shortwave radio network that connected ANS schools and hospitals with each other and with the headquarters in Juneau. By mid-1946, some seventy facilities were tied into the system.[28] The Clinic of the Air (or Radio Medical Traffic, as it came to be known) became increasingly important, and by FY1950 hospitals in Bethel, Kotzebue, Kanakanak, and Tanana were in touch with numerous schools on a daily basis.[29]

FY1950 was a historic year for the ANS health program, with the opening of the new 200-bed tuberculosis sanatorium at Mt. Edgecumbe, and the construction of twenty-four-bed Quonset huts for tuberculosis at Bethel, Kanakanak, and Kotzebue. In August 1949, ground was broken in Anchorage for a state-of-the-art tuberculosis/general hospital projected to cost $7 million. By the end of that year, ANS had 486 tuberculosis beds available in its own facilities and, in addition, contracted for 65 tuberculosis beds at the Seward Sanatorium.[30] With the opening of the long-awaited hospital at Anchorage on November 23, 1953, the ANS Medical Service reached its apogee of 701 tuberculosis beds, only to go out of business a mere eighteen months later.[31] (Tuberculosis hospitals are discussed in the following chapter.)

Screening Surveys and the Tuberculosis Registry

In April 1945 Dr. Rudolph Haas, a consultant from the Public Health Service and later director of the Skagway Sanatorium, drafted a four-point tuberculosis control program for Alaska, the first principle of which was the discovery of all tuberculosis cases. Tuberculosis case finding, in his view, aimed to discover every case of tuberculosis, including infection unknown to the victim. In that period the primary method for case finding was x-ray surveys of large groups of people at risk, using the recently developed small-film technology. This approach, Haas felt, was not practical in Alaska because of the great distances and scattered population. Instead, he recommended x-raying all hospital admissions, hospital personnel, persons newly employed, teachers, students entering and leaving high school, and all food handlers. Where x-ray equipment was not available he suggested tuberculin testing or, in patients with cough and chest symptoms, examination of the sputum for tubercle bacilli.

As the second principle of case finding, Haas recommended that all schoolchildren be routinely tuberculin tested and those with positive reactions x-rayed. Household members of each positive reactor should then be examined, with those under age twelve being tuberculin tested and x-rayed if positive, and those over twelve x-rayed regardless.[32] Dr. Albrecht, when he became commissioner in July 1945, endorsed Haas's plan. Almost immediately, however, ADH found itself with a film shortage and a request from the PHS in Washington not to conduct tuberculosis surveys until further notice.[33]

Around the same time, Dr. James A. Smith, medical director of ANS, was also casting a big net for tuberculosis. At the six ANS hospitals, x-rays were being performed on all inpatients and on outpatients with histories of contact with the disease, as well as on students applying for admission to its boarding schools and for placement in foster homes. The twenty ANS public health nurses were also active in tracing contacts and having them x-rayed.[34]

When Dr. Gehrig arrived in Juneau in March 1946, he agreed that case finding should be the number-one priority, although he favored the more traditional approach of mass x-ray surveys. Instead of using fixed equipment in hospitals and urban centers, he fostered the use of portable photoroentgen equipment carried on ships, trucks, and airplanes. This unit took four-by-five-inch films that were read immediately by the physicians. Patients with "definite" or "suspicious" tuberculosis were referred to their own physician for follow-up. Gehrig also announced a program of chest x-rays by private physicians, the cost to be borne by ADH.[35]

The ADH survey began with the schoolchildren in Juneau in May 1946 and went on to Wrangell and Petersburg, where the entire populations were x-rayed. In June and July, nearly 8,000 individuals were screened in Anchorage, an additional 1,555 in Palmer in August, and 4,200 more in Fairbanks in August and September. Nenana was not on the itinerary, but many letters and telegrams "demanding" a survey led to a visit there also. The navy then flew the team to Barrow, and in October the survey visited Nome, Kotzebue, and Unalakleet, later followed by Bethel, Seward, and Kodiak. In the winter the rest of Juneau's population was surveyed, and then it was on to Sitka.[36]

One of the striking examples of public cooperation and support was evidenced by the hundreds of female volunteers who assisted in preparing communities for their surveys. Prior to the June 1947 survey in Anchorage, for instance, more than

100 members of the Anchorage Women's Club fanned out across the city ringing doorbells and urging men, women, and children to participate. They began their work several weeks before the x-ray unit came to town, explaining the purpose of the x-rays, making appointments, and sending reminders. When the actual survey took place, volunteers manned the tables at the grade school, where the equipment operators were able to take some 7,465 films at a rate of nearly 100 per hour.[37] Both the *Anchorage Daily News* and the *Anchorage Daily Times* encouraged the campaign in enthusiastic lead editorials.[38] A similar level of enthusiasm was shown in Fairbanks, Juneau, and other communities.[39]

The first report on the extensive surveys carried out in 1946 and the first half of 1947 was released in October. A total of 15,234 individuals were x-rayed on the M/S *Hygiene*, the mobile truck unit along the Glenn, Richardson, and Alcan highways (see below), and by the new portable photoroentgen unit, but only 36.7 percent were Natives. Moreover, most of the Natives examined were from Southeast Alaska, where the standard of living was significantly higher than in most western and northern villages. Among the 8,854 whites x-rayed, only 3 percent showed evidence of tuberculosis, while 12.9 percent of the 5,592 Natives showed evidence of the disease. Although the surveys had made a solid start, health officials knew that the real tuberculosis problems were among the people of western and northern Alaska not yet reached by the survey.[40]

In 1948 the surveys were expanded to some areas of northern and western Alaska. The figures were most revealing: in Bethel 17.3 percent of x-rays showed observable lesions, in Unalakleet 15.8 percent, and in Kotzebue 23.2 percent, while in Seward the figure was 3.3 percent and in Douglas 4.3 percent—both communities with a relatively small Native population.[41]

By the end of the following fiscal year, when the survey emphasis was on Bristol Bay and the Arctic, Albrecht could report that 70 percent of all Alaskans had been x-rayed at least once. Among the 12,000 films taken that year, 1,800 (15 percent) showed proven or suspected tuberculosis.[42]

To keep track of the huge amounts of tuberculosis information being collected, a central case registry was essential. Although it got minimal publicity relative to the more newsworthy health ships and sanatoriums, it was in a sense the very foundation of the overall effort.

Dr. Gehrig took the first steps toward developing such a registry. This was to be an active file of all reported cases of tuberculosis in the territory, to include for each patient demographic data, type of disease, stage, results of x-ray and sputum tests, and what sort of care had been given. Besides being a reliable source from which epidemiological data could be derived, such a central registry also alerted health officials to where the hot spots of tuberculosis were in the territory. Its value, of course, depended wholly on the accuracy and timeliness of information provided by public health nurses, physicians, and other health officials in the field, especially the staff of ANS, whose federal status made them naturally suspicious of officials from local jurisdictions. Considerable effort was devoted to making the reporting as easy as possible, and in general the response was good. ADH even made an attempt to notify local health officials when a case of tuberculosis, at whatever the stage, moved into their jurisdiction.[43]

By mid-March 1950 the case registry had 5,279 names. Of these, only 489 were hospitalized either in Alaska or in contract hospitals outside the territory, leaving at home 3,184 individuals needing hospital care, most of whom were going about their normal daily activities as best they could and interacting with other susceptible persons. The remainder of the names included 568 patients with arrested or inactive diseases in their homes, and 1,042 "suspects," whose activity status was unknown.

The registry was not simply a permanent list of all known cases. At the end of the previous calendar year, the names of sixty-three "suspects" had been removed and another 583 cases closed because of cure or arrest of the disease. The registry totals were the highest ever, but, as Albrecht pointed out, these numbers did not necessarily represent more tuberculosis, but rather the identification of more cases by x-ray surveys and follow-up.[44]

The ADH "Navy" and the Highway and Railway Health Units

The army surplus vessel obtained by the Territorial Department of Health in 1944, appropriately named M/V *Hygiene* (or *Hy Gene*, as some wags called it), sailed from Juneau on its first health cruise on April 4, 1945, and over the next seven months visited the ANS boarding schools at Sitka and Wrangell and fifteen other communities of Southeast Alaska. The staff offered not only case finding for tuberculosis and crippling conditions but many other types of public health services and even emergency medical care.[45]

During the winter, ADH decided that a larger vessel was needed—one not restricted to the sheltered waters of Southeast Alaska, but able to visit the remote villages of Kodiak Island, the Aleutian Islands, and the Bering Sea coast. Dr. Albrecht contacted the Army Service Forces and found a suitable surplus vessel, the *FS-35*, which was to be loaned to ADH at no cost to see whether it would meet the needs of the department.[46] The wooden ship was 115 feet in length and weighed in at 280 gross tonnage. In January 1946 the deal was done, and ADH then bore the cost of extensive refitting at a Seattle dry dock to modify the ship for use as a clinic. The annual cost of operating the ship in Alaska was estimated at $70,500.[47]

On April 3 the special session of the legislature authorized the sale of the M/V *Hygiene*, with the proceeds to offset the cost of alterations on the new marine unit, dubbed the M/S *Hygiene* (sometimes called *Hygiene II*).[48] The vessel, capable of operating year-round in stormy Alaskan waters, was equipped with a modern photoroentgen unit, powered by a generator on the deck and capable of taking several hundred large or small films a day, including those necessary for diagnosing tuberculosis of the bones and joints. The ship sported a doctor's office, nurse's office, secretary's office, clinic room, compact laboratory, and large waiting room that could be used for group discussions and health education movies. The professional staff included a field physician—initially Dr. Ann Kent—a public health nurse, bacteriologist, dentist, dental assistant, and secretary.[49]

The staff and crew set off on their shakedown cruise in early June 1946, visiting two villages and three canneries near Juneau before proceeding to Ketchikan, where some 3,300 x-rays were taken. Later that year the *Hygiene* visited the villages of the Alaska Peninsula and Aleutian Islands, then the next year returned to Southeast Alaska before heading north as far as Norton Sound.[50] Patients were initially screened with four-by-five-inch films, but if the doctor noted suspicious lesions, the patient was called back for a full-size film.[51] Sometimes, in more remote communities where the ship had to anchor offshore, the doctor read the film while it was still wet, so that the patient and his or her family would know the good (or often bad) news before setting out on the dangerous journey home in a small open boat or canoe.[52]

Catherine ("Kitty") Smulling was a public health nurse on the *Hygiene* during its early voyages. Many years later (as Kitty Gair) she and medical officer Dr. Elaine Schwinge collaborated on x-ray and laboratory technician Susan Meredith's book, *Alaska's Search for a Killer*, describing in detail their day-to-day adventures visiting the remote coastal communities of Alaska.[53] The expected arrival of the ship would be radiogrammed ahead whenever possible. The ship would usually anchor near a town, then the staff would go ashore in a dory to meet with village leaders, send messengers through the town, and set up a clinic schedule. The villagers then came out to the ship in family groups in small boats and underwent x-rays, blood tests, immunizations, and physical examinations throughout a seemingly endless day. The ship would then weigh anchor and move through the night to a new village, where the process began again. The staff had its emotional highs and lows: "We'd gripe and howl one minute, and grin the next. When we'd hit a big port, after mail-less months of isolation, there'd be an explosion of spirits." The living conditions, tough as they were, led to many shipboard romances and six marriages, including Smulling's own.[54]

Although the ship offered a wide range of health services, its primary mission was tuberculosis case finding and education. Between April 4, 1945 and July 1, 1948, the staff of the two *Hygienes* x-rayed 13,341 people, discovering 756 cases of active tuberculosis.[55] A special contribution of the M/S *Hygiene*'s program was the examination of families as a group, an approach that allowed the nurse and doctor to see how families interacted when confronted by a disruptive and disturbing disease like tuberculosis.[56]

The second marine health unit was the M/V *Health,* acquired in November 1948. It was a 104-foot seagoing barge designed for use by the army in the Aleutians

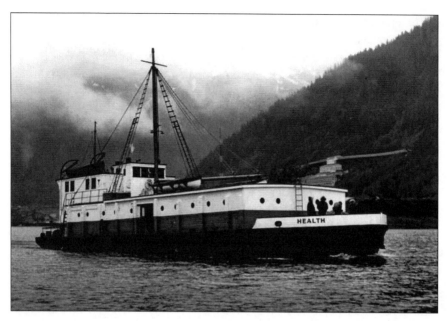

:: M/V *Health*, marine unit for the Alaska Department of Health. ::
(Courtesy of Margery Albrecht)

during World War II. Because of its shallower seven-foot draft, it was able to operate in coastal waters, such as river deltas, inaccessible to the *Hygiene*. The vessel was
remodeled that winter and provided with a new 200-milliampere x-ray unit capable
of taking both four-by-five-inch plates and standard fourteen-by-seventeen-inch
films. A clinical laboratory allowed the staff to make immediate examination of
sputum specimens. The new vessel was commissioned on April 19, 1949.[57]

During the 1949 cruise, Dr. Hazel Blair reported optimistically on the efforts
of some of the villages to deal with the tuberculosis problem. Writing of Elim, a
Norton Sound community, she noted:

> The village council is interested and cooperative about the care of these people [with
> tuberculosis]. At the time we left they were willing to assist tuberculous families in
> building an extra room on their houses so that the infected people might be isolated.
> One family offered to adopt the baby of one young woman whom [*sic*] we found to
> have active tuberculosis. The offer, incidentally, was accepted. The people are intel-
> ligent with regard to their tuberculosis problem and are beginning to handle it them-
> selves in their own way. . . .[58]

In addition to its regular public health work, the staff of the *Health* carried out
extensive tuberculin testing and administered BCG.[59] The enthusiasm of the villagers about the arrival of the floating clinic was impressive. At Sheldon's Point (now

called Nunam Iqua), people visiting the ship had to travel eighteen miles at sea in an outboard motorboat. The village chief provided transportation for the doctor and nurse to be able to visit bedridden patients in the village. Sometimes villagers held an Eskimo dance for the benefit of the visitors. At Kwiguk, near the mouth of the Yukon, most of the transient cannery workers remained two weeks after the close of the canning season in order to take advantage of the ship's visit.[60] Over the next two years, the *Health* remained largely in the Aleutians and the Bering Sea, including a visit to East Cape, Siberia. In 1952 work was concentrated in the Aleutians, Norton Sound, St. Lawrence Island, and the Bering coastal villages.[61]

The third marine unit, the *Yukon Health*, was an eighty-six-foot former navy supply power barge, purchased in Seattle in late 1948 and refitted there and in Juneau. The vessel had an unconventional design, being thirty feet wide, with only thirty inches of draft, allowing it to pass over many of the treacherous and shifting sandbars on the Great River.[62] The emphasis of its program was tuberculosis case finding, but the staff offered a full range of public health services.[63]

In 1949 the *Yukon Health* visited eight lower Yukon Yup'ik villages, and the following year stopped at ten permanent river communities and a number of smaller camps before going into winter quarters. Besides general health services, the public health nurse administered tuberculin tests and vaccinated those who were negative with BCG, although as many as 93 percent of those tested were already positive.[64] During the 1951 and 1952 seasons, the vessel again visited villages of the Lower Yukon, wintering both years at Holy Cross. A notable event occurred there when the majority of the people from Holikachuk came 110 miles downstream in open boats and those from Shageluk made a sixty-mile journey to be examined.[65]

Drastic cuts in federal funding caused all three health ships to be deactivated at the end of the 1952 navigation season. Personnel on the units, to the extent possible, were assigned to unfilled positions elsewhere in the department.[66] The following spring Dr. Albrecht testified in Washington about the importance of the ships in the tuberculosis program, suggesting darkly that "the health gains won in the past few years will be lost and to regain the losses will mean a larger appropriation for tuberculosis hospital beds [and] more beds for orthopedic cases." Despite support from many, including the governor, his efforts failed.[67] The *Yukon Health* and the *Health* were sold a few years later without returning to service, but in August 1954 a special appropriation allowed the *Hygiene* to be reactivated for duty in the Bering Sea. It continued its operations through the summer of 1957, primarily serving the Aleutian Island communities.[68]

The marine health units had accomplished much in bringing general public health services to parts of Alaska that had rarely, if ever, seen a health professional. The visits of the ships reduced the isolation, relieved many anxieties, and let the people of far-flung communities know they were part of something larger and, for once, benevolent. It is difficult to measure in any scientific way just what the

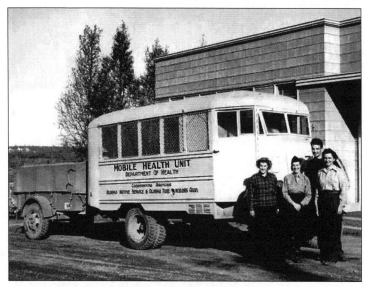

:: ADH mobile health unit, 1940s. ::
(Courtesy of Alaska State Library, Alaska Department of Health and Social Services Collection, D.C. Knudsen, PCA 143-1282)

marine units contributed to tuberculosis control, but it is evident that many new cases were discovered and brought to treatment, and other individuals were given solace and reliable advice on how to make the best of the situation until the call to the hospital arrived.

Other types of mobile units were land-based. In the summer of 1946 the health department converted an army surplus truck into a mobile clinic. The unit contained clinic space, health education facilities and supplies, and portable x-ray equipment powered by a gasoline generator pulled behind in a trailer. X-ray films were developed in the truck, so that they could be read before the truck left the village. Sometimes the staff even had to string a "film line" between two trees to hang the x-ray films out to dry. The unit was staffed by a physician, nurse, and driver-technician. The clinic stops were announced ahead by radio, usually on a Fairbanks station. When the truck reached a community, the first priority for the staff was to find living quarters and then some type of facility in which the clinic could be set up. Typically this was an Alaska Road Commission camp, roadhouse, the home of an ANS teacher, or a Native home. Volunteers from the community, including teachers, missionaries, village chiefs, and children, often assisted in rounding up the families for their x-rays and examinations.

Beginning in October 1946, the highway unit traveled the Glenn, Richardson, Tok, and Alcan (Alaska) highways, concentrating particularly on x-ray surveys in areas where no health services were available. By the time of its return to Anchor-

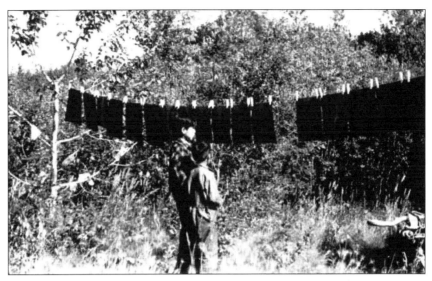

:: Boys viewing x-rays hanging out to dry, ADH mobile truck unit, 1940s. ::
(Courtesy of Alaska State Library, Alaska Department of Health and Social Services Collection, PCA 143-999)

age on December 9, the staff had found 88 active cases of tuberculosis among 896 persons x-rayed (9.8 percent).[69]

In the earlier years, when tuberculosis beds were in drastically short supply, the team identified patients with active disease and put them on a waiting list, then concentrated on teaching the family how best to care for the patient at home, not only to give the victim the best hope of survival while awaiting treatment, but also to protect other members of the household from infection. In many homes this was an empty hope, because of poverty and crowding. In several Athabascan villages the prevalence of active disease reached nearly 10 percent, and in one community the team found only two families without evidence of the disease.[70] The unit continued its seasonal operations until 1949, when it too became the victim of budget cuts.[71]

Encouraged by the success of the truck unit, Commissioner Albrecht was quick to see the potential of a railway unit to serve the railway section houses and rail communities between Seward and Fairbanks. Many of these areas were inaccessible by road and inhabited mainly by rail workers or Alaska Natives, both groups at special risk for tuberculosis. In the spring of 1949, ADH was able to obtain two railway cars, with the cooperation of the Alaska Railroad, for use as a mobile rail unit.[72] The rail unit began operations in November 1949, and during its single season it visited some twenty-eight communities—large, small, and even flag stops—many of them with no other access to health services. The program was scuttled after the winter of 1949–50 because of budget constraints.[73]

BCG Vaccination Program

Each year, even through the war years, Dr. Joseph Aronson's team visited Alaska to follow up on the participants in his study of BCG vaccine, as discussed in chapter 3. By 1948 he was able to report that of a total of 1,550 Southeast Alaska Indians given the vaccine, only 6 had died of tuberculosis, whereas among the 1,457 people serving as controls, no fewer than 52 had died of the disease. Among 123 newborns vaccinated, none died of tuberculosis, compared with 4 tuberculosis deaths among 139 newborns serving as unvaccinated controls. The tuberculin test remained positive after ten years in about 90 percent of those vaccinated.[74]

These rather impressive results caught the eye of Commissioner Albrecht in early 1947, and he expressed the hope that the vaccine might be suitable for more general use in Alaska. At that time, BCG was available only on an experimental basis in the United States.[75] In January 1948 Albrecht traveled to Washington and gained the support of Surgeon General Parran, Dr. Ralph Snavely, medical director of OIA, and Aronson himself. At that time, the vaccine was being produced in the United States in a single laboratory in Chicago, and had to be administered no more than ten days after its preparation. The logistics and expense of the proposed program were formidable, but the cost was moderate compared with that of treating and rehabilitating individuals with active disease.[76]

In the summer of 1948 Aronson and a couple of ADH physicians began vaccinating around Barrow and in Southeast Alaska with BCG from the Chicago laboratory. The team recommended that newborns and other infants should be given the vaccine, since a large majority of Native children under twelve were known to have a primary infection.[77] In September, with Washington's guarded blessing, Albrecht established the first of several ADH teams to carry out vaccinations in the areas of Alaska with the highest tuberculosis incidence. The teams were to administer BCG to all individuals with negative tuberculin tests living in those areas, whether Native or white, as well as to all contacts of tuberculosis patients, and, to the extent possible, all newborns. In the interest of economy, the teams had other health functions, including case finding and treatment of venereal disease, and the provision of emergency treatment in isolated areas.[78]

Beginning in October two BCG teams, each consisting of a physician and a nurse, gave about 5,000 vaccinations. Local physicians were also taught the technique for administering the vaccine, since plans called for a continuing program of administering BCG to newborns and to those not previously immunized. The ADH teams would then be able to concentrate their efforts on larger communities.[79]

The marine health units were especially effective for carrying out the program, since the vessels usually remained at a village for a week or more. Getting the vaccine from the Chicago laboratory to those who administered it in the villages, however, could be quite an adventure. The vaccine had to be preserved in special containers to keep it cold. Because of the vaccine's limited shelf life, the health team, whenever possible, scheduled the arrival of the BCG after it had already tuberculin tested the local population. The airlines cooperated magnificently. They flew the vaccine to Seattle and then on to Anchorage, where Alaskan pilots took it to the field either on the regular mail planes or by small chartered aircraft. On occasion, when airplanes couldn't land because of weather or other adverse conditions, the vaccine was even dropped into the water by parachute in a specially wrapped container and recovered by skiff.[80]

One of the department's most experienced field nurses, Ruth Grover Hudson, wrote an account of the vagaries of the BCG program. This deserves to be quoted at some length, even allowing for its sentimentality and the patronizing attitudes of the era, because it gives a realistic picture of the routine followed by many nurses and doctors in the field, whether in the BCG program or not.

"You going to poke me?" little dusky skinned, rosy cheeked Alaskan natives ask the BCG nurse as they peer out from the furred ruffs of their winter parkas. Even though the nurse has just crawled out of a tiny bush plane that is still sitting on the ice of the small lake bordering the village, news somehow gets around quickly in these isolated Eskimo, Aleut or Indian villages and a crowd of children and grown-ups greets her and accompanies her up the path to the mustard-colored Alaska Native Service school building which is the center of community activity....

The teacher and villagers have been expecting the arrival of the BCG nurse if they have heard her itinerary broadcast over Mukluk Telegraph or Tundra Topics (nightly radio programs originating in Anchorage and Fairbanks which broadcast items of special interest to small villages). Perhaps the Alaska Native Service doctor has publicized the route over his daily radio schedule....

Within a few minutes, the schedule is arranged and the clinic starts. At an extra long peal of the school bell, people seem to appear from nowhere. As many as 15 come pouring out of one small shack or sod hut. They gather in the school room and listen as the nurse tells them of the program. Then an interpreter translates for those who do not understand English.... Everyone...looks forward, eagerly, to the "pokes"—their favorite term for injection with a hypodermic needle....

Tuberculin tests are read 48 or 72 hours later and the negative reactors are then vaccinated with BCG. During the waiting period, the nurse finds herself doing varied tasks. If there is no teacher in the village, she is sometimes asked to read and write letters for those unable to do so for themselves. In areas where medical assistance is not available, she may be asked to help with emergencies and to inspect chronic conditions such as draining glands, running ears and infected eyes....[81]

Although the stated goal of the BCG program was ultimately to vaccinate all Alaskans who were tuberculin-negative, efforts to accomplish this end were concentrated in isolated areas with a high incidence of the disease and in larger cities where the service could be provided with relatively little expense. Although the ADH staff was small, the program was able to accomplish what it did by the support and cooperation of many physicians, nurses, educators, the airlines, and the armed services. Activity reached its peak during 1948 and 1949, but in January 1950 budget constraints reduced the BCG unit to a nurse and a clerk in the ADH Anchorage office.[82] Congress made further cuts in tuberculosis control funds for FY1952, causing the suspension of the program during the winter of 1951–52. By then some 30,000 tuberculin tests had been administered and 13,000 vaccinations given.[83]

Meanwhile, Dr. Aronson was continuing his follow-up studies on the original group of children he had vaccinated in the 1930s. On a visit to Juneau in June 1951, he reported that over a fourteen-year period, more than four times as many individuals had died of tuberculosis and more than three times as many had contracted tuberculosis among the unvaccinated group as among those who had received the vaccine.[84]

In March 1952 Dr. Albrecht was able to reactivate the BCG program because the PHS loaned a nurse, Gladys Ray, to the department for four months. She set to work training the public health nurses in the technique of administering the vaccine, concentrating on those who had not had previous BCG experience.[85] One major advantage for the renewed program was that dry vaccine was now available, offering a shelf life of three months instead of the previous maximum of ten days. Special emphasis was now placed on vaccination of the newborn. By April 1953 ADH could report that over the previous thirteen months 2,486 Alaskans, mostly very young children, had been given BCG in communities stretching from the Kenai Peninsula to Barrow. The teams found the lowest tuberculin-positive rates (20 percent) in the Seward area and the highest in Barrow, where virtually everyone but the very young were tuberculin-positive.

In September 1954 Drs. Joseph B. Stocklen and James E. Perkins, tuberculosis consultants for the Parran survey team, noted that the BCG program was beginning to lag, a view acknowledged by both ADH and ANS health personnel. Physicians and local health officers rarely promoted use of the vaccine, and public health nurses working in the towns and cities often failed to include it in their regular immunization program. ANS staff acknowledged that Native newborns usually did not receive the vaccine because of a rule that such infants had to remain isolated in the hospital for six weeks. Even so, during FY1954, some 1,900 individuals were vaccinated.[86]

In August 1955 Dr. Charles R. Hayman, then ADH director of tuberculosis control, was still urging that BCG be given to all negative reactors and newborns in those areas where tuberculosis was widespread, and when the M/S *Hygiene* resumed its voyages in June 1956, BCG vaccination was still part of its general health program.[87] In April 1956 Dr. Aronson returned to Alaska to finish up his studies on BCG, and concluded that there was "ample evidence that BCG gives a significant degree of immunity against tuberculosis." A grand total of 962 children in Southeast Alaska had participated in the study, of whom 498 received the vaccine and 464 served as controls. In the former group, only four deaths from tuberculosis had occurred, compared with thirteen in the unvaccinated group.[88]

Despite continued evidence of the efficacy of the vaccine, other methods of prevention, notably INH prophylaxis (see chapter 6), were proving even more valuable, since the use of the pills, unlike BCG, did not interfere with tuberculin sensitivity. In 1959 Gentles reported that BCG had not been used to any extent during the previous three years, and thus this important element of tuberculosis control in Alaska passed into history.[89] During the period 1937 to 1956, more than 18,000 people had been vaccinated, mostly Natives living in high-risk areas of the territory. The findings of Aronson's study make it likely that many individual Alaskans were spared the development of active tuberculosis by receiving BCG vaccine.[90]

American Medical Association Surveys

In the spring of 1947 Dr. Albrecht, in consultation with the staff of the Alaska Native Service, asked the Department of the Interior for a comprehensive survey of health conditions in Alaska. Not the least of his reasons was to gain publicity on the national stage for the severity of Alaska's health problems so that he could use this information to badger Congress for further health appropriations. The survey was to be carried out by a team of eminent physicians selected by the Advisory Committee of the American Medical Association (AMA) to the Department of the Interior. The group of five physicians, all from the Cook County Hospital in Chicago, was chaired by Dr. Arthur Bernstein.

The team arrived in Anchorage on July 19 and completed its 4,500-mile tour on August 9. Guiding the team were Drs. Albrecht and Gehrig from ADH, Dr. Howard Rufus, medical director of the ANS Medical Branch, and Dr. W. T. Harrison, representing Surgeon General Thomas Parran. During their three weeks in the field, the group visited fifteen communities, including Bethel, Unalakleet, Nome, Gambell, Kotzebue, Barrow, Tanana, Hoonah, and Metlakatla. They consulted with ANS physicians, private physicians, field and hospital nurses, teachers, school administrators, local and territorial officials, and finally with Governor Gruening himself. Team members also carried out several hundred patient consultations and even performed a few operations in the field hospitals. Their report was published in full that October in the *Journal of the American Medical Association*, where it reached a nationwide readership of physicians. The hard-hitting account covered all aspects of health, but focused mainly on tuberculosis, where "the statistical data are unassailable, and these with our personal inspection served to impress the committee with the urgency of the problem...."

Pulmonary tuberculosis was everywhere they went. At Bethel the team spent a half day in the outpatient clinic and picked up six new cases of active tuberculosis, all of whom had to be sent home because no beds were available. The ANS physician

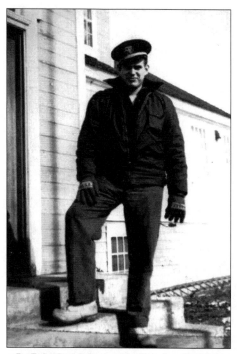

:: Dr. E. S. "Stu" Rabeau at the Kotzebue Hospital ::
in the 1950s. *(Courtesy of Mary Ann Rabeau)*

there, Dr. Fred Langsam, considered that, regardless of the diagnosis, 50 percent of cases that presented were complicated by tuberculosis. Persons with tuberculosis of the spine, both active and inactive, "were a common sight." At Kotzebue the team met with Dr. E. S. Rabeau, who had compiled statistics showing that over a four-and-a-half-year period, 54.7 percent of deaths were attributable to tuberculosis, with about half of these cases confirmed at autopsy. In a period of seventeen months, he had treated forty cases of tuberculous meningitis. At Barrow, the teacher reported that of the thirty children who had entered school between the ages of five and six years, only six had lived to finish. At Perryville, on the Alaska Peninsula, more than half of the children died before the age of six. A review of official statistics by the committee revealed that there were an estimated 4,500 cases of open tuberculosis in the territory, with some villages showing 25 percent of the population affected. Tuberculosis was causing 20 percent of all deaths in the territory, and 69 percent of all communicable disease deaths were due to the disease. About 60 percent of the cases reported to ADH in 1945 were first reported from the death certificate.

The committee noted further that the sanatorium facilities in the territory were "hopelessly inadequate to stem the tide of tuberculosis." They praised the case finding efforts of ADH, but noted with concern that there was no rehabilitation program in place for those with tuberculosis. The team optimistically predicted that tuberculosis could be controlled in Alaska in about five to eight years if the proper resources were available.

In concluding their section on tuberculosis, they stressed that tuberculosis knew no color line, that Alaska and its people were important from the defense standpoint, and that a workforce with tuberculosis was an economic liability. "Finally," they wrote rather ominously, "to the parents, relatives, and friends of those going to Alaska, both as civilians and in armed forces, the rate of tuberculosis in the territory constitutes an ever present danger." The suffering of the Native people of Alaska seems not to have penetrated their consciousness.

Their recommendations, however, proved a great boost to Dr. Albrecht's agenda. They considered tuberculosis to be the "most serious and urgent problem that faces the territory at present," and recommended a total of 1,000 beds be provided "at once" for tuberculosis. In addition to the 250 beds then available at Seward and at Alice Island near Sitka, the group recommended 100 beds be added at Mt. Edgecumbe, 400 beds in Anchorage, 100 beds in Fairbanks, and 25 beds each in Bethel, Kotzebue, Unalakleet, Fort Yukon, and Nome. Surplus Quonset huts were suggested for these latter units.[91]

The AMA report drew considerable attention to the territory, and ADH was pleased more than anyone that the report was published.[92] The Secretary of the Interior issued a press release in which he stated: "Their [the committee's] recommendations for the improvement of these conditions cannot be ignored. The American people must provide sufficient money to eradicate the evils that are menacing the development of our great Territory or must be willing to accept the blame for our failure to heed the warning that is contained in this penetrating report...."[93]

On his January 1948 trip to Washington, Albrecht had far-ranging talks with federal officials about health plans for Alaska. En route he stopped in Chicago to see the members of the team that had visited Alaska the previous summer and to work out plans for them to present Alaskan health problems to Congress when it next convened.[94] Dr. Bernstein did indeed testify and was instrumental not only in restoring cuts made to the ANS health budget but also in obtaining some $1.2 million in additional funds for public health work in Alaska.

In the summer of 1948 Secretary Krug again asked the AMA Advisory Committee to name a team to visit Alaska to report on health conditions and, especially, to provide consultative clinical services to the Alaska Native hospitals. This team of five physicians included specialists in pediatrics, ophthalmology, dental medicine, orthopedics, and diseases of the chest. Once more tuberculosis was confirmed as the foremost health problem of Alaska.[95]

The desperate tuberculosis situation they attributed to many factors, among them crowded homes, the unwillingness of Natives to enter hospitals, the impracticality of BCG vaccination, and the lack of money for sanatoriums and tuberculosis-control programs. The team recommended an expansion of tuberculosis beds to 1,000, including twenty-four-bed tuberculosis units at eight field locations. In addition, they suggested that small custodial units of four to twelve beds be constructed in some of the larger Native villages for isolation and terminal care of tuberculosis patients who refused to go to the hospital.

Many other recommendations were made relating to tuberculosis, including better use of streptomycin, more home care, financial assistance to dependents, tuberculosis education, rehabilitation, and BCG vaccination. They found "reason for optimism" in the present spirit of cooperation between ANS and ADH, manifested especially at the Mt. Edgecumbe Medical Center, the Seward Sanatorium, and the public health nursing program, as well as in the operation of the health ships. And, in high tribute from representatives of the private sector of medicine, they wrote: "We did not see evidence of inefficient or wasteful operation in either agency. On the contrary, the administrative abilities of the men in these agencies, working as they have with limited funds, have helped to insure efficient use of tax dollars."[96]

The AMA survey came at a critical time and accomplished much good. Its members were all respected physicians, and they were affiliated with the professional organization that represented all American physicians. Moreover, their report was published in what was at that time probably the most widely read medical journal in the nation. Members of the group that toured Alaska were profoundly affected by the health conditions they saw firsthand, and over the next few years several actively lobbied for additional health funding for the territory.

An Army of Volunteers

In 1945, the Alaska Tuberculosis Association (ATA) continued its generous support of the tuberculosis effort by contributing $11,625 to the new health department to match federal funds, but henceforth followed much more closely how the money was being spent. Among other projects, it paid for social services and occupational therapy for Alaskan patients in Seattle-area hospitals and set aside $3,000 to treat Alaskan children with pulmonary tuberculosis admitted to Seattle hospitals under the Crippled Children's Program. The organization also continued to expand its program of providing "extras" to the patients at the new ANS sanatorium at Skagway with the purchase of a phonograph and record collection, a movie projector, and a screen. Smaller items, such as magazine subscriptions, art goods, yarn, and beads were also made available to the patients.[97]

By 1948, the ATA was funding occupational therapists at Mt. Edgecumbe and Seward, and a medical social worker at Seward. These new directions were aimed at gaining the confidence and trust of the patients, with the ultimate goal of helping them to survive the hospital experience and return home. The occupational therapist provided work for the fingers, to distract the patients from their cares, while the social workers listened to the patients, tried to allay their anxieties, and explained the importance of hospital care.[98]

During its 1948–49 fund-raising drive, ATA raised an all-time high of $28,483, largely from the sale of Christmas Seals, which that year were purchased in 211 Alaskan communities from Afognak to Yakutat. The military services also contributed generously, as did several large corporations, such as the Alaska Packers' Association. ATA spent $6,399 in various ANS hospitals, especially Mt. Edgecumbe, an additional $7,797 at the Seward Sanatorium, and $1,360 in various private hospitals in the territory. The money was largely directed toward areas where federal and territorial funds were inadequate, such as Christmas gifts, transportation for patients, spending money for patients for toiletries, movie rentals, and occupational therapy supplies, but it was also spent for major items such as specialized medical equipment and the partial support of professional salaries.[99] In June 1950 ATA sponsored a series of thirteen radio dramas over KINY titled *The Constant Invader,* based on stories of people who had fought personal battles against tuberculosis. Each episode was fifteen minutes in length and featured Henry Fonda, among other Hollywood actors.[100]

On June 10, 1949, the ATA's energetic and ubiquitous executive secretary, Bess Winn, died following surgery for a brain tumor.[101] Her successor was Frances L.

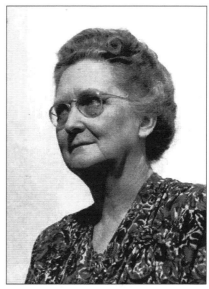

:: Frances Paul, longtime executive secretary :: of the Alaska Tuberculosis Association.
(Courtesy of Ben Paul)

Paul, who had been a member of the board since 1934 and recently served as president. In 1950 the bylaws were changed to allow local Seal-sale chairpeople to become representative members of the board of directors, and the thirty members-at-large, raised from fifteen, were elected to three-year terms. As a result, the ATA became a full-constituent member of the NTA, with a seat on its board of directors.[102]

In the summer of 1950, Paul accompanied Agnes E. Gerding of the NTA staff in New York on a tour of Alaska. They spent ten days in Anchorage, then went on to Bethel, McGrath, Kodiak, Seward, Sitka, Palmer, Cordova, and Wasilla. A major outcome was NTA's recognition that a territory-wide rehabilitation plan for tuberculosis patients was urgently needed.[103] During her trip, Paul was especially discouraged with the tuberculosis situation at Bethel, where 900 active cases were on the waiting list, most of them poorly nourished and living in one-room huts with little ventilation. Just a few miles up the Kuskokwim at Kwethluk, however, she took comfort in the very positive attitude of the people, the teachers, and the Moravian missionaries toward isolation, tuberculosis education, and rehabilitation.[104]

The Christmas Seal drive for 1950 netted $35,732, mostly in small contributions of two to five dollars each. Six percent of the proceeds went to the national office, 20 percent remained with the local community committee, and the remaining 74 percent was returned to the ATA office in Juneau.[105] By 1951, the operations had grown to the extent that the association hired Nel Middleton as a part-time executive secretary to serve the Anchorage branch and the rail-belt region. Each year the

Seal-sale receipts continued to climb, and in 1952 reached $40,015, second only to Hawaii in per capita giving (28.3 cents per person).

In her 1953 message, the ATA president spoke rather pessimistically of "mountains . . . so high that their summits are not even in sight" still to be overcome in the struggle against tuberculosis. Challenges included "lack of sufficient hospital beds, lack of isolation facilities for home care, difficulties in securing and keeping trained professional personnel, inadequate casefinding, extreme poverty and malnutrition, crowded and unsanitary housing, ignorance of the simplest precaution against infection, an inadequate rehabilitation program, and lastly and basically, too much ignorance and indifference to responsibility on the part of the general public."[106] Less than a week before, however, there was a new cause of optimism—the opening of a 400-bed hospital, with 300 tuberculosis beds, in Anchorage (see chapter 5).

A few words on the subsequent history of ATA would be appropriate here. In 1962 ATA was still providing a wide range of tuberculosis services to patients, physicians, and the public. Education, case finding, prevention, and rehabilitation were the mainstays of the program, which for the most part was funded by the sale of Christmas Seals ($36,455 in 1960), supplemented by grants from NTA. The organization had only three paid employees in the state, but could still raise and motivate a battalion of volunteers from all walks of life. No longer did ATA provide basic equipment, drugs and supplies, or the support of professional salaries, as it had done in the 1940s; instead, the organization focused more on the development and distribution of educational materials and on organizing training courses for physicians and nurses.[107]

In 1968 the organization refined its objectives further to reflect recent changes in its bylaws. These objectives included education, support of research, and coordination with other official and voluntary health agencies, not only for tuberculosis but also for other chronic respiratory diseases, particularly emphysema, asthma, bronchitis, bronchiectasis, and hay fever. Areas of program emphasis included chemoprophylaxis, school health, inpatient and outpatient service, legislation, rehabilitation, and public relations.[108] In 1970 the association changed its name to the Alaska Tuberculosis and Respiratory Disease Association, to reflect this evolving mission. Three years later the name was changed again, this time to the American Lung Association of Alaska, a name that, despite a brief one-year flirtation with Alaska Lung Association, has continued until the present time.

The other great volunteer player in the struggle against tuberculosis was the Alaska Crippled Children's Association (ACCA), which was formally launched in Anchorage in January 1946, due largely to the enthusiasm and commitment of one individual, Margot Hoppin. She not only recognized the magnitude of the need for medical care of the many Alaskan children with disabilities, but also saw that ordinary citizens had an essential role in supporting the efforts of the new and underfunded Alaska Department of Health. She formally presented her ideas to the community in a meeting at the Anchorage City Council chambers in mid-January. Only twelve people showed up, but it was enough to establish the association and draw up its articles of incorporation. Hoppin was elected president and then the members and trustees got down to work to establish chapters throughout Alaska. Their first project was to make handicrafts for sale with the proceeds contributed directly to ADH, where they could be matched by federal funds. Hoppin firmly believed that since the organization was serving Alaska's children, every person who lived in the territory should become a supporter by paying a one-dollar annual membership. Within a few months, about half the people of Alaska had joined the enterprise.

The response of the women making handicrafts was overwhelming, and soon the need for space became urgent. Hoppin spied an unused triangular area in the foyer of the principal office building on Fourth Avenue in Anchorage and appropriated the area, which became known as the Gilded Cage, since it was enclosed by heavy wire. There the organization collected and stored all the crafts and "white elephants" that had been donated by the community. Sometimes husbands found their favorite objects mysteriously whisked away, only to have them offered back at a slightly higher price at the Gilded Cage. Soon this little corner was overwhelmed with objects for sale and ACCA had to find a permanent home. Finally, through fund-raising efforts throughout the territory and much volunteer labor and donated materials, a new headquarters was constructed in 1948 at Third Avenue and E Street.

By 1950 there were more than thirty ACCA chapters around the territory. Not only did the members continue to provide crafts and other items for sale, they also contributed cash and personal time. For example, some volunteers helped by meeting at the airport the children attending the orthopedic clinics and offering them temporary housing. Others worked in the Chronic Disease Unit based at St. Ann's Hospital in Juneau. By 1950 ACCA had raised some $68,225 for ADH, a sum matched in full by the federal government.[109]

Dr. Philip Moore, director of the Mt. Edgecumbe Orthopedic Hospital (see chapter 5), was in a position to appreciate the services of ACCA more than anyone. Hoppin, in fact, was indirectly responsible for bringing Moore to Alaska, since by the force of her personality she had originally persuaded Dr. Albrecht of the need for an orthopedic hospital in Alaska, and he in turn had sought out Moore. In his later years Moore characterized Hoppin as "the most dynamic individual I have ever run into." "Bankers would give her $1000," he remembered, "just to get her out of their office—she really browbeat them."[110] The volunteers took on the responsibility for purchasing specialized surgical instruments and equipment for the hospital. A later project was the brace shop, for which ACCA purchased much of the equipment and even supported the training of a former patient in the art of brace-making. Finally, the Orthopedic Fund was a small account ACCA set up at a Sitka bank to be used for the purchase of any small needed item for which the governmental requisition process was too cumbersome.

In 1948 ACCA placed a full-time representative, Kate Robertson, at the hospital, and her caring presence did much to integrate the services of the hospital and make life more tolerable for the children who had to bear such heavy burdens so far from home. ACCA provided most of the equipment and decorations for the schoolroom, radios and phonographs, and toys and equipment for the playroom and outdoor playground. A very popular item was a tape recorder used to record the voices of the children to be played on local radio stations in the communities where they lived. ACCA also furnished most of the physical therapy and photographic equipment used at the hospital. Since children often remained in the hospital for more than a year, during which time their own clothes either wore out or were outgrown, ACCA made available a large selection of donated clothes, including a special set of "traveling clothes" for the great day when the child could finally return home.

ACCA volunteers arranged parties for the children for birthdays and holidays. Members also came to read to the children and otherwise entertain them. Moore summed up the work of ACCA thus: "We have many visitors here at the orthopedic hospital and one of the most common remarks heard is, 'The children seem to be so happy here.' We believe that this happiness may be a measure of the success of the Alaska Crippled Children's Association in its work for the crippled children of Alaska."[111]

Besides the exceptional and lasting contributions of ATA and ACCA, many other organizations and individual volunteers contributed selflessly to the tuberculosis campaign. Most, but by no means all, volunteers were women. Especially in "sanatorium towns" like Seward, Sitka, and Anchorage, women from local clubs or as individuals spent hours writing letters for patients, reading to them, sponsoring parties, decorating for the holidays, playing games with children, and in other ways trying to make life more bearable. Individuals helped in the occupational therapy programs, sharing their skills, providing supplies, or offering to sell crafts for the patients. Among the women's clubs, the Soroptimists were especially active, but Women of the Moose, VFW Auxiliary, Beta Sigma Phi, Business and Professional Women, United Council of Church Women, and many other church-related groups made valuable contributions. Businesses offered magazines, books, films, and supplies for the patients. Men's service clubs, notably the Kiwanis, Lions, and Rotary, also devoted a great deal of members' money and time to promoting the programs of ATA. In November 1953 fifteen churches in Juneau got together for a combined Thanksgiving service attended by Governor Frank Heintzleman, and donated the entire offering to ATA. When the x-ray surveys were in town, volunteers appeared from all walks of life to help with the publicity, registration, and housing of staff.[112]

The tuberculosis effort seemed to bring out the best in people, sometimes in unexpected ways. In 1952 a fire in the nurses' quarters at Seward Sanatorium caused fourteen nurses to lose all their clothing and possessions. Several volunteer groups in Anchorage immediately collected sufficient clothing for all of them. The local Red Cross took the donations to the railway depot and the Alaska Railroad shipped them free to Seward.[113]

During the 1940s, especially, volunteer organizations were essential to the tuberculosis campaign. ATA, ACCA, and other organizations mobilized the time and treasure of hundreds of people who, although they lacked professional training or special skills, wanted to contribute something to the struggle against tuberculosis. Alaskans turned out to be remarkably generous in this regard. Their efforts were particularly directed toward providing tuberculosis victims and their families with what impersonal government agencies were sometimes unable to offer—the human touch.

The Propaganda War: Teaching About Tuberculosis

Nearly everyone agreed that tuberculosis education was the foundation of any program to prevent tuberculosis. In the 1930s and 1940s, ATA had directed much of its energy toward teaching the public about tuberculosis and how to prevent it, treat it, or simply live with it safely. Public health nurses considered health education about tuberculosis one of their core tasks, especially in the villages. Clinical physicians devoted much of their effort in treating patients with tuberculosis to instructing them about the need for rest, routine, good diet, and the proper care of sputum. Not just the patient and his or her family had to be informed: everyone, beginning with schoolchildren, had to know the dangers of tuberculosis and how to avoid them.[114]

Despite these efforts, most tuberculosis education was carried out by individuals who had other responsibilities. There was little money designated for the purpose of education, nor was there much professional backup. Dr. Albrecht clearly saw the need for a departmental focus on health education activities. As discussed previously, Lois M. Jund was assigned to the department in February 1946 with the help of NTA and became the first member of the newly established Division of Tuberculosis Control.[115] She soon laid out her tuberculosis education philosophy:

> The fundamental objective of all tuberculosis and health education is to change the attitudes, motives and conduct of the public.... Facts are important but an emotional basis for action is also imperative. A great portion of the populace has been lulled into an attitude of indifference because of the lack of knowledge about and

familiarity with tuberculosis. A tuberculosis education program, therefore, cannot be predicated on the assumption of rationality of the people.

She followed with a ten-point plan of action, the first principle of which was that each community should have an active health-education subcommittee.[116] Jund then set to work, concentrating on local health councils, public health nurses, voluntary agencies, and official agencies such as VA and ANS. All of ADH's educational literature, radio scripts, and the monthly bulletin *Alaska's Health* were also put under Jund's direction. Albrecht recognized the importance of unifying this work by establishing a separate Health Education Unit in May 1946.[117]

One of Jund's early projects was to prepare a series of "Teaching Aids on Tuberculosis and Its Prevention," later issued jointly by the Territorial Department of Education and ADH. The six "aids" were distributed as a series of *Bulletins* for teachers, providing them with authoritative information about tuberculosis. Some of the materials were specifically designed as reference information for teachers, while others were prepared for students at different levels, from the second grade through high school. Materials included games, quizzes, stories, discussion guides, tuberculosis statistics, nutritional guidance, and reference lists. Each guide integrated tuberculosis education into established sections of the curriculum, such as literature, history, public speaking, drama, journalism, science, mathematics, and physical education.[118]

In March 1947 Jund left for a nine-month field trip, armed with one suitcase, a duffel bag, a movie projector, and a briefcase filled with promotional materials. ATA agreed to contribute $3,000 toward her travel and per diem. She was to carry out preliminary organizational work for the territory-wide x-ray survey, traveling by small and large plane, boat, car, truck, dog team, and Sno-cat from Ketchikan to Barrow and most points in between. Once, when she was flying in a navy aircraft over the Brooks Range, ice formation on the wings led the pilot to consider jettisoning the heavy x-ray equipment to stay aloft. She returned from this odyssey in November, then in March 1948 took a new position with ADH as administrative director and personnel officer.[119] She left the department in 1956 to become the executive officer of the PHS Arctic Health Research Center.

Although the scope of the tuberculosis education consultant's job had broadened, tuberculosis continued to be the principal focus as long as it remained an important health problem. The principal areas of concentration included informational posters for schools and public buildings, additional educational resource materials for teachers in the classroom, informational booklets for adults and children entering sanatoriums, and tuberculosis information pamphlets for the general public.

Perhaps the most ambitious tuberculosis education project of all was the production in 1947 of a colorful booklet titled *Home Care of the Tuberculous in Alaska*, carried out by ADH in cooperation with ATA and ANS. This publication was designed by Frances Paul and produced by her son William L. Paul, Jr., who was a professional photographer. ANS provided most of the funding and arranged for the printing at their Haskell Institute in Kansas. The 117-page book was put together at the ANS school in Juneau. The purpose of the book was to assist in the proper home care of a tuberculosis victim when hospitalization was either unavailable or inappropriate. Through photographs and dialogue, the book told the story of a sixteen-year-old Native girl named Sally Brown who developed tuberculosis, was briefly hospitalized in a sanatorium, and then returned home early to allow another patient to be

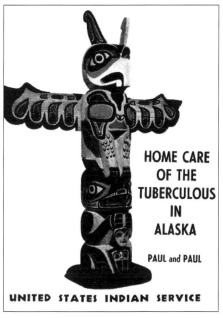

HOME CARE OF THE TUBERCULOUS IN ALASKA

PAUL and PAUL

UNITED STATES INDIAN SERVICE

:: Educational booklet on home treatment :: published jointly by ADH, ANS, and ATA, 1948. *(Author's Collection)*

admitted in her place. The book related how Sally's mother, Emma, her father, and her siblings all contributed to her care in a middle-class home presumably located in Southeast Alaska. The book ends with a picture of the smiling family, including Sally, and the caption, "Emma Brown's hard work has paid off. Here is her healthy, happy family!" Sally takes a business course and gets a job as a secretary in an office.[120]

The cast of characters was thoroughly Alaskan, with the photographs depicting Juneau resident Katie Villoria and her real-life daughter Jessie Villoria Greenwald. The publication was distributed widely to all nurses, teachers, and ANS and private doctors in the territory, as well as to public libraries.[121] Although professionally produced, it must not have seemed entirely relevant to those living in the more remote areas of Alaska.

In 1952 the Health Education Division produced two series of posters about the prevention of tuberculosis, which were sent to all schools, health centers, and clinics, together with a teaching guide. The first series was titled "Cleanliness Fights Germs and Sickness" and was intended for the young, telling about germ theory through the cartoon character "Herm the Germ." The second series, called simply "Tuberculosis," was directed at children at the third-grade level and depicted how the disease was spread and how it could be prevented.[122]

Notes

1. William R. Hunt, *Alaska, A Bicentennial History* (New York: W.W. Norton, 1976), 112.

2. *Session Laws, Resolutions and Memorials 1945* (Juneau: 1945), 80–85, 177–78.

3. Letter from C. Earl Albrecht to Ernest Gruening, March 13, 1945, Albrecht Collection.

4. Memo to Adjutant General, US Army, from Conrad E. Albrecht, April 11, 1945, Albrecht Collection.

5. C. Earl Albrecht, "To Promote and Protect the Public Health," *AH* 3, no. 7 (July 1945); "Members of the Board of Health," *AH* 3, no. 8 (August 1945).

6. It is noteworthy that Governor Gruening did not accept any of Albrecht's nominations for the board.

7. "Board of Health Asks More Funds," *AH* 3, no. 9 (September 1945).

8. "Gov. Gruening Issues Special Session Call," *ADT,* November 17, 1945.

9. C. Earl Albrecht, "The Challenge of the New Year," *AH* 4, no. 1 (January 1946).

10. Lois M. Jund interviewed by M. Walter Johnson, April 17, 1996, at Sitka, Alaska; Lois Jund, 1955; "Dog Sled Nurse," *Wellesley Alumnae Magazine* 40, no. 4 (November 1955): 22–24.

11. Dr. Gehrig went on to a distinguished Public Health Service career, attaining the post of deputy surgeon general.

12. "Dr. Gehrig Joins Staff," *AH* 4, no. 4 (April 1946); ADH and USPHS, "Public health progress," 21.

13. "Sanatoriums for Alaska," *AH* 4, no. 2 (February 1946).

14. "Campaign Started to Secure TB Sanatorium for Southeast Alaska," *JAE,* January 8, 1946; "Sanatoriums for Alaska."

15. "TB Control Bill First to Be Passed, Signed," *JAE,* March 16, 1946.

16. *Laws of Alaska, 1946* (Juneau: 1946), chap. 1: 37–39.

17. *Laws of Alaska, 1946,* chap 5: 42–44. The special session also passed the Hospital Survey Act, permitting the territory to participate in the federal Hill-Burton Hospital Construction Bill, established a Division of Vocational Rehabilitation, and strengthened the authority of the Board of Health to enforce health regulations; C. Earl Albrecht, "Extraordinary Session," *AH* 4, no. 4 (April 1946), 1.

18. *Session Laws, Resolutions and Memorials Passed by the Extraordinary Session of Seventeenth Territorial Legislature* (Juneau: Territory of Alaska, 1946), 37–39.

19. "Dr. Albrecht Visits Washington," *AH* 4, no. 6 (June 1946).

20. C. Earl Albrecht, "A New Year's Message," *AH* 5, no. 1 (January 1947).

21. "Dr. Albrecht's Trip Profitable," *AH* 6, no. 2 (February 1948).

22. C. Earl Albrecht, "The Alaska Health Plan," *AH* 6, no. 7–8 (July–August 1948).

23. Statement by Governor Ernest Gruening, February 7, 1948, Governor Correspondence, roll 247.

24. "For Second Year Accidents Were Chief Cause of Death in Alaska," *AH* 10, no. 5 (October 1953).

25. C. Earl Albrecht, *Biennial Report of the Office of the Commissioner of Health for the Period July 1, 1948 to June 30, 1950* (Juneau: ADH, 1950), 41–42.

26. James A. Smith, "Tuberculosis Program of the Alaska Native Service," *Annual Report, July 1, 1945 to June 30, 1946, Alaska Tuberculosis Association* (1946), 8–11.

27. Ernest Gruening, *Annual Report of the Governor of Alaska to the Secretary of the Interior, Fiscal Year Ended June 30, 1945* (Washington, DC: GPO, 1945), 22–23.

28. Ernest Gruening, *Annual Report of the Governor of Alaska to the Secretary of the Interior, Fiscal Year Ended June 30, 1946* (Washington, DC: GPO, 1946), 45–46.

29. Dr. E. S. "Stu" Rabeau, a PHS officer detailed to ANS in Kotzebue from 1946 to 1957, was one of the pioneers of these radio clinics. Virtually every night he sat down at the radio at 6:00 p.m. and spent the next several hours diagnosing and treating illnesses and injuries, prescribing

medications from the school medical supplies, or simply reassuring anxious patients, families, and teachers. During some periods when the Barrow and Tanana hospitals were unstaffed, he took radio calls for these areas as well. Dr. Rabeau later went on to become the director of the Indian Health Service in Washington, D.C. He returned to Alaska in the 1980s to become director of the Division of Public Health, Alaska Department of Health and Social Services, in Juneau. *See* "Progress Being Made by Doctors with New 'Clinic of the Air,'" newspaper article (1950), scrapbook #2, Alaska Tuberculosis Association Collection; Ernest Gruening, *Annual Report of the Governor of Alaska to the Secretary of the Interior, Fiscal Year Ended June 30, 1950* (Washington, DC: GPO, 1950), 57.

30. Gruening, *Report, 1950,* 61.

31. B. Frank Heintzleman, *1954 Annual Report for the Fiscal Year Ended June 30, Governor of Alaska to the Secretary of the Interior* (Washington, DC: GPO, 1954), 79.

32. Rudolph Haas, "A Tuberculosis Control Program for Alaska," *AH* 3, no. 4 (April 1945).

33. "Tuberculosis Control Program," *AH* 3, no. 11 (November 1945).

34. Smith, "Tuberculosis Program of the A.N.S."

35. Gehrig, "Problems in Tuberculosis Control."

36. "Dept. Of Health Will Conduct Mass X-ray Program in Concerted Battle Against TB; Wide Cooperation Shown," *Alaska Sunday Press,* October 26, 1947.

37. "100 Women Launch City-wide Survey for X-rays," *ADT,* June 3, 1947.

38. "Join the Army Against TB," *ADN,* June 7, 1947; "The X-ray Program," *ADT,* June 9, 1947.

39. "Organizations Unite to Aid X-ray Survey" and "Mass X-ray Program," unidentified newspaper clippings in the Albrecht Collection.

40. Donald J. McMinimy, "Preliminary Report on Tuberculosis Incidence in Alaska," *AH* 5, no. 10 (October 1947).

41. Richard L. Neuberger, "Alaska's White Scourge," *Rocky Mountain Empire Magazine,* (November 14, 1948).

42. *Annual Report of the Alaska Department of Health, July 1948–July 1949,* ADH (Juneau: ADH, 1949), 8.

43. "Tuberculosis Control Program," typescript, revised October 1946, Albrecht Collection.

44. "Latest TB Report Shows 5,279 Cases in Alaska; Brings Ratio to 1 in 20," *AH* 8, no. 3–4 (March–April 1950).

45. Ann P. Kent, "The Mobile Unit's First Season. A Preliminary Report," *AH* 3, no. 10 (October 1945).

46. Letter from Clifford Starr to Ernest Gruening, December 21, 1945, Governor Correspondence, roll 248.

47. "Health Fleet Invades Alaska," *Pacific Motor Boat* (September 1949), 34–36; George W. Grupp, "M/S *Hygiene* Carries Medical Aid to Thousands in Alaska," *Modern Hospital* (October 1948), 24.

48. *Session Laws, 1946,* chapter 26: 109–10.

49. Don Luke, "The Good Ship *Hygiene,*" *Alaska Life* 11, no. 9 (September 1948): 8.

50. Gruening, *Report, 1947,* 47.

51. Bob Callan, "Alaska's Floating Hospital," *Alaska Life* 9, no. 9 (September 1946): 50.

52. W. J. Granberg, "Alaska's Floating Clinic," *Seattle Times,* August 29, 1948.

53. Susan Meredith, with Kitty Gair and Elaine Schwinge, *Alaska's Search for a Killer, 1946–1948: A Seafaring Medical Adventure* (Juneau: Alaska Public Health Nursing History Association, 1998).

54. Catherine Smulling, "The M/S *Hygiene.* Alaska's Floating Health Unit," *Public Health Nursing* 39 (May 1947): 258.

55. Helen Johnson, "The Nursing Consultant in the Tuberculosis Control Program in Alaska" (essay in support of degree of MPH, Yale University, 1950), 14.

56. Catherine Gair, "Review First Six Years Aboard M.S. *Hygiene,*" *AH* 9, no. 5 (October 1951).

57. "New Marine Units," *AH* 6, no. 11 (November 1948); "Health Fleet Invades Alaska," 34–36; "New Marine Unit Arrives," *AH* 7, no. 5 (May 1949).

58. "Spring Signals Mobile Units to Summer Operations," *AH* 8, no. 5–6 (May–June 1950).

59. "M.V. *Health* Is Scheduled Here after 18 Months," unidentified newspaper clipping, scrapbook #2, ATA Collection; Ernest Gruening, *Annual Report of the Governor of Alaska to the Secretary of the Interior, Fiscal Year Ended June 30, 1951* (Washington, DC: GPO, 1951), 48; "M.V. *Health* Views Siberian Hills While Holding Clinics," *AH* 8, no. 9–10 (September–October, 1950); "Health Ship Back after Long Voyage" (1951), unidentified newspaper clipping, scrapbook #2, ATA Collection.

60. "On Public Health Services," 6–9.

61. Gruening, *Report, 1952*, 61; "M.V. *Health* Sets Sail for Far North Again," *AH* 9 (April 1952): 5.

62. "Health Fleet Invades Alaska," 34–36.

63. "New Marine Unit," *AH* 7, no. 7–8 (July–August 1949).

64. "Spring Signals Mobile Units"; Ernest Gruening, *Annual Report of the Governor of Alaska to the Secretary of the Interior. Fiscal Year Ended June 30, 1951* (Washington, DC: GPO, 1951), 51; William H. Kiloh, "Eskimos Are Quick to Welcome 'Hospital Ship' as Yukon Health Barge Goes up Big River to Offer Chest X-rays and General Health Service," *AH* 8, no. 9–10 (September–October, 1950).

65. Gruening, *Report, 1952*, 61; *Seventh Biennial Report, July 1, 1950–June 30, 1952*, Alaska Department of Health (Juneau: ADH, 1952), 46–47; *Eighth Biennial Report, July 1, 1952–June 30, 1954*, Alaska Department of Health (Juneau: ADH, 1952), 52.

66. "Health Ships Tied Up as Result of Fund Slashes," *AH* 9 (October 1952), 1–2; Memorandum from C. Earl Albrecht to all Alaska Department of Health Staff, September 11, 1952, Governor Correspondence, roll 350.

67. "Health Ships Tied Up"; "On Public Health Services," 9.

68. Memorandum from Charles R. Hayman to all offices, Alaska Department of Health, August 16, 1954, Governor Correspondence, roll 350; ADH Press Release, Juneau, Alaska, September 27, 1957, Governor Correspondence, roll 350.

69. Florence O. Eby, "Riding a Mobile Health Unit," *Public Health Nursing* (July 1947); Johnson, *Nursing Consultant*, 14.

70. Gruening, *Report, 1948*, 41; Leo Gehrig and Elaine A. Schwinge, "Must We All Die of the TB?" *AH* 6, no. 10 (October 1947).

71. Gehrig and Schwinge, "Must We All Die?"; *Annual Report of ADH, 1948–49*, 13; "Spring Signals Mobile Units"; *Alaska Department of Health Annual Report, 1950–1951* (Juneau: ADH, 1951), 30.

72. Gruening, *Report, 1949*, 39.

73. Gruening, *Report, 1950*; "Spring Signals Mobile Units"; Gruening, *Report, 1950*.

74. Joseph D. Aronson, "BCG Vaccination among American Indians," *American Review of Tuberculosis* 57, no 1 (January 1948): 96–99.

75. C. Earl Albrecht, "Streptomycin and BCG," *AH* 5, no. 7 (July 1947).

76. "Dr. Albrecht's Trip Profitable," *AH* 6, no. 2 (February 1948).

77. Frank H. Douglass, David B. Law, W. Charles Martin, Austin T. Moore, and John E. Tuhy, "Medical Conditions in Alaska: A Progress Report" (typescript, October 29, 1948).

78. ADH and USPHS, "Public Health Progress in Alaska" (Juneau: January 1949).

79. Elaine Schwinge, "Alaska's Population Receiving Benefits of BCG Vaccination," *NTA Bulletin* (May 1949): 69.

80. C. Earl Albrecht, transcript of interview with Kenneth Kastella, in Anchorage, Alaska, May 6, 1983; "M.V. *Health* Views Siberian Hills While Holding Clinics," *AH* 8, no. 9–10 (September–October, 1950).

81. "Alaska's Tuberculosis Vaccination Work Is Resumed," *AH* 9 (June 1952).

82. Jack C. Haldeman, "Tuberculosis Control, Program Review Fiscal Year 1950, Conducted by Representatives of the Public Health Service and the Children's Bureau, Federal Security Agency, Region IX" (typescript, 1950), AHRC Papers.

83. "Alaska's Tuberculosis Vaccination Work Is Resumed," *AH* 9 (June 1952): 2.

84. "Dr. Aronson Comes to Follow Work on BCG Vaccinations," *AH* 9, no. 4 (August 1951): 2.

85. "Alaska's Tuberculosis Vaccination Work Is Resumed."

86. Joseph B. Stocklen and James E. Perkins "Tuberculosis Control in Alaska" (typescript, September 22, 1954), 34–35.

87. Charles R. Hayman, "Tuberculosis Problem Is Studied from Territorial Standpoint," *AH* 12 (August 1955): 1–2; "Sale of M-V *Yukon Health* Leaves M-S *Hygiene* Sole Survivor of ADH Marine Health Centers That Pioneered Isolated Areas," *AH* 13 (October 1956).

88. "Dr. Aronson Checks 19-year BCG Study," *AH* 13 (October 1956): 8.

89. E. W. Gentles, "Tuberculosis in Alaska," *Alaska Medicine* 1 (June 1959): 53–54.

90. In a rather remarkable long-term follow-up study, Aronson's daughter and her colleagues found that, after fifty years or more, the tuberculosis rate of the Alaska Indians who had taken the vaccine in the study was only 59 percent of the rate of those who had taken placebo. *See* Naomi E. Aronson, et al., "Long-term Efficacy of BCG Vaccine in American Indians and Alaska Natives: A 60-Year Follow-up Study," *Journal of the American Medical Association* 291 (June 5, 2004): 2086–91.

91. Harry Barnett, Jack Fields, George Milles, Joseph Silverstein, and Arthur Bernstein, "Medical Conditions in Alaska: A Report by a Group Sent by the American Medical Association," *Journal of the American Medical Association* 135, no. 8 (1947): 500–10.

92. Barnett, et al., "Medical Conditions in Alaska," 500–10.

93. "Alaska Medical Care Is Judged 'Appalling,'" *Alaska Life* 10, no. 11 (November 1947): 15.

94. "Alaska Health Report Released," U.S. Department of the Interior, Information Service (October 23, 1947), Governor Correspondence, roll 247.

95. "Dr. Albrecht's Trip Profitable."

96. Frank H. Douglass, David B. Law, W. Charles Martin, Austin T. Moore, and John E. Tuhy, "Medical Conditions in Alaska: A Progress Report" (typescript, October 29, 1948), 1.

97. Douglass, et al., "Medical Conditions in Alaska," 3–10, 19–27.

98. Bess Winn, "Christmas Seal Sale—1945," *AH* 3, no. 11 (November 1945).

99. Bess Winn, "The ATA In-Hospital Services," *AH* 6, no. 11 (November 1948).

100. "Alaska TB Association Broadens Attack on Public Enemy No. 1," *Forty-Ninth Star*, August 28, 1949.

101. "New series of TB broadcasts, KINY," unidentified newspaper clipping, June 4, 1950, scrapbook #2, ATA Collection.

102. "In Memoriam: Bess Anderson Winn, Executive Secretary 1943–1949," *Annual Report, Alaska Tuberculosis Association, For the Year Ending March 31, 1949* (1949).

103. Frances L. Paul, "Administrative History of the Alaska Tuberculosis Association," typescript (n.d.), ATA Collection.

104. "Officials of National TB Association Visit Several Alaskan Towns," *Alaska's Weekly*, September 15, 1950.

105. Transcript of radio interview of Frances Paul by Helene Johnson, November 1950, scrapbook #2, ATA Collection. Ironically, only a few days later the Bethel Hospital burned down and was a total loss.

106. "Christmas Seal Sale Is Starting Here Next Week," unidentified newspaper clipping, October 27, 1951, scrapbook #2, ATA Collection.

107. "Alaska's Christmas Seal Sale," editorial, unidentified newspaper clipping, November 28, 1953, scrapbook #2, ATA Scrapbook.

108. Mildred Mantle, "Alaska Tuberculosis Association," *Alaska Medicine* 4 (March 1962): 51.

109. *Annual Report, Alaska Tuberculosis Association, April 1, 1967 to March 31, 1968.*

110. "Alaska Crippled Children's Association Makes Great Progress in First 5 Years of its Energetic Life," *AH* 8, no. 11–12 (November–December 1950): 2; Philip H. Moore, "ACCA Lends Great Aid to Mt. Edgecumbe Orthopedic Center," *AH* 8, no. 11–12 (November–December 1950): 1, 3.

111. Sandy Poulson, "Dr. Moore Begins Retirement after 23 Years in Sitka," *Alaska Medicine* 12 (June 1970): 33–35; Philip Moore, transcript of interview by Kenneth Kastella in Sequim, Washington (1983), 9.

112. Moore, "ACCA Lends Great Aid."

113. "Thanksgiving Community Services," unidentified newspaper clipping, November 19, 1953, scrapbook #2, ATA Collection.

114. "Seward Nurses All Outfitted," unidentified newspaper clipping, scrapbook #2, ATA Collection.

115. Rudolph Haas, "A Tuberculosis Control Program for Alaska," *AH* 3, no. 4 (April 1945).

116. "Lois Jund Comes Here," *JAE*, February 15, 1946; Lois Jund, "Dog Sled Nurse," *Wellesley Alumnae Magazine* 40, no. 4 (November 1955): 22–24. Jund remained in Alaska for the rest of her distinguished professional career and retired in the state.

117. Lois M. Jund, "The Tuberculosis Education Program," *AH* 4, no. 10 (October 1946).

118. *Biennial Report of the Office of the Commissioner of Health, for the Period July 1, 1946 to June 30, 1948*, Alaska Department of Health (Juneau: ADH, n.d.), 44.

119. Lois M. Jund, "Teaching Aids on Tuberculosis and Its Prevention: Territorial Schools of Alaska," *Bulletins* no. 1–6 (Juneau: Dept. of Education and Department of Health, 1946).

120. Jund, "Dog Sled Nurse."

121. Frances L. Paul, *Home Care of the Tuberculous in Alaska*, Alaska Native Service (Juneau: US Indian Service: 1953).

122. "Pamphlet on Care of the Tuberculous Is Published by ANS," *Alaska Sunday Press*, November 2, 1947.

122. "Ten Original Posters Tell Things to Do to Prevent Tuberculosis," *AH* 9, no. 1 (February 1952).

: 5 : **Taking Prisoners**

The Sanatorium Campaign

Preparations for the Campaign

Dr. Carl Buck's report on the public health needs of Alaska listed as its second-highest priority, behind tuberculosis case finding, "much more adequate hospital facilities, particularly for the care of tuberculosis, available to all persons in the territory who need such services regardless of race, color, or creed."[1] He concluded that approximately 900 sanatorium beds were needed: 200 in the North, perhaps at Nome, 200 in Southeast Alaska, and 500 in south-central Alaska.[2] All hospitals, he stressed, should care for both whites and Natives on a "pavilion plan," that is, separation of the races. Costs would be borne by individual patients, or by various federal and territorial agencies.

Dr. Rudolph Haas also endorsed the idea of three or four large sanatoriums, preferably at Juneau, Anchorage, and Fairbanks, although he also considered Nome a possibility. In any event, the hospitals had to be in large communities and sufficiently close together for easy travel from one to another by a small number of specialists in medicine and surgery who would provide consultative services. Doctors specially trained in pneumothorax and pneumoperitoneum should be stationed at each hospital, he felt, with at least one itinerant chest surgeon capable of major thoracic surgery. Larger communities would also make it easier to recruit and retain professional nursing staff. Patients and visitors needed ready access to the hospitals initially and a place where they could stay nearby for follow-up when they became well enough to work part-time. To avoid hardship, he urged that families left behind be provided for.[3]

Patients eligible for Alaska Native Service (ANS) care were referred to that agency for hospital care as appropriate. In contrast, those referred to the Alaska Department of Health (ADH) for hospitalization were expected to pay part or even all of the cost of their treatment if they were able to do so, although no one was to be denied treatment on the basis of inability to pay. The daily rate for the cost of sanatorium care was set by ADH at $5 per day, to include subsistence, nursing care, usual medications and supplies, laboratory, and x-rays, but not professional fees. The latter were set at $1 per day for the first month, $0.50 per day for the second month, and $7.50 per month thereafter.[4]

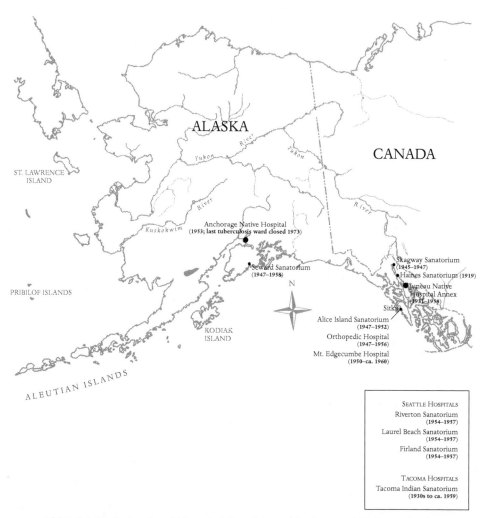

:: Map showing the location of tuberculosis hospitals used for the care of Alaskan patients. ::

Around this time the newly constituted Tuberculosis Control Division of ADH set forth some criteria on the priority for tuberculosis hospital admission, since the number of active cases greatly exceeded the available beds. Admission to a sanatorium had two main functions: 1) care and treatment of the individual, and 2) isolation of contagious patients so that their disease would not spread to others. These goals were often in conflict with each other, since the minimal and moderately advanced cases had the best hope for recovery, while the far advanced cases were the most infectious for others. Where many people were at risk in a household, hospitalization was more urgent, but sometimes, if conditions were suitable, a case in the early stages could be effectively treated at home. Patients with advanced disease were to be referred for hospital admission as a public health measure, but only after all options were exhausted for isolation outside the hospital.

Somewhat later, in September 1951, a new interagency committee was established to review cases for hospital admission every six months and assign a priority based on the diagnosis and prospects for gaining the greatest benefit from sanatorium care. The committee included thoracic surgeons and medical directors from Mt. Edgecumbe and Seward, two ADH tuberculosis consultants and the director of the Division of Tuberculosis Control, and the ANS area medical director. In late February 1952, some 300 applications for sanatorium treatment were reviewed and classified by the committee, and in April 1953 another 300 applicants were classified.[5]

An Army Pig in a Poke: The Skagway Sanatorium

As noted in chapter 3, Governor Gruening had been successful in 1944 in obtaining the army hospital at Skagway for ANS. The hospital campus sat in a wooded grove and consisted of some seventeen framed barrackslike buildings sprawled along the bank of the Skagway River, about three miles from town over a rocky unsurfaced road. Five of the buildings were used as wards, each with thirty beds, plus an administration building, mess hall, recreational hall, various maintenance facilities, and quarters for the physician, nurses, and attendants. The wards were long open rooms with visible trusses. All the facilities were connected by closed walkways, with the main corridor no less than 640 feet long. The whole complex had its own water supply, electric plant, and sewage disposal unit. At the time of the transfer of the property, in the fall of 1944, the buildings were in poor shape, drafty, and some had suffered damage from frozen pipes. A team of workers swarmed over the buildings during the winter to repair and recondition them, and the facility was finally more or less ready for occupancy by spring.[6]

Since there was a significant nursing shortage near the end of the war, the governor asked Bishop Crimont for a religious congregation to staff the hospital. After some negotiation, the Sisters of St. Ann, who had operated a hospital in Juneau since Gold Rush days, agreed in February 1945 to a temporary contract for nursing services at the hospital. The nurses arrived at the hospital on March 24 with Dr. E. W. Norris, medical director of ANS, and found the buildings in a run-down condition. The sisters went to work scrubbing the floors and walls and readying the buildings for the first patients.[7]

Dr. Rudolph Haas was detailed from the Public Health Service to ANS to serve as hospital superintendent. He arrived in Skagway on April 10, and the hospital officially opened four days later. By the end of June, the hospital had already admitted forty-five patients in two wards, but by September no further progress had been made because of shortages of nurses and hospital attendants. The Sisters of St. Ann sent additional help to assist with the nursing duties, and by January 1946 four wards were open.[8] In the spring of 1946, the contract between ANS and the Sisters

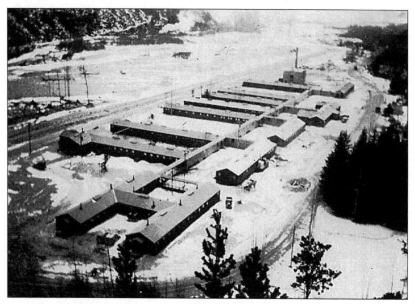

:: Military hospital at Skagway, which became Skagway Sanatorium in 1945. ::
(Courtesy of Skagway Museum & Archives, Everson Collection, 94.16.85)

of St. Ann was renewed for a second year, but the provincial superior, Mother Mary Mildred, advised the government that this would be the last. Plans went forward to open another ward and close in the screened porches.

Although the hospital was rated at 150 beds, nursing and attendant staff shortages allowed only 100 beds to be open during that first year. The average daily census was sixty-three patients, but by June 30, 1946, the hospital was at full capacity with a census of ninety-nine. For the next six months the wards continued to be full.[9]

Because of budget constraints, the hospital initially could offer little more than bed rest and a balanced diet. The Alaska Tuberculosis Association saw the need for improving morale, especially for the Native patients who were so far from home, and contributed a radio and loudspeaker system that permitted music to be piped into all the rooms. The volunteers purchased a phonograph and a "well-selected assortment" of records, a movie projector, a screen, and magazine subscriptions for the hospital. To keep idle hands busy, they also provided art goods, yarns, beads, and other materials that could be used for making crafts.[10]

Ethel Pederson, a nurse who worked at the hospital, had vivid memories of the conditions under which the staff worked:

Because towering mountains were so near, the rising and setting sun was never in our view. At times the winds blew down the valley in gusts of 60 to eighty miles per hour. The entire frame building would rock or shake. The heating system was inadequate, the windows and doors were loose in their frames. The air was so dry we had to improvise coffee cans full of water to set on the radiators as humidifiers.

Our food was army surplus. Of distinct memory to sight, smell and taste was the old canned butter more like cheese than butter, dehydrated potatoes and eggs and powdered milk. Our meat was mostly reindeer, so old and tough we felt sure it must be Santa's first team and refrozen since their demise in antiquity. . . .

During the severe winds of cold spells the nurses added long johns buttoned to the neck and two or three tee shirts to their usual attire. On top had to be two or three sweaters and as many wool anklets as shoe size would permit. We were a colorful lot indeed, as no one owned sufficient of these various articles in the prescribed white.[11]

In early January 1947 Governor Gruening, ANS Superintendent Foster, and Commissioner Albrecht decided that the Skagway Sanatorium was "useless because of high operating cost and should be abandoned." With only one boiler working, temperatures in the ward were about 40°F and those in the connecting corridors were reported as -7°F. Some staff wore parkas as they went about their work.[12] The officials agreed on a plan to transfer all patients and staff to Alice Island, near Sitka, where both the Skagway patients and additional ones could be cared for more satisfactorily.

The reaction from the community of Skagway was predictably swift and fierce. Not only had large amounts of federal taxpayers' money gone into the reconditioning of the facility only two years before, but the community had developed many new services in support of the sanatorium and its staff. The government had supply contracts with many local merchants with large inventories, and a number of new businesses, including a theater and a laundry, had sprung up specifically to serve the hospital. When they realized that the decision to move had already been irrevocably made, city officials felt justified in protesting the decision by pointing out that it was unwise to remove bedridden tubercular patients by sea in the dead of winter, and that Skagway, with the sunniest climate in Southeast Alaska, provided much more cheery and healthful weather than dark, rainy Sitka.[13]

The decision to move came not a moment too soon. As a nurse described it:

About five days before the [ship] *North Sea* arrived, the snows came, the wind blew and the thermometer went as low as twenty-eight below.

In those five intervening days that we fed and panned the patients, they washed their faces and hands once a day . . . that was the extent of the nursing care. As soon as the chilling winds increased in force, the water in our coffee can humidifiers froze solid. The Bendix washer froze. Our wash cloths froze as soon as they were hung up. Each day added some new freeze up.

The pipes froze and the entire crew at the hospital were limited to one wash bowl.[14]

Despite all efforts of the community to delay the departure, the *North Sea* docked at Skagway on February 6. Some ninety-one patients were bundled up against the cold and transferred to the ship, where they had bunks in steerage. After a sixteen-hour trip, the ship berthed at Japonski Island, connected to Alice Island, where the new sanatorium was located. Once the patients had left the ship, the *North Sea* was thoroughly disinfected, including fumigation, as required by the ship's owners.[15]

ADH Joins the Fray: The Seward Sanatorium

The territorial health department, as noted in chapter 3, had begun negotiations with the army for the transfer of the hospital at Fort Raymond, near Seward, well before the end of the war. The property, together with supplies and equipment, was finally transferred to the health department on December 9, 1944, contingent upon the legislature's willingness to acquire and operate the hospital.[16] In senate Bill 32, passed March 24, 1945, the legislature authorized negotiations with the army and appropriated the sum of $14,500.[17]

Albrecht hoped to have the territory contract with a religious organization to operate the facility, as at Skagway. He had preliminary discussions with several church-related organizations, but selected the Methodists both because of their experience in operating hospitals and because they were already operating charitable institutions in Seward.[18] The Board of Missions representatives were none too pleased, however, when they saw the conditions at the hospital site, where they found doors open, snow on the floors, many pipes frozen, and one heating unit totally inoperable.[19] In February 1946 Albrecht telegraphed Governor Gruening in Washington, suggesting that since the army had gutted the hospital of linens, x-ray equipment, refrigerators, ranges, and an ambulance, the territory offer only $1,000 for the plant and use the rest of the $14,500 appropriation to replace equipment and supplies. Gruening then sent a strongly worded message to the army engineers at Fort Richardson, calling on them to undertake the necessary repairs since the frost damage had occurred while the property was still under their control.[20]

Finally, on May 10, Albrecht was able to announce that the War Assets Administration had transferred its hospital at Fort Raymond to the health department for lease to the Methodist Mission Board as a tuberculosis sanatorium. The buildings included the hospital itself, which had cost $361,000 to build, and the adjoining warehouse area, which had been constructed for $209,000.[21] The hospital compound was a rambling, 150-bed complex of seventeen single-story wooden buildings connected by passageways, not unlike the facilities at Skagway and Alice Island. The site included fifty-four acres of land along the Alaska Railroad and the Seward Highway just 500 feet north of the city limit of Seward.[22] The territory leased the property to the Methodist Mission Board for the token amount of $1 per year.

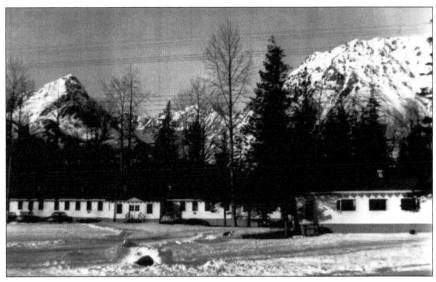

:: Seward Sanatorium. ::
(Courtesy of Margery Albrecht)

In preparation for taking over the compound, territorial officials made a thorough investigation of the heating and plumbing and were dismayed to learn that indeed both had been severely damaged by frost. The army agreed to make the necessary repairs, which cost approximately $25,000 and delayed the actual transfer about sixty days. The handover finally occurred in June 1946, at which time the army unexpectedly gave the territory a 100 percent rebate on the $14,500 that had been appropriated by the legislature at the special session. The value of the property transferred was conservatively estimated to be $190,000.[23]

In its new incarnation as the Seward Sanatorium, the refurbished hospital accepted its first patients on July 6, 1946. Albrecht saw it as fulfilling a major part of his dream for the tuberculosis program—a facility that would serve all Alaskan patients, Native and non-Native, private and public.[24] The hospital opened under the professional direction of a thoracic surgeon, Dr. A. R. Valle. During the hospital's first year of operation, Valle performed a variety of surgical procedures, including bronchoscopy, thoracoplasty, phrenic nerve crush, pneumonolysis, lobectomy, and even two pneumonectomies.[25]

The hospital was funded from several sources. The majority of patients were indigent whites whose care was paid for by the territorial Department of Public Welfare, while other patients were supported by ANS or the Veterans Administration, or by paying their own way. The financial break-even point was said to be a census of 125, a level that could not be achieved without ANS supporting the cost for approximately forty Native patients.[26] By February 1947 Albrecht could report that the Seward Sanatorium had cared for ninety-two patients, either at the expense of the territory or of ANS, since it had opened the previous July. More would have been admitted but for a three-month maritime workers' strike that necessitated paying air freight charges for essentials such as eggs.[27]

In late April, however, the program suffered a severe blow when the overall ANS budget for FY1948 was slashed some $501,000 below its FY1946 level. These cuts made it necessary for the ANS to withdraw its support from the Seward Sanatorium, the M/S *Hygiene*, the highway unit, and all other cooperative projects except the contract for public health nursing services. Albrecht asserted that, without the ANS support for Native patients, the sanatorium would have to close, and offered to go to Washington to testify before Congress on the appropriation.[28] At that time, the hospital had a patient census of eighty-five, with thirty-four supported by the territory, forty-seven by ANS, and four by the VA.[29]

Albrecht tried every argument he could muster to prevent the transfer of Native patients from Seward to Alice Island (the ANS facility at Sitka that had replaced the Skagway facility), citing as reasons that the patients were not well enough to leave, that they were being transferred yet further from their homes in western and northern Alaska, that they would no longer have access to a chest surgeon, and finally, and most important to him, that the transfer would necessitate closure of the Seward facility.[30] ANS, however, could not spend money it didn't have. It did agree that no patients would be moved if their lives were in danger, and officials expressed the hope that Valle could provide itinerant surgical care for the tuberculosis patients at Juneau and Sitka.[31]

By early October ANS owed more than $75,000 in back payments for the care of Native patients at Seward, and on October 5 ANS Superintendent Don Foster announced that all forty-eight of the Native patients at Seward would be transferred to Alice Island within the next two weeks. Anyone refusing transfer would have to become financially responsible for his or her own care. Albrecht hurried to Seward to discuss the situation with Methodist officials, who assured him that they would try to keep the hospital open despite the pullout. Thirty-three Native patients had already been transferred, however, and the remainder were scheduled to depart the following week, leaving a total of only sixty-two patients in the hospital.[32]

After conferring with Methodist officials, Congressional Delegate Bob Bartlett announced that the Seward Sanatorium would be forced to close in two weeks unless the ANS paid its debt in full. Indian Service officials in Juneau and Washington frantically tried to find a way to reshuffle their budgets to make the funds available, but the outlook seemed bleak.[33] Ten days later, however, Bartlett was able to announce that the Indian Service had scraped together $30,000 to cover the deficit it owed up to July 1, 1947, a gesture that persuaded the Methodist Missionary Board to keep the hospital open at least until December.[34] By mid-November the old debt was paid and new Native patients were being admitted to the hospital, causing ADH officials to scurry to bring their own obligations to the Methodist Church up to date. By mid-December both houses of Congress accepted Bartlett's amendment to add $176,000 to a supplemental appropriation bill for foreign aid, and the hospital was saved.[35]

The Seward Sanatorium remained the main focus of the ADH tuberculosis treatment program, gradually introducing new services as opportunities presented, including a rehabilitation program. In 1952 a total of seventy-seven patients were admitted to the sanatorium, which then had a staff of about 100 employees. In June 1950, Dr. Francis J. Phillips arrived as director of the hospital and thoracic surgeon, and remained until the hospital closed in 1958. He and Dr. Richard Chao made up the regular medical staff, and Dr. Joseph Deisher, an orthopedist, attended part-time.

Serving Crippled Children with Tuberculosis: The Orthopedic Program

Although tuberculosis of the lungs posed by far the greatest threat by its infectiousness and progressive nature, other forms of tuberculosis were also causing death, disability, and suffering in Alaska, especially in children. Indeed, among children fourteen years old and younger with tuberculosis, approximately 25 percent were affected primarily in sites other than the lung. Tuberculous meningitis and miliary tuberculosis were often fatal, even with prompt treatment. Scrofula was also a widespread problem among Alaskan schoolchildren during the early part of the twentieth century, and was often remarked upon by the teachers, nurses, and physicians. A more destructive and lasting form of tuberculosis, also found mainly in children but not limited to them, was tuberculosis of the bones and joints, often leading to progressive destruction of the large weight-bearing joints such as the hip and knee. A particularly crippling form was tuberculosis of the spine, or Pott's disease, which not only caused a sharp angulation of the spine but often led to neurological complications due to pressure on spinal nerves.[36]

The treatment for these conditions, at least prior to effective drugs, was long-lasting and unsatisfactory. A tuberculosis manual from the era described the ideal principles: "Complete bodily rest, pleasant surroundings, nutritious diet, graduated exposure to sun and outdoor air, combined with local rest to the affected part by means of adequate apparatus and competent trained nursing care are the basic essentials...." Rest involved immobilization of the joint by extensive casting, sometimes for years. Some surgical procedures were also used, mainly bone grafts to immobilize, or "fuse," a joint permanently, and drainage of abscesses.[37]

Since the time of World War I, the Bureau of Education, followed later by the Office of Indian Affairs and the Office of the Governor, had been sending a few children out of the territory for the specialized treatment of crippling conditions, more often than not due to tuberculosis of the bones and joints.[38] The federal Children's Bureau also provided funds through the health department not only for hospitalization but also for screening, transportation, and aftercare. By June 30, 1939, the territorial registry had reached 175 cases, two-thirds of them due to bone and joint tuberculosis, with the remainder largely cases of poliomyelitis, congenital defects, and birth injuries.[39] The program was administered by a part-time physician under the direction of the part-time commissioner of health.[40] Even with the addition of matching territorial appropriations, the Crippled Children's Service helped only a few Native children each year, despite the fact that 75 percent of the children on the territorial register were Native.[41]

The law establishing the health department in 1945 provided that the board of health cooperate with the federal government "in matters of mutual concern pertaining to...crippled children." That year, for the first time, all the thirty-four Native children receiving hospital care for crippling conditions were funded by ADH. During its first formal meeting in September 1945, the board passed a resolution encouraging the formation of a territorial Crippled Children's Association, since the federal government agreed to match dollar for dollar any funds raised.[42] In January 1946, Commissioner Albrecht announced that the newly established Alaska Crippled Children's Association (ACCA) would sponsor the territorial program (see chapter 4).[43]

In June and July 1946 the Division of Crippled Children of the health department conducted a survey in Fairbanks, Kotzebue, Nome, Bethel, Anchorage, Juneau, and Ketchikan. In addition to the local children at each site, many others were brought in from outlying communities, mostly by air. The team evaluated 228 children, 63 percent of them Native, and found most of the urgent and severe cases to be caused by tuberculosis of the spine or major joints. For some, their condition had progressed for years untreated and soon would be beyond help. Many of these children also had pulmonary tuberculosis, which precluded them from being cared for in the Seattle orthopedic hospitals.[44] Dr. N. Berneta Block, head of the Division of Crippled Children, was so discouraged by the huge numbers of children urgently needing care that she asked the consultant, Dr. Moffatt, to make his recommendations for individual patients on the assumption that the territory already had a sixty- to eighty-bed orthopedic hospital. When the team's 5,000-mile odyssey was finally over, she promoted a four-point program: 1) develop an educational program to prevent crippling conditions; 2) secure funding for an orthopedic hospital within the territory; 3) support the efforts of ACCA; and 4) support a program of specialized vocational training.[45]

By mid-1946 Albrecht was negotiating animatedly with Dr. Ralph B. Snavely, director of health for BIA, about using the old naval hospital on Japonski Island for a territorial orthopedic hospital. Snavely had other plans for the building, but was willing to allow the use of the wooden barracks on Alice Island for the orthopedic program. This controversy prompted a heated reply from Governor Gruening to the Director of Territories in Washington, in which he called the proposal to use the Alice Island barracks "utterly unthinkable and amazing."[46]

As a result of a meeting in Washington, D.C., on November 20, 1946, Gruening, Albrecht, and Snavely finally hammered out a plan that was to establish a fifty-bed orthopedic hospital at Sitka under a cooperative agreement. The site would indeed be the former naval dispensary on Japonski Island, a one-story reinforced-concrete structure consisting of two twenty-two-bed wards and seven single rooms, plus space for offices and x-ray and operating rooms.[47] ADH was also to provide specialized consultants, specifically an orthopedic surgeon and an orthopedic surgical nurse. These consultants were also to serve as advisors to the department's Crippled Children's Division.[48]

On this same trip east, Albrecht succeeded in persuading Dr. Philip H. Moore, a well-trained orthopedic surgeon in Greeley, Colorado, to come to Alaska and set up the orthopedic program. According to Moore, Albrecht turned on his awesome powers of persuasion and convinced him within two hours to give up his newly established practice and move to a very uncertain future in Sitka.[49] When he arrived in Alaska with his wife in March 1947, he found some twenty-five children, most of them Natives with bone and joint tuberculosis, already waiting for him in the new orthopedic unit. He had vivid second thoughts about his decision to come to Alaska when he saw the dilapidated condition of the hospital and realized how little experience he had in tuberculosis. After three weeks he was so discouraged by the magnitude of the task before him that he wrote a letter of resignation, only to tear it up when he found himself bonded with the children in a special way. "The little rascals hooked me—just couldn't resist them," he admitted many years later.[50]

The hospital was indeed in poor shape, with the floor badly damaged. The navy had taken away the supplies and most of the useful equipment in the hospital, including the main operating room lamp, a loss that left a gaping hole in the ceiling.[51]

The funding for the new hospital was byzantine in its complexity. The 1947 operating budget of $140,000 included $35,000 from territorial health funds, $35,000 from ACCA, and matching federal funds of $70,000.[52] The hospital was open to all, regardless of race, with ANS paying ADH a daily rate for the hospitalization of Natives and non-Native patients paid for through Crippled Children's funds.[53]

In May and June 1947, shortly after he settled in, Moore organized a series of orthopedic clinics throughout Alaska to bring the crippled children's registry up to date and to get a clearer idea of the dimensions of the problem throughout the territory. The ADH team screened for new cases, offered consultation to local physicians, and provided follow-up for those children previously identified. They examined 275 children on the trip, including 55 flown in from outlying villages. When the trip was completed, the registry contained the names of 440 critically ill children needing immediate hospitalization.[54]

Since funding allowed care for only approximately one-seventh of those on the register, some children with orthopedic problems continued to be sent out of the territory to the University of Chicago Hospital and to Swedish Hospital in Seattle.

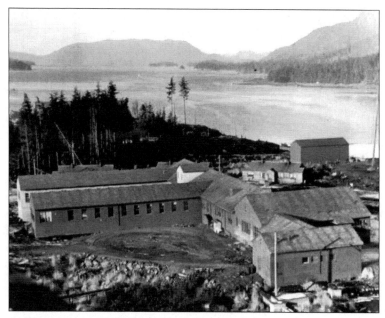

:: Mt. Edgecumbe Orthopedic Hospital. ::
(Alaska Department of Health and Social Services Collection, George A. Dale, PCA 143-509)

In 1949, eighty-eight patients were cared for at Mt. Edgecumbe and another nine in the Chronic Disease Unit at St. Ann's Hospital in Juneau.[55]

After a shaky start, Moore could claim within a year that orthopedic care at Mt. Edgecumbe was second to none in the United States. Surgical equipment was of the latest design, a full-service physiotherapy program had been established, and a brace shop was under development. A research and training program was also being actively pursued. The hospital maintained an active outpatient clinic on site, and its staff periodically held clinics in other communities around the territory. In 1948 Moore performed major surgery on about twenty patients at the Bethel ANS hospital and the following year extended this work to Kotzebue.[56]

In August 1948 the bed capacity of the unit was raised from fifty to sixty-five beds and the hospital remained full. Ranging in age from five to fourteen years, the children came from Metlakatla to Unalaska to Barrow. Tuberculosis accounted for about half of the crippling conditions, the most common type being tuberculosis of the spine, followed by tuberculosis of the hip and the knee.[57]

In view of the massive backlog of cases, Moore visited major medical centers in New York, Chicago, Seattle, San Francisco, and Columbia, South Carolina, to explore new and more efficient methods of treatment. He also persuaded a number of eminent orthopedic specialists to come to Alaska to perform surgery and assist in field clinics. As a result of these consultations, he began performing earlier and more radical surgery. Fusion of the spine and the major joints usually required an autolo-

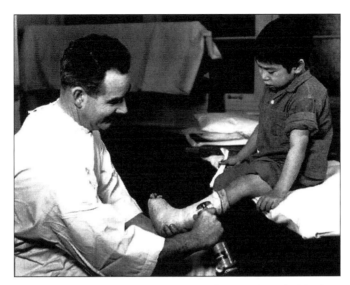

:: Dr. Philip Moore cutting the cast from the leg of a small tuberculosis patient. ::
(Courtesy of Margery Albrecht)

gous bone graft, that is, a segment of bone removed from the individual, usually from the iliac crest. In very young or debilitated children, this procedure was often dangerous; as an alternative Moore began experimenting with the idea of a "bone bank" using homologous grafts, or bone material removed from another person. Initially he used bone segments taken from ribs removed during the thoracoplasties regularly performed by Dr. Fred Coddington at the Mt. Edgecumbe sanatorium. Fresh bone was ideal, but after some experimentation he found that frozen bone seemed to work almost as well.[58]

The first "deposit" in the bank came on February 26, 1951. When a transplant was contemplated, the bone was freshly ground up to a specified fineness under strict aseptic conditions, then used to pack the cavity where the patient's diseased bone had been removed.[59] In June 1952 Moore was able to transport frozen bone specimens, using dry ice and an insulated cabinet, all the way to Kotzebue, where it was used for seven successful fusions in patients ranging in age from sixteen months to nineteen years. For the return trip he filled his "bone box" with eighteen units of blood that had been donated by the people of Kotzebue.[60] On the way to Kotzebue on another trip, he told of being stuck in Fairbanks with the dry ice in his bone bank cabinet rapidly evaporating. With the help of a bush pilot, he sprayed carbon dioxide from an airport fire extinguisher over his bones, which kept them frozen until he reached Kotzebue. Once there he buried the bone bank in the snow, only to have the sled dogs try to dig it up.[61]

After a notable career at the Orthopedic Hospital, Moore resigned his post in 1956 and established a private practice in Sitka, where he continued to attract patients from a wide area. He was dismayed by the lack of support for the orthopedic program, as evidenced by reduced numbers of clinics, the discontinuation of the residency program he had established, and by the fact that no full-time orthopedist was hired to replace him. The large database on over 7,000 orthopedic cases which he had developed was also being neglected, in his opinion. He remained on as a consultant, however, and continued to conduct some clinics in the field.[62]

By 1961 new cases of bone tuberculosis were being diagnosed infrequently, although the orthopedic program still had to continue follow-up on many cases throughout the territory. Instead, the program was devoting more time in its periodic clinics in the bush and in larger towns to helping the victims of poliomyelitis and other crippling conditions. In Anchorage, the state Division of Public Health was cooperating with the Alaska Native Health Service to hold monthly clinics at the Alaska Native Hospital. In 1960 some 524 children were treated as outpatients and another 34 hospitalized for anywhere from a few days to a few months.[63]

Alice Island and the New Sanatorium at Mt. Edgecumbe

Since two entire military bases at Sitka were transferred to ANS—a value estimated at $50 million—there were many available buildings, including ample and well-appointed quarters for staff and recreational facilities within a short distance. By early 1947, the Skagway Sanatorium had proven unsatisfactory and the patients had to be moved elsewhere. Since Congress had already approved the construction of a large new facility at Mt. Edgecumbe, ANS decided to use some of the army buildings on Alice Island as a temporary hospital.

The Alice Island hospital, like the one at Skagway, was a complex of barracks-style buildings that could accommodate 150 patients.[64] The facility became one of three units then comprising the Mt. Edgecumbe Medical Center, the other two being the Orthopedic Hospital and a fourteen-bed infirmary serving the students at the new Native boarding school. The center was under the overall direction of Dr. M. M. Van Sandt, formerly the assistant medical director of ANS. There he was assisted by Dr. Moore, already on duty as head of the Orthopedic Hospital, Dr. David J. Shulman, head of the general hospital, and later Dr. A. J. Wehler, who became head of the Alice Island Sanatorium.

The sanatorium consisted of a number of single-story wards, some with storm porches, connected by long closed-in corridors. The heating system, mercifully, was more efficient than that of the Skagway facility, and the buildings were later provided with concrete foundations and firewalls to make them safer. Although Alice Island itself was originally a true island, it had become incorporated into Japonski Island by fill and causeways during the war years. The hospital facility was located at the site where an elementary school now stands.

The ninety-one patients from Skagway arrived in February 1947, followed in August by a second large contingent from the Seward Sanatorium, as a result of

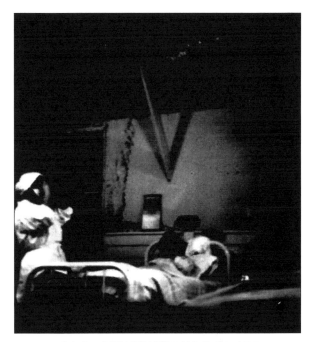

:: Interior of Alice Island Sanatorium, showing ::
stark surroundings, circa 1948.
(Photo by Pat Sarvela, courtesy of the Sitka Historical Society, Sitka, Alaska)

the ANS budget crisis. By early 1949 the sanatorium had five wards open, with a capacity of 140 beds, although the space had been designed for 120. Two additional wards were planned, to bring the official capacity to 150.[65]

Mother Mary Mildred visited the Sisters of St. Ann, who had accompanied the Skagway patients, and reaffirmed that the order would not renew its contract after July 1, 1947, in part because of the difficulty in recruiting nurses. Upon their departure, Dr. Rufus, medical director of ANS, was quoted as saying, "The sisters worked under terrific handicaps due to the personnel shortage and difficulty in obtaining materials and supplies during the war. Their efforts were undaunted day and night to see that the tuberculosis patients received every needed attention."[66]

Conditions at the new facility were not a great improvement over those of the previous institution, but at least there was heat. As early as January 1948, the patients complained that they were unable to eat the food they described as "over-ripe" reindeer meat and "uneatable fish gaffed from spawning creeks," not to mention dehydrated vegetables.[67] Stung by the criticisms, ANS Superintendent Foster challenged any "disinterested parties" to come and investigate the situation for themselves, adding that the food for the hospital was prepared in the same kitchens that served the school and Orthopedic Hospital—all under the supervision of two "well-qualified and capable dietitions [sic]."[68]

When the AMA survey team visited in the summer of 1948, they reported that the building was a well-equipped 150-bed facility, but recommended that it should be immediately expanded by 100 beds, with the addition of a thoracic surgeon, physician-anesthetist, staff physician, dentist, and additional nurses. Four physicians were at the Mt. Edgecumbe complex at that time, but at least two spent the majority of their time at the Orthopedic Hospital. The report also stressed the need for ANS to allow for the care of white patients at their facilities, but federal policy was not ripe for change on this issue. Another suggestion, which ultimately came to fruition, was the idea of using medical students and residents at the Mt. Edgecumbe facility, not only as a wonderful training experience but also as a help to the overburdened doctors.[69]

Certainly the Alice Island Sanatorium was better equipped than Skagway, and its medical staff qualified to provide additional treatment options, including pneumothorax and pneumoperitoneum, for its patients. In March 1949 a chest surgeon, Dr. Frederick L. Coddington, was recruited for the hospital from Portland, Oregon. Since Coddington was dissatisfied with the standard government salary offered, ATA undertook to supplement it annually. With his arrival, more sophisticated surgical procedures were undertaken, particularly thoracoplasties, a procedure in which some of the upper ribs were removed to collapse the infected portion of a lung. After the move to the new hospital in 1950, Coddington was able to carry out more extensive lung surgery, including lobectomies and even pneumonectomies. In 1950 he helped establish a walking blood bank in Sitka in support of the surgical program.[70]

In May 1948 construction began on the 200-bed replacement hospital that was to adjoin the old navy infirmary, with an expected completion date of November 1949.[71] The new facility was not in fact completed until March 1, 1950, following which the Alice Island Sanatorium and the Orthopedic Hospital underwent remodeling, and no new patients were accepted for a period.[72] Finally, on April 14, 1952, some beds were again opened at Alice Island to expand capacity pending completion of the new Anchorage Hospital.[73] The facility closed a few years later, when all tuberculosis patients could be accommodated at the new hospital.

In late 1945 Commissioner of Indian Affairs William A. Brody had included in his FY1947 budget request to Congress funds to build and operate a tuberculosis sanatorium in Southeast Alaska. Once the facilities on Japonski Island became available in 1946, it seemed most appropriate and economical that the new hospital be constructed there. The hospital complex was to be state of the art and was conservatively estimated to cost $1.45 million, including renovations on the naval infirmary, construction of the new 200-bed sanatorium, and equipping both buildings.[74] The medical director of ANS expressed the hope that the hospital would be ready by December 1947, although in fact construction began only in late May 1948.[75]

The 200-bed hospital building was finally completed in February 1950 at a total cost estimated at $2 million. At the opening on March 1, patients at the Orthopedic Hospital and at Alice Island were moved to the new building, and soon the older facilities were being renovated with new flooring, better lighting, and repainting. Although the ultimate capacity of the complex depended on these renovations, it was anticipated that there would ultimately be a total of 415 beds available at Mt. Edgecumbe, of which 325 would be for pulmonary tuberculosis and another 65 for bone and joint tuberculosis. At the time of opening, an estimated 130 orthopedic patients and another 2,400 cases of pulmonary tuberculosis were on the waiting list for admission, with an additional 2,091 pulmonary cases recommended for supervised home care.[76]

Rehabilitation

Every authority on sanatorium care concurred that rehabilitation was an essential component of effective care of the tuberculous. Dr. Haas, in his 1945 plan, stressed the importance of rehabilitation and follow-up, comparing it to the assistance demobilized soldiers need in adjusting to civilian life.[77] The following year Dr. Gehrig listed "rehabilitation and after care" as one of the six major elements of his tuberculosis control program.[78] The special session of the legislature in 1946 had established a territorial program of vocational rehabilitation, but failed to fund it appropriately.[79]

ATA recognized from its beginning the importance of rehabilitation, but felt compelled in the early years to commit its meager resources to the all-important x-ray surveys. By 1947, however, ATA was placing primary emphasis on supporting rehabilitation. At Seward, ATA cooperated with the VA and the American Red Cross in establishing a rehabilitation program, with the emphasis first on occupational therapy, especially handicrafts, and second on educational opportunities for the patients. ATA also began a search for qualified people trained in rehabilitation, "capable of looking ahead and planning long-range programs."[80]

Bess Winn, who tirelessly promoted rehabilitation, pointed out that in its simplest form it meant nothing more than recreation, since many patients were too ill for anything but mild entertainment. Even the sickest could read, listen to music, or perhaps watch a movie. The next phase was education. Happy patients were usually the most likely to recover, she went on, and nothing promoted happiness like keeping the mind busy with educational opportunities. The third phase was occupational therapy, to keep the hands busy in a useful activity. The final stage was vocational rehabilitation, where patients could learn new job skills commensurate with their physical limitations.[81]

In December a newly formed ADH mental health team consisting of a psychiatrist, clinical psychologist, and psychiatric social worker spent a week at Seward assisting with the fledgling rehabilitation program. The team interviewed about ten patients from the sanatorium, making evaluations and recommendations for

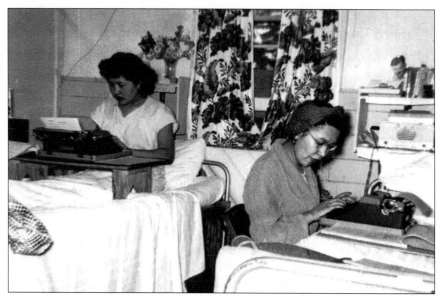

:: Patients at Seward Sanatorium learning typing as part of the rehabilitation program. ::
(Courtesy of Margery Albrecht)

vocational training. It also devoted time to meeting with the hospital professional staff to help them better understand and deal with patients' problems.[82] Rehabilitation was considered to begin on the day of admission and to continue after discharge until the patients had safely met the problems of adjustments to life outside the hospital. Many with tuberculosis had previously led independent, strenuous, outdoor lives of hunting, fishing, or trapping—activities incompatible with lungs or bones severely damaged by the disease. Some could no longer live in a village setting far from medical help when it was needed. Rehabilitation involved preparation of such patients intellectually, emotionally, and physically for a new line of work and a whole new outlook on life.

The program required the cooperative efforts of the medical team, the social welfare–mental health team, and the vocational rehabilitation team. The task of the physicians was to make the patient as well as possible and to set any necessary physical limits on his or her future activities. The social welfare–mental health team was to help the patient keep in touch with family and solve personal and financial problems. The psychiatric social worker helped the patient deal with the many emotional issues that arose from sanatorium treatment, while the psychologist was responsible for psychological testing and assessing personality traits. A consultant psychiatrist integrated all this information and made recommendations for vocational training, while personally treating the more severe emotional problems. Members of the vocational rehabilitation team used the recommendations of the other teams to work with the patients to determine a future vocation compatible with the patient's skills and interests, while at the same time realistically addressing any physical limitations the patient might have. Vocational counselors, armed with up-to-date information on vocational schools and skills needed, were then able to make arrangements for further training either at the hospital or after discharge.[83]

By 1954 a Rehabilitation Center at Seward Sanatorium had been established. Under the supervision of a commercial enterprises officer, training in at least ten different trades and skills was made available to patients.[84] The Parran survey group visiting that year (see chapter 6) strongly supported vocational rehabilitation and felt it would in the long run reduce tax expenditures for care for the chronically disabled, increase their purchasing power, and train workers from the villages. The average tuberculosis patient, moreover, was an ideal candidate because of his or her need to develop new skills.[85]

A report from the Seward Sanatorium in February 1955 showed just how far these principles were being realized. The patient was assessed as soon as possible after admission for interests and abilities, and even brought to the Rehabilitation Center to observe as soon as his or her treatment plan permitted. The first enterprise the center developed was a photo-finishing shop, followed shortly by a shoe repair shop, a gift shop for merchandising crafts, skin sewing, key making and saw filing, a gas and service station, and a grocery store. Other ideas under development included a small greenhouse and outdoor summer garden, institutional cooking instruction, and commercial driving. During the winter of 1954–55, the center had seventeen trainees who were earning their own room and board, but as their studies progressed, they could also go on the payroll to earn personal wages. Some patients in the late stage of their training and treatment were even able to move into comfortable private quarters on the grounds of the hospital. Several "graduates" had already gone on to full-time jobs following discharge, either at the sanatorium itself or in the private sector.[86]

In September 1952 a rehabilitation program was initiated at the Mt. Edgecumbe Orthopedic Hospital, with Elaine Corke assigned to the hospital to work on vocational needs in close cooperation with the territorial vocational rehabilitation program.[87] In December a clinic of specialists in different aspects of rehabilitation, financed by ATA and the Alaska Office of Vocational Rehabilitation, met at the Seward Sanatorium to provide direct services and to assist in setting up a rehabilitation program. The Mt. Edgecumbe Hospital, however, never developed a full vocational rehabilitation program. As the inpatient census declined, the need and justification for a major rehabilitation program receded. Moreover, the average length of stay for those few tuberculosis patients who still required hospital treatment became so short that an elaborate in-house program was not cost-effective. By the late 1950s, nearly all Native tuberculosis patients had been transferred to Anchorage.

In 1965 at the Anchorage Native hospital (as discussed below), a group of concerned professionals, led by Dr. Martha Wilson, recognized that Alaska Natives crippled by tuberculosis and other disabling conditions had special rehabilitation needs. Accordingly, they established a research-demonstration project, funded by the federal Office of Vocational Rehabilitation (OVR), to evaluate such patients in a holistic manner and prepare them for a productive future. The patient was helped primarily by referral and job placement, with the only actual job-training opportunity being the operation of the staff cafeteria as a sheltered workshop by a group of about fifteen former patients. The project continued until June 1969.[88]

Magic Bullets at Last

As the work of many came to fruition and Alaska at last attained the necessary tuberculosis beds to address the problem effectively, the whole concept of sanatorium treatment became obsolete. By 1952 three anti-tuberculosis drugs—streptomycin, para-aminosalicylic acid (PAS), and isoniazid (INH)—had become available and these changed forever the treatment of tuberculosis. No longer did those afflicted with tuberculosis have to spend many months in a hospital, suffering boredom, a monotonous diet, regimentation, and painful procedures.

In mid-1946 ADH published an informational article on the new drug streptomycin, noting that it was available only in small quantities, with its use restricted by the National Research Council to a few federal agencies. All the available drug was being channeled into research trials involving nine types of infectious disease. Curiously, tuberculosis was not on the list.[89]

In January 1947 Dr. Gehrig announced that a very limited supply of streptomycin was available in the territory. Although the drug had shown promise, he warned that tuberculosis patients and their families should not expect miracles. He also pointed out that although the streptomycin could retard the progress of pulmonary tuberculosis in some cases, the disease often flared up when it was discontinued. The drug was also associated with serious side effects, including balance problems and hearing loss.[90]

In October 1948 the follow-up report of the AMA team concluded that streptomycin therapy in Alaska was "sadly neglected" because of lack of funds. ANS had purchased enough of the drug for about thirty patients at Mt. Edgecumbe, but other Natives on the drug had to pay for their own. The National Institutes of Health provided enough dosages to treat forty patients at the Seward Sanatorium in a controlled trial, and the Orthopedic Hospital obtained enough to treat twenty-three patients as part of a research project. At Kotzebue Dr. Rabeau obtained a small amount to treat scrofula patients, with good results. The AMA consultants concluded that ANS should ask for sufficient funds to treat at least 20 percent of its hospitalized tuberculosis patients with the new drug.[91]

Dr. Moore at Mt. Edgecumbe received a grant of $10,000 from the National Research Council that year for a trial of streptomycin in the treatment of bone and joint tuberculosis. Beginning in April 1949, some 100 patients were given the drug. In his summary of the study, Moore noted:

> At least three amazing results were produced by the use of streptomycin. Most important, the use of streptomycin definitely saved the lives of some patients. Furthermore, we established the fact that use of streptomycin effected arrest of tuberculosis of bones and joints in all patients treated and its use definitely reduced the hospitalization period needed to arrest the disease.

He gave details of one boy who had been given streptomycin over a period of time to prepare him for major surgery. The child improved so markedly that surgery was found to be unnecessary and he was discharged with an anticipated total restoration of function.[92]

By June 1952, INH was in limited use both at Seward and Mt. Edgecumbe, and streptomycin and PAS, the latter introduced in Alaska about 1950, were also being supplied to all patients at the Seward Sanatorium.[93] One of the staff physicians there, Dr. Shih-Shun (Richard) Chao, evaluated the clinical response of fifty patients receiving INH. At the end of six months, 75 percent of those on the drug had shown improvement in their sense of well-being, but only three had sputum conversions and four showed striking improvements in their x-rays. Other patients taking the medication, moreover, showed side effects, and one had a massive spread of his disease. These unimpressive results led Dr. Phillips to conclude that the new drug was of questionable value: "That INH may be an adjunct in the hospital or sanatorium treatment of the tuberculous is not questioned, but the experience with it thus far at this sanatorium does not make INH seem useful as a specific outpatient medication. In fact, we suspect that it could be very harmful. It does not supplant proper bed rest."[94] Just why the Seward experience with the drug was so poor remains unclear.

By 1954 Moore was using a combination of two of the three anti-tuberculosis drugs then available, namely streptomycin, PAS, and INH, and claimed he had seen no significant adverse reaction from any drug or combination of drugs.[95]

Over the next decade, Phillips, Chao, and other skeptics in Alaska would prove to be spectacularly wrong about the chemotherapy of tuberculosis, especially INH, which became not only the mainstay of treatment but also a godsend for the prevention of tuberculosis. Within a few short years, the hard-won sanatoriums would close or be turned to other uses.

The Last Sanatorium: The Anchorage Hospital Opens

In 1947 the AMA Survey group had suggested a 400-bed tuberculosis hospital in Anchorage. Commissioner Albrecht had much bigger plans, however, asserting that a 700-bed facility was needed, with 300 tuberculosis beds and 100 general beds for Alaska Native beneficiaries, but in addition 100 tuberculosis beds for non-Natives, 100 general beds for federal workers, 75 orthopedic beds for all Alaskans, and 25 contagious disease beds for all Alaskans. Anchorage seemed ideal for the largest hospital in the territory because it was centrally located and served by air, sea, and railroad, thus reducing transportation costs. It was also the headquarters for most federal agencies in Alaska, and all signs pointed to the city's rapid future growth.[96] Albrecht considered a large hospital in Anchorage his highest legislative priority, but given the political climate in Washington and the realities of private-sector medicine, the Federal Hospital Board was not willing to go beyond the original 400-bed Native hospital, including 100 general medical and surgical beds.[97]

Construction bids for the hospital went out in April 1949 and ground-breaking began on August 9. In November 1950, further bids were put out for the construction of a quarters building on the hospital campus, a three-story complex to be used for rooms and apartments to house some 197 single nurses and other hospital staff.[98] The grand opening of the hospital took place with much local fanfare on November 29, 1953. The final cost was $7.2 million, almost exactly the amount the United States paid Russia for the territory in 1867.[99] The final staff for the 400-bed facility was expected to be about 450, including 20 physicians, with an annual payroll of $1 million—a considerable infusion into the economy of Anchorage.

The overall hospital design was that of a sanatorium, and indeed 300 of its beds were allotted for that purpose. The 100 remaining beds were divided among neuropsychiatry, general pediatrics, obstetrics, and acute contagious diseases. Originally, only a tiny suite of offices on the first floor was reserved for outpatient services, with no provision for a chest clinic or the primary-care needs of the constantly increasing number of Alaska Natives who were settling in Anchorage during the postwar employment boom.

On the other hand, the hospital had state-of-the-art features for patient comfort, a far cry from the drab surroundings at Skagway, Alice Island, and even Seward. The six-story building had three tuberculosis wards on each of the third, fourth, and fifth floors. Most of the sixth floor was taken up by a large, bright common room called the Solarium, where convalescing patients could meet and talk, work on crafts, and even, it was thought, absorb some therapeutic sunlight through the windows on three sides.

Each ward, which made up one floor of one wing, had approximately thirty-two beds, and the walls were painted in "optimistic hues," such as rosy pink, sky blue, and aqua. Every bed had a radio control panel that permitted the patient to select either music from the hospital's own record collection or a live feed from a local radio station. The fifth floor included a patient library, barber shop, beauty salon, occupational therapy shop, and later a school. Features for the modern treatment of tuberculosis showed how far Alaska had come since the makeshift Skagway Sanatorium had opened only eight years before. The hospital had three modern operating rooms, an obstetrical suite, and a contagious ward, as well as a pneumothorax room and a minor surgery unit.

The hospital began admitting patients on November 30, and thereafter patients were called in as rapidly as possible according to the priority list that had been previously developed by an interagency team. Of the first 100 patients admitted to the hospital, nearly all for tuberculosis, 53 came from the Yukon-Kuskokwim region and another 22 from northwest Alaska.[100] The first death from tuberculosis was an infant who died of tuberculous meningitis in April 1954. Over the first four full years of the hospital's operation, only 3 more deaths out of 136 were attributed primarily to tuberculosis, although another 20 deaths listed tuberculosis as a contributing cause.[101] Thus, by 1954, death was no longer the inevitable or even the expected outcome of tuberculosis in Alaska.

The new Anchorage hospital, with its central location, modern equipment, ample staffing, and pleasant patient environment boded well for the future of the tuberculosis program. When it opened, more than 2,000 patients were still awaiting a hospital bed, yet by the end of the 1950s, widespread use of anti-tuberculosis drugs had radically altered its role as a sanatorium. Most hospital patients no longer required a long course of bed rest and isolation, but instead could be discharged after a few months with medication continued at home. Many others received supervised drug treatment from the time of diagnosis. Thoracic surgery also significantly reduced the length of hospital stays. As the tuberculosis census declined, the flagship sanatorium began its evolution into a general hospital.

Wings to Washington

Because of an intensive postwar anti-tuberculosis campaign, Washington State's tuberculosis death rate declined from 32.4 per 100,000 in 1946 to 6.3 per 100,000 only seven years later, leaving its sanatoriums running at less than half of capacity. At the request of three hospitals facing closure in the Seattle area, the Washington State Health Department proposed that beds be made available at cost to the federal government for care of Alaska Natives, a plan that seemed to benefit everyone. The scheme would virtually eliminate the waiting list for admission in Alaska, thus taking many potentially infectious patients out of circulation.

In February 1954 Commissioner Albrecht took up the idea with the Washington State Health Department, and soon these discussions expanded to include the Washington congressional delegation, Alaska Governor Frank Heintzleman, Delegate Bob Bartlett, and Surgeon General Leonard Scheele. In mid-summer these negotiations resulted in a bill in Congress adding $1.18 million to the ANS budget for the care of approximately 400 Alaska Natives during FY1955.[102]

The hospitals selected for the program included the state-owned Firland Sanatorium, with a total capacity of 1,310 beds, and two private facilities: Riverton and Laurel Beach, each with a capacity of 100 beds. Under the plan, about 300 Native patients would be treated at Firland, and another 100 at the other two hospitals combined. Although the plan seemed to have many advantages, there were some opponents, including the medical director of the Firland Sanatorium himself, who felt that since Native patients sent to Seattle would be thousands of miles from home and thrust into an alien culture and climate, their recovery might actually be impeded. Other officials were concerned that Native patients might be discharged in Seattle and remain there, thus becoming a burden on the health and welfare services of the city, county, and state.

A memorandum of understanding was finally signed on September 9, 1954. Alaska pledged to pay all transportation costs and to screen all patients, to be sent in groups of twenty to thirty, for their ability to adapt to the situation. Washington state health laws and regulations would apply to Alaskan patients just as they would to Washington patients.[103]

The first group of sixty-eight Native patients, mostly Eskimos, arrived in Seattle by chartered plane on October 14, 1954, and were distributed between the Riverton and Laurel Beach hospitals. They were followed a few days later by a group of thirty, who were sent to Firland. By the end of December Native patients were pouring into the Seattle airport. The new arrivals, mostly from the Yukon-Kuskokwim Delta, were dressed in their mukluks and parkas, and some brought guitars and mandolins. They made such a colorful impression that a few of the regular patients at Riverton thought they were an entertainment troupe. The majority seemed, at least to outsiders, to be apprehensive and excited by the long trip but to be adjusting well to their new surroundings, including new foods, but soon the deadly routine of the hospital asserted itself and they settled in for the long haul.[104] By spring 1955, there were a total of 431 Alaska Native patients hospitalized in the Seattle area. In early May the first of the initial group were pronounced "cured" and were on their way home, and more were expected to be discharged within the next few weeks.[105]

The airlift to Seattle continued through the following year, and the new Anchorage hospital effectively became the control and staging center. Patients flown in from the villages stopped there briefly, usually for a day or two, until transportation could be arranged and paperwork completed. On a single day in 1956, forty-eight patients were discharged from the Anchorage Hospital to catch the plane to Seattle. Although many flew with escorts on commercial flights, the medical officer-in-charge also made arrangements with the air force to make use of Military Air Transport System (MATS) flights to McChord Air Force Base in Tacoma. Some nurse escorts of that period recall that since Alaska was then a territory, they had to show proof of citizenship before they could enter the state of Washington.

Periodically, critics from both Alaska and Washington noted that Alaska was sending Native patients all the way to Seattle for care when there were empty tuberculosis beds at Seward, Mt. Edgecumbe, and the new hospital in Anchorage. ANS explained this anomaly by reminding its critics that Congress had not appropriated enough money to maintain the Alaskan sanatoriums at full capacity, and that at any rate, the daily cost of care was less in Washington.[106] They might have added that it was the heavyweight political influence of the Washington State congressional delegation that had obtained the appropriation for the use of Seattle beds in the first place.

Dr. Daniel W. Zahn, medical director of the Firland hospital, was the guest speaker at the ATA convention at Juneau in 1956 and warmly praised the work of ADH and ATA in beating back the tuberculosis epidemic. He had originally been strongly opposed, as he confessed, to bringing Alaska Native patients to Seattle, but admitted that Alaskan patients had responded better than expected to the radical changes in their lives. He particularly singled out Ray Hruschka, the Alaskan vocational counselor, for his enthusiasm and devotion. One problem, Zahn observed, was that the Alaskan patients received much less spending money for incidentals than the Washington patients. They did, however, receive blood for transfusion and various gifts, not to mention personal visits, from various service groups in the Seattle area.[107]

In November 1956 Dr. T. E. Hynson, area medical officer for the new Alaska Native Health Service (see chapter 6), also praised the work of the Seattle hospitals, noting that a total of 510 Alaskan patients, many with far-advanced disease, had been served in the first two years of the program. The average length of stay for Alaskan patients was just under a year.[108]

The following April Dr. Joseph Gallagher, director of the PHS Anchorage Hospital, announced that the backlog of tuberculosis cases had shrunk to the extent that all new patients could henceforth be treated in Alaskan hospitals, adding that by December 1, 1957, all the Alaskan patients in Seattle hospitals would be returned to the territory for any further care needed.[109] The contract between the Washington State Health Department, ADH, and the Alaska Native Health Service officially terminated on December 31, 1957.

Thus ended a curious chapter in the tuberculosis story in Alaska. The program brought many people to treatment much earlier than would have been possible with the facilities then available in Alaska. For the duration of the program, the tuberculosis death rate in Natives dropped from 221.6 per 100,000 in 1954 to a mere 36.6 per 100,000 in 1958. Other factors were at work as well, particularly the home treatment program described in the next chapter, but the availability of hundreds of new beds in Seattle to draw down rapidly the backlog of active cases requiring treatment played a significant part in breaking the back of the tuberculosis epidemic in Alaska.

As we have seen, sanatoriums played an essential role in the Alaska tuberculosis control program in the decade or so after 1945. In the absence of effective anti-tuberculosis drugs, hospitalization offered the best hope for individuals with the disease. In the hospital patients could rest, eat a nutritious diet, be treated for symptoms and complications, and even learn new skills for coping with life after discharge. Perhaps most important, hospitalization kept the patient with active disease from infecting others in the household and in the community. Through much of the decade, however, hospital care was unavailable to most individuals because of the huge backlog of active cases that were identified but not yet under treatment. It was only in the final stages of the planned building program in Alaska, and with the unexpected availability of additional beds in Washington State, that the waiting list finally dried up. The introduction and use of effective anti-tuberculosis drugs greatly hastened the process, as did the use of drug treatment in the home (see chapter 6).

Although sanatorium care was indispensable to the overall tuberculosis campaign in Alaska, it is easy to overlook its impact on individual patients, particularly Alaska Natives, all of whose lives were changed by the experience of a long hospitalization far from home. Some aspects of the hospital patients' point of view are described in appendix A.

Notes

1. Carl E. Buck, "Public Health Needs in Alaska," *AH* 1, no. 1 (June 1943): 3. The top priority, incidentally, was for a "single, medically directed health service" available to all citizens of Alaska.

2. Memorandum from Earl D. McGinty to E. L. Bartlett, December 22, 1943, Governor Correspondence, roll 248.

3. Rudolph Haas, "A Tuberculosis Control Program for Alaska," *AH* 3, no. 4 (April 1945); Rudolph Haas, "Tuberculosis Can Be Conquered," *AH* 3, no. 11 (November 1945).

4. "Tuberculosis Control Program" (typescript, revised October 1946), Albrecht Collection, 2–8.

5. "TB Workshop Meetings Review Applications for Hospitalization," *AH* 9, no. 2 (April 1952); "Tuberculosis Medical Conference Studies Applications of 400 Cases Awaiting Hospitalization; 277 Get Class I Priority for First Beds," *AH* 10, no. 6 (December 1953).

6. Bess Winn, "287 Beds Must Do for Alaska's 4,000 T.B. Cases. Ex-army Hospital to Serve 150," *Chicago Sunday Tribune*, September 2, 1945.

7. Margaret Cantwell and Mary George Edmond, *North to Share: The Sisters of Saint Ann in Alaska and the Yukon Territory* (Victoria, BC: Sisters of St. Ann, 1992), 187–91.

8. Cantwell and Edmond, *North to Share*, 190.

9. James A. Smith, "Tuberculosis Program of the A.N.S.," *AH* 4, no. 10 (October 1946); C. Earl Albrecht, "A New Year's Message, *AH* 5, no. 1 (January 1947).

10. Bess Winn, "Christmas Seal Sale—1945," *AH* 3, no. 11 (November 1945).

11. Ethel Pederson, with assistance from Ernie Fuess and Lillian and Max Workman, "Reminiscences" (unpublished typescript, 1949[?]).

12. Cantwell and Edmond, *North to Share*.

13. "Skagway Makes Strong Protest to Removal of Sanatorium to Sitka," *JAE*, January 28, 1947.

14. Pederson, "Reminiscences," 2.

15. Cantwell and Edmond, *North to Share*; telegram from Northland Transportation Company to Ernest Gruening, January 22, 1947, Governor Correspondence, roll 248.

16. Letter from Henry L. Stimson to Harold L. Ickes, December 9, 1944, Governor Correspondence, roll 248.

17. *Session Laws, Resolutions and Memorials, 1945* (Juneau: 1945), chapter 52: 134–35.

18. C. Earl Albrecht, "Another Step Forward," *AH* 4, no. 6 (June 1946).

19. Letter from Mrs. Robert Stewart to E. L. Bartlett, undated, Governor Correspondence, roll 248.

20. Telegram from C. Earl Albrecht to Ernest Gruening, February 6, 1946, Governor Correspondence, roll 248; telegram from Ernest Gruening to C. Earl Albrecht, February 6, 1946, Governor Correspondence, roll 248.

21. "Army Hospital Given to Alaska," *Alaska Life* 9, no. 6 (June 1946): 30.

22. "Notice of Sale. Surplus Government Real Property. Fort Raymond Hospital and Warehouse Projects. Accepted August 19, 1946," Governor Correspondence, roll 248.

23. C. Earl Albrecht, "Budget Report to the 18th Session of the Alaska Territorial Legislature, February 1, 1947," typescript, Albrecht Collection.

24. Albrecht, "Another Step Forward."

25. "Seward TB Hospital Will Stay Open, Says Albrecht," *Forty Ninth Star* (Anchorage), October 5, 1947; *Alaska Department of Health. Biennial Report of the Office of the Commissioner of Health, for the Period July 1, 1946 to June 30, 1948* (Juneau: ADH, 1948), 45.

26. Harry Barnett, Jack Fields, George Milles, Joseph Silverstein, and Arthur Bernstein, "Medical Conditions in Alaska. A Report by a Group Sent by the American Medical Association," *JAMA* 135, no. 8 (1947): 500–10.

27. Albrecht, "Budget Report to the Legislature, 1947," 9.

28. Telegram from Governor's Office to Ernest Gruening, April 24, 1947, Governor Correspondence, roll 248.

29. "Lack of Funds May Close Tuberculosis Sanatorium at Seward, Says Albrecht," *JAE,* April 24, 1947.

30. Telegram from Ernest Gruening to Edwin G. Arnold, September 11, 1947, Governor Correspondence, roll 248.

31. Telegram from Edwin G. Arnold to Ernest Gruening, September 17, 1947, Governor Correspondence, roll 248.

32. "Seward Patients Sent to Edgecumbe," *Forty-Ninth Star* (Anchorage), October 5, 1947.

33. "Hospital at Seward May Close Soon," *JAE,* October 15, 1947.

34. "Seward T.B. Hospital Remains Open," *Ketchikan Chronicle,* October 25, 1947.

35. Letter from E. L. Bartlett to C. Earl Albrecht, December 19, 1947, Governor Correspondence, roll 248.

36. Michael D. Iseman, *A Clinician's Guide to Tuberculosis* (Philadelphia: Lippincott Williams and Wilkins, 2000), 152–53, 162–63, 257–58,.

37. J. Arthur Myers, *Tuberculosis among Children and Adults*, 3rd ed. (Springfield, IL: Charles C Thomas, 1951), 220.

38. George A. Parks, *Report of the Governor of Alaska to the Secretary of the Interior, 1925* (Washington, DC: GPO, 1925), 63.

39. John W. Troy, *Annual Report of the Governor of Alaska to the Secretary of the Interior for the Fiscal Year Ended June 30, 1939* (Washington, DC: GPO, 1939), 54.

40. Ernest Gruening, *Annual Report of the Governor of Alaska to the Secretary of the Interior, Fiscal Year Ended June 30, 1940* (Washington, DC: GPO, 1940).

41. Ernest Gruening, *Annual Report of the Governor of Alaska to the Secretary of the Interior, Fiscal Year Ended June 30, 1941* (Washington, DC: GPO, 1941), 51.

42. "Crippled Children's Associations," *AH* 3, no. 11 (November 1945).

43. C. Earl Albrecht, "The Challenge of the New Year," *AH* 4, no. 1 (January 1946).

44. N. Berneta Block, "Tuberculosis . . . Crippler of Children," *AH* 4, no. 8 (August 1946).

45. N. Berneta Block, "Alaska's Crippled Children," *Alaska Life* 9, no. 12 (December 1946): 10–15.

46. Telegram from Ernest Gruening to Acting Director of Territories, August 1, 1946, Governor Correspondence, roll 273.

47. James A. Smith, "Proposed Sitka Tuberculosis Sanatorium," *AH* 4, no. 8 (August 1946).

48. "Orthopedic Hosp. Is Now Certain, Says Don Foster," *JAE*, December 3, 1946.

49. Philip Moore, transcript of interview by Kenneth Kastella in Sequim, Washington (1983), 7.

50. Sandy Poulson, "Dr. Moore Begins Retirement after 23 Years in Sitka," *Alaska Medicine* 12 (June 1970): 33–35.

51. Moore, interview.

52. "Dr. Albrecht Cites TB Problem," *Ketchikan Chronicle*, October 23, 1947.

53. Philip H. Moore, "History of the Orthopedic Program for the State of Alaska," *Alaska Medicine* 1, no. 1 (1959): 29–30.

54. "Orthopedic Clinics," *AH* 5, no. 6 (June 1947); Gruening, *Report, 1947*, 50–51; Moore, "History of Orthopedic Program"; "Orthopedic Center Was Opened at Mt. Edgecumbe in March 1947 with Only 50 Beds," *AH* 8, nos. 11–12 (November–December 1950), 2.

55. "Alaska's Little Cripples," pamphlet (n.d. [1949?]), Alaska State Library, Historical Collection, MS 113-1-73.

56. Moore, "Alaska Progresses in Care."

57. "Orthopedic Center Was Opened."

58. Poulson, "Dr. Moore Begins Retirement"; Moore, "History of Orthopedic Program."

59. "Bone Bank Is Newest Aid in Orthopedic Surgery," *AH* 9, no. 4 (August 1951): 5.

60. "Kotzebue ANS Hospital Used in Pioneering Medical Step," unidentified newspaper clipping, June 9, 1952, scrapbook #2, ATA Collection.

61. Poulson, "Dr. Moore Begins Retirement."

62. Moore, "History of Orthopedic Program."

63. "Orthopedic Clinics Offer Wide Service," *AHW* 18 (June 1961): 3.

64. "Skagway Makes Strong Protest to Removal of Sanatorium to Sitka,"*JAE,* January 28, 1947.

65. This information is from Mr. Walter Dangel, a lifelong resident of Sitka, in an interview with M. Walter Johnson, at Sitka, April 18, 1996; Druxman, "Mt. Edgecumbe," 11–13.

66. Cantwell and Edmond, *North to Share.*

67. "Sitka Sanatorium," *JAE,* January 12, 1948; "Communication," *JAE,* January 12, 1948.

68. "ANS Head Asks Inspection at Mt. Edgecumbe," *JAE,* January 13, 1948.

69. Douglass, et al., "Medical Conditions in Alaska," 4–6, 9–12.

70. Dorothy Bronsema Thomsen, untitled and undated typescript in author's possession; "Dr. Coddington, Chest Surgeon, to Mt. Edgecumbe," unidentified newspaper clipping, September 24, 1949, scrapbook #2, ATA Collection; Frederick L. Coddington, "Walking Blood Bank Need Explained by Island Doctor," *Daily Sitka Sentinel*, May 8, 1950.

71. Ernest Gruening, *Annual Report of the Governor of Alaska to the Secretary of the Interior, Fiscal Year Ended June 30, 1948* (Washington, DC: GPO, 1948), 60.

72. Ernest Gruening, *Annual Report of the Governor of Alaska to the Secretary of the Interior, Fiscal Year Ended June 30, 1950* (Washington, DC: GPO, 1950), 61–62.

73. *Alaska Department of Health 1951–1952, Twelfth Annual Report* (Juneau: ADH, July 1, 1950), 29–30.

74. Smith, "Proposed Sitka Sanatorium."

75. Smith, "Tuberculosis Program of A.N.S."; Bob Callan, "Sitka Sanitorium [*sic*] Approved," *Alaska Life* 10, no. 1 (January 1947): 15.

76. "Mt. Edgecumbe Sanatorium to Open Here for Patients by March 1st," *Daily Sitka Sentinel*, February 13, 1950.

77. Haas, "Tuberculosis Control Program."

78. Leo J. Gehrig, "Problems in Tuberculosis Control," *AH* 4, no. 10 (October 1946).

79. *Biennial Report, 1946–48*, 47–48.

80. Bess Winn, "Rehabilitation for the Tuberculous," *AH* 5, no. 10 (October 1947).

81. Bess Winn, "What Rehabilitation Can Do," unidentified newspaper clipping, scrapbook #3, ATA Collection.

82. "Mental Health Team to Aid T.B. Patients," unidentified newspaper clipping, December 5, 1953, scrapbook #2, ATA Collection.

83. Francis J. Phillips, "Hospitalization and Rehabilitation Carried on as Parallel Programs for Tuberculosis Treatment at Seward Sanatorium," *AH* 10, no. 2 (April 1953): 2–3.

84. *Annual Report, Alaska Tuberculosis Association, April 1, 1953 to March 31, 1954*, 14.

85. Thomas Parran, *Alaska's Health, A Survey Report* (Pittsburgh: University of Pittsburgh Graduate School of Public Health, 1954), VI-47, IV-51.

86. "Rehabilitation Center at Seward Sanitorium Offers Practical Training in Several Varied Crafts, Trades and Businesses. Methodist Church Group Operates Project," *AH* 12 (February 1955).

87. "Rehabilitation Program Is Started at Mt. Edgecumbe," unidentified newspaper clipping, September 5, 1952, scrapbook #2, ATA Collection.

88. See Robert Fortuine, *Alaska Native Medical Center: A History 1953–1983* (Anchorage: Alaska Native Medical Center, 1986), 68–70.

89. "Streptomycin," *AH* 4, no. 7 (July 1946).

90. "Dr. Gehrig Makes Statement about Drug Streptomycin," *JAE*, January 9, 1947.

91. Douglass, et al., "Medical Conditions, Progress Report," 22.

92. "Dr. Moore Reports on Streptomycin Treatment for TB of Bones, Joints," *AH* 9, no. 4 (August 1951), 5.

93. Ernest Gruening, *Annual Report of the Governor of Alaska to the Secretary of the Interior, Fiscal Year Ended June 30, 1952* (Washington, DC: GPO, 1952), 57.

94. Francis J. Phillips, "Seward Sanatorium Uses New TB Drug," *AH* 9, no. 6 (December 1952): 1, 4.

95. Philip H. Moore, "Tuberculosis of the Bones and Joints as Found in the Alaskan Native," typescript in the files of the Alaska Department of Health and Social Services, Division of Public Health, Epidemiology Section (n.d. [1954?]), 7–8.

96. C. Earl Albrecht, "Hospital Needs in Alaska (Non-Military) and Congressional Legislation Pertinent to Alaska Health Program," ADH (Juneau: 1947), Albrecht Collection.

97. "Dr. Albrecht's Trip Profitable," *AH* 6, no. 2 (February 1948).

98. "To Call for Bids on $1,750,000 Bldg. ANS Anchorage Hospital," unidentified newspaper clipping, November 28, 1950, scrapbook #2, ATA Collection.

99. Detailed information on the planning and construction of the hospital can be found in Fortuine, *Alaska Native Medical Center*, chapter 2.

100. Admission log of the Alaska Native Medical Center, 1953.

101. Death log of the Alaska Native Medical Center, 1954–58.

102. "Supplemental Monies Asked to Hospitalize 400 More TB Patients," *AH* 11 (August 1954); "What Goes on Behind the Scenes," *ATA News* 7, no. 3 (September 1954). A last-minute crisis arose when BIA tried to withhold $820,000 from the Alaska budget to fund other Indian hospitals, a move that would have led to the closure of 200 tuberculosis beds in Alaska. The funds were restored, however, and by late July the supplemental appropriation had been signed into law.

103. "Memorandum of Understanding Between the Alaska Native Service, Alaska Department of Health, and the State of Washington Department of Health Regarding Hospitalization of Alaska Native Tuberculosis Patients, September 9, 1954," Governor Correspondence, roll 349.

104. "Firland Greets 40 Eskimos, Indians," *Seattle Post-Intelligencer*, December 30, 1954; "Eskimo TB Victims Flown Here," *Seattle Times*, October 31, 1954 [incorrectly marked "1955" in ATA Collection].

105. *ATA News* 8, no. 1 (May 1955); "First Alaska TB Patients Sent Home," unidentified newspaper clipping, May 3, 1955, scrapbook #1, ATA Collection.

106. "Native TB Treatment Going Okay—Says Official," unidentified newspaper clipping, March 18, 1955, scrapbook #1, ATA Collection.

107. "Alaskans Praised for Decrease in TB Rate by Seattle Director," *JAE*, March 9, 1956. ATA provided $2 per patient per month for incidentals.

108. "Hynson Praises Seattle Sanatorium for Care Given Alaska TB Patients," unidentified newspaper clipping, November 8, 1956, scrapbook #3. ATA Collection.

109. *Annual Report, ATA, April 1, 1956 to March 31, 1957,* 4.

:6: The Juggernaut

Tuberculosis in Retreat

PHS Takes Over Alaska Native Health Care

Since at least 1919 the Bureau of Indian Affairs (BIA) had been urged by Congress and various health organizations to transfer its health responsibilities to the US Public Health Service. The BIA, deeply involved in education and trust-land responsibilities, had never been completely comfortable with the administration of its medical care program. Recruitment of health professionals was a particularly difficult task, and many vacancies were the rule of the day in Alaska and elsewhere.

After reviewing the 1947 American Medical Association report, Hugh J. Wade, the regional director for the Alaska Native Service, wrote a confidential memorandum to the commissioner of Indian affairs on November 21, 1947. In it he confessed his doubts about the BIA's efforts in health. "This Federal agency has made little progress in the health field," he wrote. "Long ago I came to the conclusion that the principal reason for lack of progress was the agency administering it. The medical field is foreign to the Department of the Interior.... I have often asked myself why the US Public Health Service should not be administering the medical care in the Territory, even if Federal aid was to be confined only to the native population."[1]

Although the transfer to PHS had wide support nationally, both the Interior Department and the new Department of Health, Education, and Welfare balked at the idea, as did the Bureau of the Budget and some congressional delegations. In August 1954, however, the bill authorizing transfer was passed as PL 83-568 calling for an effective date of July 1, 1955.[2] Under its provisions, all facilities and programs relating to health of the Indians and Alaska Natives were transferred to a new entity of the Public Health Service, to be known as the Division of Indian Health (DIH). In 1969 DIH was renamed the Indian Health Service (IHS).

The Alaska program became known as the Alaska Native Health Service (ANHS). With the transfer, it became part of a nationwide Indian health program with considerable health expertise and resources. PHS offered its professional staff better salaries and benefits, training opportunities, and more chances for career advancement. It also comprised other health agencies with vast technical resources that could be brought to bear on the problems of Indian health, including the National Institutes of Health, Centers for Disease Control, Bureau of State Services, and Bureau of Medical Services (at that time operating the marine hospitals).

As part of PHS, moreover, DIH would be able to command higher appropriations from Congress, particularly for preventive work. The transfer of all health facilities, personnel, and services from BIA to PHS took place as scheduled on July 1, 1955.[3]

The transition went smoothly in Alaska and neither patients nor staff probably noticed much change right away, except for the new yellow flag with the blue fouled anchor and caduceus flying at all Native hospitals in the territory. Gradually, however, the program developed a new look among its professional staff. BIA civil service physicians, often in mid-career, were replaced as they resigned or retired with young PHS commissioned officers, most of them serving a two-year military obligation. In September 1957 the ANHS area office was moved from Juneau to Anchorage. At the time of the transfer, Native hospitals were located at Mt. Edge-cumbe, Juneau, Anchorage, Kanakanak, Bethel, Kotzebue, Barrow, and Tanana.

The Parran Report

In the early months of 1953, both the governor and the legislature had asked the Department of the Interior to authorize a comprehensive survey of the health conditions, resources, and programs serving the people of the territory. Officials of ADH and the federal Department of Health, Education, and Welfare both expressed their support for the idea, and they were soon joined by the Department of Defense. The Interior Department, which had ultimate responsibility for both the ANS medical program and ADH, selected the Graduate School of Public Health at the University of Pittsburgh for the task. Its founding dean, Dr. Thomas Parran, had served from 1936 to 1948 as surgeon general of the US Public Health Service and at the time was one of the most respected figures in public health in the world. The initial proposal called for the survey to be completed during the summer of 1953, but after reviewing the scope and complexity of the project, Parran recommended that only a preliminary survey be conducted that year, followed by part-time consultation over the following year with the definitive field survey taking place during the summer of 1954.

The purpose of the survey was to assess health programs conducted by the federal and territorial governments and by voluntary and private organizations, with special attention to the health problems of the Alaska Natives. The survey team was to collect detailed data on disease problems (particularly tuberculosis), including the socioeconomic conditions contributing to these problems, and evaluate existing programs, facilities, and services. Finally, the team was called upon to make immediate and long-term recommendations on the programs, facilities, and services required to address the health problems identified. The investigation was funded by a grant of $90,000 from the Department of the Interior.

In 1953 four senior faculty members visited Alaska, led by Dr. Parran. The *Anchorage Daily Times* editorialist was impressed with Parran's comment on arrival

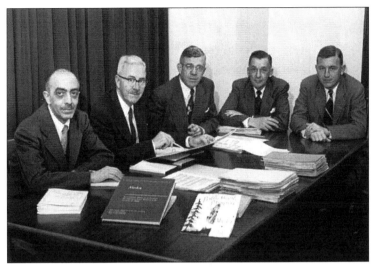

:: Members of the Parran Survey Team, 1953. L-R: Dr. Antonio Ciocco, Dr. Thomas Parran, :: Dr. Albrecht, Dr. James A. Crabtree, Dr. Walter J. McNerney. *(Courtesy of Margery Albrecht)*

in Juneau: "We do not go to Alaska with answers, but with questions."[4] A conflicting view was that of Dr. Milo Fritz, a local physician, who took the occasion to blast the survey as a waste of money because no action had been taken as the result of previous surveys. He acknowledged that some progress in tuberculosis had been made, but now felt it was time to deal with dental problems, mastoiditis, and eye disease, the latter two being his special area of expertise.[5]

Over the next six weeks members of the team logged some 6,000 miles and interviewed some 300 people from all walks of life. Upon their return to Juneau in mid-September they presented a series of recommendations to Interior Department officials. The team urged that the new tuberculosis hospital, then in the final stages of construction in downtown Anchorage, be staffed, opened, and operated at full capacity at the earliest possible date. The survey team also recommended that PHS health professionals be assigned to the hospitals of northern and northwestern Alaska, and that training programs for Native health workers be initiated at the Anchorage hospital and the newly opened hospital at Bethel. A final recommendation was the pre-hospital treatment of tuberculosis with the new anti-tuberculosis drugs (see chapter 8).[6]

In 1954 Parran's team, which comprised a select group of nine consultant specialists, again traveled widely in Alaska, visiting several remote villages. This time the team included two tuberculosis specialists, Drs. James E. Perkins, managing director of the NTA, and Joseph B. Stocklen, tuberculosis controller for Cuyahoga County, Ohio.

The final report, submitted in October, was unsparing in its appraisal of Alaska's health situation. It drew a stark contrast between "Native Alaska" and "White Alaska" in terms of economic development, political power, and health.

> The indigenous peoples of Native Alaska are the victims of sickness, crippling conditions and premature death to a degree exceeded in few parts of the world. Among them, health problems are nearly out of hand.... If other Americans could see for themselves the large numbers of the tuberculous, the crippled, the blind, the deaf, the malnourished, and the desperately ill among a relatively small population, private generosity would dispatch shiploads of food and clothing for Alaska,... doctors and nurses would be mobilized and equipped with the urgency of the great hospital units in wartime; the Alaskan missions would not need to beg for support.

This scathing indictment went on to contrast prompt American generosity to flood victims in Europe and famine victims in India with our attitude toward "our year-in-year-out victims of hunger, disease, and exposure."[7]

Under "Emergency Actions" the report baldly stated:

> Tuberculosis is the Alaskan scourge. Only by a "crash" attack carried on with increasing intensity during the next five years will it be possible to break the back of this Number 1 killer of young men and women and crippler of children. Such a program involves not only the full-scale employment of all proven methods such as systematic case finding, the hospitalization of every person needing it, but the immunization of infants and the extensive use of anti-tuberculosis drugs....

The report presented figures for 1950, which, taken at face value, indicated that overall tuberculosis mortality was eight times greater in Alaska as a whole than in the States, but that in Natives the mortality was approximately thirty times greater. The mortality for Native children under fourteen years of age was over 100 times that of a comparable group from the States, and in the group over forty-five years of age the mortality was twenty times as great. The highest rates were in the Eskimo population of the western and northwestern parts of the territory, with the lowest rates in Southeast Alaska and in the southern Railbelt.[8] Mortality trends were difficult to assess, but the Native tuberculosis mortality had seemingly fallen from 841 per 100,000 in 1943 to 673 per 100,00 in 1950, and to a provisional figure of about 300 per 100,000 for 1953, a rather remarkable decline of nearly 64 percent in a decade. The team was dubious about the accuracy of the earlier figures, but conceded that the extensive efforts toward hospitalization of patients with active disease had probably made an important difference.

Even accepting the 1953 figures at face value, however, the Alaska Natives still had a severe tuberculosis problem. Some of the most striking evidence was the tuberculin survey of Weiss, which showed that in the period 1948 to 1951, 89 percent of five-to-eight-year-old Yup'ik children in the Yukon-Kuskokwim Delta, 67 percent of the Eskimos in northwestern Alaska, and 65 percent of Athabascans in the Interior had positive tuberculin tests. The Parran team called the proportion of positive reactors among the Eskimos and the Indians of the Interior "higher than has ever been reported for any population group anywhere." In contrast, 7 percent of all high school children in Anchorage were infected, a figure comparable to that of the United States at large.

The report also quoted figures from the ADH tuberculosis register report of March 15, 1954, which showed 2,606 persons with active or probably active tuberculosis, a rate of 1,785 per 100,000 for the territory as a whole. If only the 2,363 Native cases were considered, the rate jumped to 6,474 per 100,000—that is, nearly 6.5 percent of the Natives had active tuberculosis. This rate, according to the Parran team, was "outside any range ever observed."

The Parran team concluded this section thus:

Apparently the problems [of tuberculosis] are located almost entirely in the native groups of west and north of the Railbelt, and the disease apparently has assumed epidemic proportions in some villages. The problem is essentially a native one, but we cannot say that it is or will be limited to this group and will not effect [sic] the white population should closer contact be established.[9]

The consultants then carefully evaluated every aspect of the tuberculosis programs of the territorial government, ANS, other agencies of the federal government, voluntary agencies, and the private sector, and made specific recommendations for improvements. Duplication of services was a special concern, particularly the overlap of responsibilities for tuberculosis control between ANS and ADH. Tuberculosis had to be accepted as a single territorial health problem, not a Native problem or a white problem. A "logical solution," according to the report, would be the appointment of a single tuberculosis control officer to correlate case finding, hospitalization, and follow-up throughout the territory.

The team emphasized that a hospital was still the best place for treatment for the "vast majority" of cases of active disease, especially when home conditions were poor. The newer antimicrobials, however, should be employed for all patients for whom no hospital bed was available. In late 1954 some 933 beds were available for the treatment of Alaskan tuberculosis patients, but despite these numbers the team felt there was still a deficit of at least 400 beds in Alaska. They recommended no new construction but instead fuller utilization under contract of the surplus sanatorium beds in the state of Washington.

The report addressed many other issues of tuberculosis control in Alaska, with specific recommendations, among them:

- Sanatorium beds should be filled even in the face of staff shortages, so that patients could at least be isolated and given good food and shelter
- Patients should be placed on the priority list for hospital admission based on "public health menace," not curability
- All new active cases of tuberculosis should be started on INH and PAS on an outpatient basis while awaiting a hospital bed
- Too little attention was being given to rehabilitation programs, except at the Seward Sanatorium, where a start had been made
- All Natives who were tuberculin-negative should be given BCG vaccine
- Special attention should be paid to the nutritional needs of tuberculosis patients
- New research was needed in the design, construction, and maintenance of Native housing, in order to reduce transmission of tuberculosis and other infectious diseases
- Both public and professional education about tuberculosis should be increased, this being especially the province of ATA
- Too much of the tuberculosis control budget (92.6 percent) was being directed toward hospital care, whereas at least 15 percent should be spent on case finding and follow-up[10]

The Parran Report represented a turning point in the battle against tuberculosis in Alaska. Although by the time of the team's first visit in the summer of 1953 much had already been accomplished in tuberculosis control, the helpful attitude and practical suggestions of a group of well-respected experts infused new enthusiasm into the struggle, together with state-of-the-art information in the evolving field of tuberculosis prevention and treatment. The tone of the report is sometimes harsh, but the venom was directed toward Congress and the American people at large for their neglect of Alaska, not toward the tired, overworked, and underpaid health workers on the Alaskan battlefield.

Over the next decade, many of the recommendations of the Parran Report were put into practice to strengthen the tuberculosis program. Furthermore, for years the report became a kind of scripture used by many health professionals to justify increased budgets for tuberculosis and other disease problems.

The Ambulatory Chemotherapy Program

After their first visit to Alaska in 1953, the Parran team convened a conference in Pittsburgh to consider the use of anti-tuberculosis medications on an ambulatory basis in Alaska. The group, including Dr. Albrecht, Dr. Hynson, and some twenty-five specialists in tuberculosis and health administration, reviewed a number of recent studies on the use of the new chemotherapy drugs in an urban outpatient setting, all of which showed that under favorable conditions medication alone

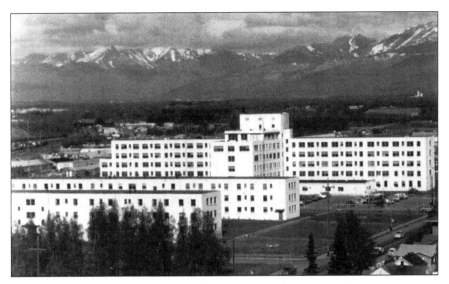

:: Alaska Native Hospital at Anchorage, at the time it opened in 1953. ::
The building in the foreground is the nurses' residence.
(Courtesy of Margery Albrecht)

could convert sputum status to negative and arrest the progress of the disease. The participants then drew up a detailed program addressing the feasibility of home drug treatment outside the hospital under Alaskan conditions. Initially, the idea was to use INH alone, and although the group recognized the risk of emergence of resistant strains, it concluded that patients could ultimately be treated with multiple drugs if necessary when a hospital bed became available. The group further stressed that the experimental program should not undermine or interfere with the tuberculosis programs already under way.

The goal was to reduce the number of infected individuals in Alaska to a point where the problem could be managed with standard tuberculosis control methods. The chemotherapy program would be restricted to the northern and western parts of the territory, where conditions were at their worst, and be limited to communities with a Native hospital or those with access to one. A population estimated at 13,437 people living in seventy-five villages around Barrow, Bethel, Dillingham, Fort Yukon, Kotzebue, and Tanana were selected for the program. Initially, the plan called for three groups to receive daily INH for six months: 1) those on the tuberculosis register; 2) those with positive sputum; and 3) children under six with a positive tuberculin test and no history of BCG vaccination. Participants would be evaluated after six months to determine whether they should receive the drug for another six months, be sent to the hospital, or be treated in some other fashion. The effects of the program would be assessed after twelve months to see whether it should be continued for a second year. Evaluation was intended to measure the effect of INH on the community-wide load of tuberculosis infection, and how well the drug was able to convert sputum under "the primitive Alaskan conditions." Moreover, it was hoped, the study would determine the relative value of x-rays and sputum surveys in identifying active cases.[11]

The Ambulatory Chemotherapy Program (ACP), as it came to be called, was to be directed by the Arctic Health Research Center (AHRC), with the cooperation of the Alaska Native Service and the Alaska Department of Health. AHRC had been established in Alaska by the Public Health Service in 1948 to undertake studies of the relation of heath to the special conditions of northern latitudes. The unit of the AHRC involved with ACP was the Epidemiology Section, located in Anchorage.[12] The estimated cost of the entire program was $150,000, but the Department of the Interior came up with only $100,000, to become available July 1, 1954.[13]

On their 1954 visit to Alaska, Parran and his team found skepticism "within some circles" whether any measures other than more hospital beds would be useful in tuberculosis control. In the field, however, everyone interviewed favored the idea of outpatient drug treatment. Parran himself was convinced that the plan could work because of the Natives' sterling record of participation in x-ray surveys and their low rate of discharge against medical advice from tuberculosis hospitals.[14]

In Alaska, home treatment was not a completely new idea. Dr. Francis Phillips, director of the Seward Sanatorium, remembered the concept beginning in 1950 with a group of doctors returning on the train from Mt. McKinley after a meeting of the Territorial Medical Association. Because of the tremendous pressure for tuberculosis beds, the doctors felt that if a hospital patient's condition could be stabilized by means of pneumoperitoneum and a course of dihydrostreptomycin, he or she could be discharged for follow-up care by a local physician, thus freeing up a bed. With the introduction of PAS in 1951 and INH the following year, the idea seemed even more practicable.[15] Young ANS physicians at Tanana and Bethel embraced the concept and soon were undertaking similar outpatient treatment.[16]

When ACP actually got under way, it was decided to limit it to seventy villages north and west of the Alaska Railroad in an area of about 400,000 square miles, roughly the size of Texas and California combined. This district was sparsely populated with about 25,000 Yup'ik and Inupiaq Eskimos and Athabascan Indians who had little access to medical care and were known to suffer the highest tuberculosis rates in the territory. Most lived subsistence lifestyles—hunting, fishing, and gathering their food—in villages that averaged about 200 people organized into thirty to forty households. Most health care in the villages was carried out by the school-teacher, with the help of radio consultation from the nearest hospital.[17]

The isolation and lack of local health resources precluded the use of strepto-mycin, a drug given only by injection. Instead, both INH and PAS were employed in order to reduce the likelihood of drug resistance. The dosage of INH was set at five milligrams per kilogram, requiring the adult patient to take six to eight fifty-milligram tablets daily. PAS was another story, since at a daily dosage of 200 milligrams per kilogram, the average adult had to take twenty-five to thirty large tablets divided into three doses.[18]

The program began in the villages of the Bethel Hospital service area in January 1955 and was extended to Barrow, Tanana, and Kotzebue over the course of the year. By July 1956 all seventy villages were included. Physicians (and sometimes other health staff) from these hospitals made visits to the villages one to four times a year and were in almost daily contact with the schoolteachers by shortwave "radio medical traffic." Since the hospitals already had medical records on most of the residents in the study villages, it was natural for the local hospital physicians to supervise the medical aspects of the tuberculosis treatment.

ADH managed the public health aspects of the operation, including laboratory studies, x-ray surveys, and public health nursing services. During the demonstration phase, AHRC retained responsibility for the design and technical supervision of the program, including the analysis and evaluation of data.[19] Although most of the staff were based in Anchorage, the "chemo nurses" were initially assigned to the field hospitals, plus one at Fort Yukon and one at Fairbanks. In the Barrow area and on St. Lawrence Island, ADH public health nurses (PHNs) assumed the function of chemotherapy nurses.

The nurses made regular visits to the villages in their areas and supervised the program at the local level, sharing records with the territorial PHNs. In addition to their responsibilities under the new program, they were also expected to attend medical emergencies, refer patients for other needed health services, and deal with social problems. Once the program was fully under way, the nurses visited each village an average of every three months for about three to five days to replenish pill supplies, distribute sputum cans for mailing back specimens, review records, give classes, and make home visits. The field nurses selected for the program were all experienced in public health, and as part of their orientation they learned small-group dynamics and studied the culture of the Natives of the region.

The extent of the tuberculosis problem in some of the study villages is demonstrated by a review conducted by AHRC in September 1956 in a community upriver from Bethel. The population was 188 plus newborns, distributed among only thirty households. Fifteen people in the village had been discharged from tuberculosis sanatoriums and ten more were currently hospitalized. A total of thirty-two people were taking home treatment, nineteen of whom had never been hospitalized. An additional eleven from the village were on the top priority list for hospitalization.[20]

By mid-1955 ACP was expanded to the treatment of positive tuberculin reactors and patients awaiting hospitalization, the delay being then about six months.[21] By July, 1,625 persons, or about 9 percent of the people in the seventy study villages, were receiving chemotherapy at home. That year the supply of tuberculosis beds became equal to the demand, and as a consequence pre-hospital ambulatory chemotherapy declined in importance in favor of post-hospitalization care and follow-up. In September 1956 ADH took over administration of ACP, as planned, in the thirty-seven northern villages, leaving AHRC to continue its research program in the Bethel area.[22]

Louise Lear, a PHN working in the program, described her experiences in 1957:

> If you should step from a bush plane into certain small Eskimo or Indian villages of Alaska, you would find a strange outpatient clinic for tuberculosis patients being conducted in a school or a store. The "chemotherapy aide"... would be making explanations in the local dialect as he weighed patients, refilled medicine bottles with isoniazid (INH), para-aminosalicylic acid (PAS), and vitamins. You would see mothers with toddlers, school children, and men climbing snowdrifts on the way to the school or store where the clinic is held every two weeks; a few dog sleds would be parked outside.
>
> Once inside the clinic, the women wriggle out of their bundlesome parkas fur tails flying, and the men remove big white National Guard boots before they are weighed; some of the young children fuss, and lumps of snow melt, on the floor....[23]

To introduce the program to the villages, the chemo nurses first sought the cooperation of the village council, elders, and other official or unofficial leaders. It is a tribute to their skill and diplomacy that they were able to present the program in such a way that every village selected for the program agreed to participate. Each village then appointed a volunteer "chemotherapy aide," who became the local representative of the program. Most of these aides were women, principally because they were more predictably available in the villages. In the earlier years of the program some schoolteachers, wives of agency officials, or missionaries—seemingly reluctant to yield authority—served as aides, but as the program developed, most villages saw the wisdom of having a local person selected by the council. Some chemo aides were former tuberculosis patients who felt a special calling to the task.[24]

Having a Native in the position was a distinct advantage. First, she or he had some official standing with the people of the community. Second, a Native aide could visit homes more easily and rouse the recalcitrant to participate in the program, dealing with individuals in a culturally sensitive way. Finally, she or he could serve as interpreter. Some aides complained about the workload and a few groused at receiving no compensation, but most seemed to enjoy the prestige of the position, and several became eloquent spokespersons in the cause of better health.[25] Not a few of these chemo aides went on to become village medical aides, and, later still, paid community health aides, when the program was formally established in 1968.[26] Lear described the aide's role:

Some of these chemotherapy aides are schoolteachers; one is the wife of a Civil Aeronautics Administration employee; one is the Canadian wife of a resident Moravian missionary; one is a 21-year-old boy with a fourth grade education; and another is a smiling little native grandmother in her sixties who attended the Catholic church school on the Yukon.

The aide of Kipnuk, Jim Anaver, is an outstanding 20-year-old, who is himself on chemotherapy. Kipnuk has a population of 200 and there are over 40 patients taking medications. Jim has an assistant, also on medications for another year, an enthusiastic patient who was recently discharged from Firland Sanatorium in Seattle. He learned little English in the hospital, but a great deal about tuberculosis, and he does not hesitate to dispense this knowledge to others. . . .

Their relationship with the chemotherapy nurse is apt to be the factor that supports and strengthens them in their work. Working with the nurse while she is in the village, the aide learns about the use of the drugs, possible toxic manifestations, how to keep records, and acquires general information about tuberculosis.[27]

The chemo aides met with all patients every two weeks, weighed them, evaluated their general health and degree of physical activity, and asked about any special problems, including adverse reactions to the medication. She or he also kept records of drug usage, dispensed a new supply of medication when necessary, and provided sputum cups for follow-up. Together the nurse and the aide worked on motivating patients to take medication three times a day, since many of them began to "forget" once they were feeling better.[28]

Sometimes directions for taking medications were confused or poorly understood, some individuals had a bizarre concept of the disease and its modes of spread, a few got fed up with taking the thirty-odd pills per day and quit. Yet on the whole people eagerly participated in the program. Although patients were normally given a two-week supply of pills at a time, they were given up to two months' supply when going on a trapline or to summer fish camp. Again Lear:

An adult patient may take . . . 10 tablets 3 times a day. . . . We know that in tuberculosis hospitals some of these medications are apt to end up in a pillowcase or paper sack at the bedside. What about these people, far out on the tundra or on the Bering seacoast? . . .

Of over 300 patients in the Kuskokwim area, only one has actually refused medication. He was a discharged sanatorium patient who "got tired of them and decided to quit." After extra encouragement from the nurse and the physician at the Bethel Hospital, he decided to take them again. Some require such encouragement, but many probably never miss a day's quota from the time the doctor, nurse, or chemotherapy aide hands them their first bottles of pills. . . .

One old man apparently determined his own dosage, faithfully taking two INH tablets every morning (instead of three times daily), eight PAS tablets at noon (instead of three times daily), and one vitamin pill every night. Another patient was found giving his son one PAS tablet every day, just as a matter of principle. There is a prevalent idea that these medications cannot be taken at the same time as certain more potent native foods, such as seal oil, frozen raw fish, or fish heads which have been buried underground. Some patients stop eating the foods; some omit the medicine.

At times the nurse wonders about her patients. How do you really know they take the pills? . . . Of course, you don't really know, but when a patient appears in fish camp having come from 100 miles away, with few personal belongings and little food, but with his bottles of medicine, you can assume he takes them. When a patient, visiting in another village, brings nothing with him but a big bottle of PAS, a small bottle of INH tablets, and a bottle of vitamin pills, you are reassured. When a man who has been out hunting on the frozen tundra with a patient says, "He stops and takes the pills even if he has no water to drink with them," you think he's doing pretty well.[29]

During the course of the program, new case finding as well as evaluation went on through tuberculin testing of children and x-ray and sputum surveys of adults. Most villagers responded to these inconveniences in good spirit, and some village councils even tried to help schedule surveys when most people would be in the village. Sputum specimens were particularly problematic. They were collected and mailed in special rigid cardboard containers to the regional ADH laboratory in Anchorage or Fairbanks, often arriving two to three weeks later, having been carried by dog team, airplane, boat, or a combination of each. Repeated freezing and thawing did not seem to make much difference, but the report "Leaked in transit" was always worrisome.

Since the ambulatory chemotherapy demonstration program itself was not a controlled study, it was not possible to measure just how effective pre-hospital treatment was. Most clinicians, however, felt that pre-hospital treatment not only prevented progression of the disease but also actually improved the patients' clinical condition. Physicians at the ANHS hospitals almost immediately reported a sharp decrease in the number of children presenting with tuberculous meningitis and tuberculous bone and joint disease.[30]

A remarkable aspect of the Ambulatory Chemotherapy Program was the manner in which it was embraced by the Native people. For the most part, it had the full cooperation of both village leaders and patients. Every village invited to participate in the program accepted the offer. The best spokespersons for the home treatment program were those who had returned to the village after their disease was arrested or cured in the hospital after drug treatment. These brought home a sense of optimism about the disease that was a far cry from the hopelessness of the pre-chemotherapy era. The idea that taking the drugs at home would greatly diminish the need for bed rest as treatment was an idea they could warmly embrace. A sense of family and community responsibility led to the widespread acceptance of the obligation to take the pills as directed.[31]

ACP was also one of the first opportunities for village leaders to become genuinely involved in the health affairs of their village. In earlier times, such responsibilities were firmly held by the white community, particularly the BIA schoolteachers, who were used to exercising their health authority through controlling access to the village medical supplies and shortwave radio. A meaningful partnership between health officials and the village elders and leaders ultimately paid handsome dividends.[32]

An example of how one Native community organized itself to participate is the village of Aniak, on the Kuskokwim River. A newsletter put out by its health council described how they first heard of the new program by a chance interception of a message on the daily radio medical traffic. Dr. Ferger, one of the physicians at the Bethel Hospital, repeated the announcement daily for about a week that two drugs were now available to treat all known and suspected tuberculosis cases in the Kuskokwim villages. ANS teachers and laypeople were requested to send in names of such cases to augment lists that were being compiled from hospital records. It was explained that home drug treatment was not intended to replace hospitalization, but that it was considered to be the best treatment for those waiting for a hospital bed, and would lessen the chance of spread in the community. The Aniak Health Council seized on the idea and submitted the names of all known and suspected cases in the village. "Soon we received dosage sheets and a shipment of two different drugs. We agreed to be responsible for dispensing the medicines, for weighing the patients at certain intervals. We also supervised the mailing in of sputum specimens, watched the patients for adverse drug reactions and kept accurate, confidential records." Aniak chose Mrs. Wayne House as its chemotherapy aide, who "devotes many volunteer hours to this important work."

In January 1955 the full chemotherapy team visited, including a PHS physician, an AHRC nurse, and a staff nurse and x-ray technician from the Bethel Hospital. The team carried out an x-ray survey, set up files for each patient, made home calls, and added several more cases to the roster. The newsletter concluded:

We have been told by workers from the Chemotherapy Program that Aniak is far from a hot-bed of Tuberculosis, yet at this writing, 23 of our people are on chemotherapy, 9 Aniak people are in TB hospitals and more are waiting for a bed to become available for them. . . .

[W]e who have worked with the TB picture, have seen great improvements in many cases. After being on drugs for a while, the people look better and they feel better. They are hopeful of shorter hospital stays and complete cures eventually. We believe the Chemotherapy Program is coping with our village's most dangerous health problem, that of the tubercular person.... We still have tubercular children of tubercular parents, but at least there is hope for their future.[33]

Summing up the positive effect of the Ambulatory Chemotherapy Program, Dr. Francis Phillips wrote that in 1950 about 85 percent of patients arriving at the Seward Sanatorium had far advanced disease. They were far from home and loved ones, lacking in physical stamina and with a sense of hopelessness and resignation. They faced a highly uncertain future, up to two years of frustrating inactivity, and the possibility of never returning home to their families. By 1957 only 15 percent of patients admitted were suffering from far advanced tuberculosis. Their morale was good, they knew they had an excellent chance of returning home cured, or at least arrested, perhaps after only a few months of treatment. The return of such individuals to the village to resume their lives encouraged others to accept hospital treatment.[34] Ambulatory chemotherapy had turned the tide of tuberculosis in rural Alaska.

INH Prophylaxis Studies

By 1957 the Ambulatory Chemotherapy Program was acknowledged to be a resounding success and shifted the emphasis in tuberculosis control from pre-hospital treatment to post-hospital follow-up. Only in the Bethel area was the tuberculosis problem still of such a magnitude that additional control measures were necessary. AHRC turned over its tuberculosis responsibilities to ADH in the rest of the territory, and now focused its attention on the Yukon-Kuskokwim Delta, where it proposed a research study using INH to prevent tuberculosis. This was not a new idea, since the PHS Tuberculosis Program had already carried out cooperative studies on the preventive value of INH in other parts of the country. The proposed trial in Alaska, to be known as the Bethel Prophylaxis Study, was designed to test the value of prophylactic INH among entire communities with a serious tuberculosis problem.[35]

As before, the study was a cooperative venture. The PHS Tuberculosis Program was responsible for the overall design and data analysis of the study, under the leadership of Dr. George W. Comstock, a world authority on the epidemiology of tuberculosis. AHRC continued the day-to-day program management in the field, using four chemo nurses who had participated in ACP. The Division of Indian Health provided some of the funding, as well as the medical support, through its hospital at Bethel, and the fourth player, as before, was ADH, which was responsible for case finding. The study got under way in December 1957. Most villages joined the program in the spring of 1958, with the last few being added in the fall of 1959.

The design was a controlled double-blind trial in which neither the patients nor the investigators knew who had received the medication and who the placebo. The study was organized around the household unit, all members of which were to receive the same medication for a twelve-month period. Households were divided randomly, with half receiving INH once daily, and the other half an inert pill that looked the same. Each household received a four-month supply of pills, equivalent to 300 milligrams per day of INH for each person over sixteen who was actually on the drug. Three groups of individuals were excluded from the study—those already on chemotherapy for tuberculosis, those with a history of seizures, and infants less than two months of age. When the public health nurses made their visits every three or four months, they asked a representative of each household how well each member was taking the pills. At the end of the study year, the nurses retrieved all unused medication and thus estimated the compliance of the household by counting the remaining pills. The clinical status of the individuals was monitored by tuberculin testing, x-ray surveys, and reports from the tuberculosis registry in Juneau.

Some 7,333 people in twenty-eight villages were included in the initial study population, 95 percent of whom were Yup'ik Eskimos. Nearly 45 percent had evidence of past tuberculosis. About 60 percent of the total population started on pills and completed the program, another 25 percent took pills for less than the prescribed time, and most of the remainder were excluded by the terms of the research plan itself. Only 197 people (less than 3 percent) of those eligible refused to participate. Of the 1,023 who stopped the medication prematurely, about half believed a rumor that the pills were being distributed by a foreign agent to ruin the stomachs of the villages and soften them up for an invasion—evidence that a Cold War mentality permeated even rural Alaska.[36]

A more realistic concern was the toxicity of INH, especially when taken by large groups of people over a long period. At the time of the study, INH was felt to be relatively nontoxic, and, indeed, side effects were relatively benign and uncommon. Only with continued use on a wide scale were the toxic effects evident on the liver, especially in higher doses, in older persons, and in those who had some prior liver damage. Very few toxic reactions were seen in the Alaska Native population, despite the fact that some individuals undoubtedly had liver damage from excessive alcohol use or viral hepatitis. A better-known side effect was peripheral neuritis, manifested by numbness of the extremities and caused by INH interfering with the biological functions of pyridoxine, or vitamin B6. In the study, a dose of the vitamin was usually given along with the INH.

A major hazard associated with any wide use of a medication is the occasional massive overdose, either accidental or as a suicide attempt. In 1972 Dr. Carolyn V. Brown reported on some forty-two cases of INH overdose in Alaska from 1956 to 1971. Most were teenagers or young adults, with the youngest two years old and the oldest forty-seven. In most cases the amount ingested was not known. Nine of the forty-two died, some in the village or en route to the hospital, and three were left with brain damage. The paper concluded with a treatment plan for INH overdose, although by that time INH was no longer used on such a massive scale in Alaska.[37]

When the results of the Bethel Prophylaxis Study were finally analyzed, forty-one new cases of tuberculosis occurred in the placebo group (1.4 percent) during the medication year, compared with only thirteen (0.4 percent) among those on INH. The reduction in active disease as a result of the drug was thus calculated at 68 percent. By November 1, 1961, an additional thirty-seven new cases were reported in the placebo group, compared with twenty-five in the INH group, suggesting that the medication offered some long-term protection against the disease.

Comstock noted with pride that the efforts of only seven people over two years—four nurses and a clerk in the field and a nurse and secretary in the central office—had prevented eighty-five cases of tuberculosis, all of which would probably have required extended hospitalization.[38] The medication also prevented much emotional and financial hardship on the part of those individuals and their families, while also saving government welfare and travel costs. The field nurses themselves, of course, contributed additional public health services to the twenty-eight villages they regularly visited. Over the next two decades Comstock and his associates continued to follow up on the experience of this original group. After six years he calculated that if all those eligible had been on INH, there would have been a 55 percent reduction in tuberculosis, or prevention of 174 cases, in the region.[39]

These impressive results led to the idea that the preventive effects of INH should be offered to those who had taken placebo in the earlier study. In the fall of 1963, therefore, the same agencies initiated a community-wide INH prophylaxis study in the Bethel area, involving twenty-six villages with an estimated population of 8,583 persons.[40] The drug administration program was phased in between October 1963 and May 1964. The nurses again consulted with local village councils, every one of which agreed to participate and to select a recorder to distribute and keep track of the medications dispensed. This individual also made notes on drug side effects in each family, and had available a small medical kit containing syrup of ipecac and a barbiturate for emergency treatment of INH overdose. Unlike the chemo aides, the recorders were paid a small amount for their work. The program was launched with a village meeting at which the nurse and the recorder explained the demonstration project in both English and Yup'ik. The nurse then showed a movie on tuberculosis and colored slides from the original project in 1958–60, followed by an audio tape in which Dr. Comstock explained that everyone who had taken a placebo in the previous study now had access to the actual drug. Sometimes children were encouraged to make tuberculosis posters to put up around the village.

Each family received enough medication in a plastic bottle for each member for one month. The nurse also provided each household with a calendar on which the head of the household could record whether or not the medication had been taken. Those known to have taken INH in the previous trial took it again during the community prophylaxis program. The nurses visited the villages every four months or so to review records, provide consultation, and encourage those on the medication. At the conclusion of the medication year, all unused pills were returned and counted, and the nurses reviewed in detail the monthly calendars and other evidence of participation. It was estimated that just under 80 percent of the eligible residents of the villages took some medication, with over half of the nonparticipants being residents of Bethel. Only 0.9 percent of the population flatly refused to participate. No serious side effects were encountered at the dosage used, and no cases of accidental poisoning of children were reported.

A comparison of the two studies showed that fewer individuals took the medication in the later program. In addition to the poor cooperation in Bethel itself, another reason was that some villagers clearly did not perceive tuberculosis as the threat it was in the 1950s. Other possible factors were a growing resistance to regimentation, and negative attitudes toward the shipment of huge quantities of medication to the villages with its distribution left to a nonprofessional person.[41]

After six years Comstock and his associates reviewed the effects of INH on the subsequent development of active tuberculosis in 1,349 individuals with untreated, nonactive tuberculosis at the onset of the controlled study. They found that those who took INH as directed had 71 percent less active tuberculosis than those who took it irregularly. Six years later they found that among 1,567 individuals with untreated, nonactive tuberculosis, those who took INH well had 89 percent less active tuberculosis than those who took it irregularly.[42] Some individuals participating conscientiously in both studies could have taken as much as twenty-four months of INH, while others, taking placebo in the first study and little or none of the prescribed medication in the second, may have taken the drug for as little as one month or so. It was found that the preventive effect seems to have peaked when approximately 70 percent of an annual dose had been taken. Taking up to 200 percent of the annual dose seemed to have had little or no additional benefit.[43]

In the next follow-up study, published in 1974, Comstock and his associates searched the state tuberculosis case registry to see what had happened to the people who had participated in the INH studies, again correlating their findings with the amount of drug estimated to have been taken by each person. They concluded that the approximately 70 percent reduction in the risk of active tuberculosis among those taking INH persisted almost without change for about fifteen years.[44] The authors originally suggested that as little as six months of INH prophylaxis offered significant protection, but on the basis of later analysis Comstock concluded that INH treatment for nine or ten months was optimal.[45] The final follow-up, nineteen years after the program began, indicated that the strength of the protective effect of INH was related to the amount taken, and that the effect was probably lifelong.[46]

Parallel to the original Bethel Prophylaxis Study, a supplementary investigation was carried out from 1958 to 1963 among a group of Native boarding school students at Mt. Edgecumbe, Wrangell, and the Sheldon Jackson High School in Sitka to determine the optimal dosage of INH. Students were invited to partici-pate on much the same basis as in the Bethel area studies, and only three among a total of 1,701 refused to participate. The study group was divided into two, with approximately half receiving five milligrams per kilogram of INH per day (the same dose as used in the Bethel area), and the other half receiving 1.25 milligrams per kilogram. Each student took medication for about six months, and about 90 percent of both groups completed their course of treatment. During the ensuing ten years, twenty, or 1.9 percent, of the students on the full dose and forty-six, or 5.7 percent, of those on the lower dose developed active tuberculosis. The smaller dose was calculated to be no more effective than a placebo.[47]

The two INH prophylaxis studies carried out in the Bethel area villages were land-marks in tuberculosis research. Several factors about the situation made the region and its people a natural laboratory. The communities were very isolated, and cultur-ally uniform. Histoplasmosis and sarcoidosis were rarely a complicating factor in the interpretation of x-rays, and there was no evidence of a non-tuberculosis *Mycobacte-rium* in the region, which could confuse the interpretation of the tuberculin test. The tuberculosis problem was severe and the people, as individuals and as communities, were highly motivated to change the situation, which had caused them such hardship and grief. The local village councils were uniformly supportive and local people were involved from the beginning in the planning and execution of the project.

The results of these studies, carried out with sensitivity and care by Dr. Com-stock and his colleagues,[48] and by a devoted cadre of field nurses, not only greatly accelerated the decline of the tuberculosis epidemic in the region but also made available new information on the usefulness of INH prophylaxis that could be applied effectively in many parts of the world. A particularly noteworthy and unusual feature of the Bethel Prophylaxis Study—rare in such studies—was that, once the results were known, all those who had taken the placebo were given the opportunity to take INH and obtain the benefits that it conferred.

The Scarred Corneas of Alaska

One of the lesser-known consequences of the tuberculosis epidemic was an eye condition known as phlyctenular keratoconjunctivitis (PKC), a problem that was not clearly defined in Alaska until the INH prophylaxis studies of the 1950s and 1960s. This disease involved a hypersensitivity response to the tubercle bacillus, causing a painful eye inflammation, which, if untreated, often led to corneal scars and visual loss. When it occurs today, PKC is thought to be caused by an altered immune reaction to certain bacterial breakdown products, generally staphylococ-cus microorganisms, the type that most commonly causes boils, impetigo, styes, and other skin infections.

PKC normally presents as a small, slightly raised, pinkish white or yellow nodule, called a phlyctenule, on the conjunctiva in the midst of enlarged blood vessels at the edge of the cornea. After a few days the nodule usually becomes gray and soft, then ulcerates, sloughs, and clears, leaving no scar. When phlyctenules occur repeatedly on the cornea, however, they heal with an opaque scar, a condition more common in children than in adults. In the active phase, the victim has intense pain, the sensation of a foreign body in the eye, intolerance to light, excessive tearing, redness, and spasm of the lids.[49]

Many of the earliest reports of health conditions among the Alaska Native made mention of red inflamed eyes, which were variously attributed to snow blindness and to the smoke-filled homes in which they lived. Indeed, these conditions may have played an important part, but it is also likely that PKC may have been a cause. Dr. Robert White, physician on the cruise of the USRC *Rush* in 1879, offered sun and smoke as explanations for the inflammatory diseases of the eyes he saw among the Indians of Southeast Alaska. In 1881 another physician observed corneal opacities among the northern Eskimos, as did a third who was stationed at St. Michael's around 1899.[50] A nonmedical visitor to Southeast Alaska observed prophetically that "an Indian in Alaska whose eyes are not diseased is an exception, while the ravages of consumption are very frequently visible to the most careless observer."[51] Dr. Krulish found many eye diseases among the Eskimos, including "trachoma, keratitis, cataracts, blepharitis, conjunctivitis, [and] corneal opacities," each of which, except for cataracts, could be due to or mistaken for PKC.[52]

In June 1946, during the first major survey for crippling conditions in Alaska, the medical team found itself stranded in Unalakleet because of weather. To pass the time the staff held an impromptu survey for corneal scarring among the children and quickly found some thirty children with corneal scars. These were said to originate with a corneal ulcer "which runs a course and terminates in a scar that leads to total or partial blindness." Such scars were already well known to the doctors and nurses working in the area.[53]

From April through June 1947 an interagency nutrition survey team conducting a survey in western Alaska considered whether the conjunctivitis and corneal ulceration found among the Eskimos was nutritional in origin. The team included an ophthalmologist, Dr. Milo H. Fritz, who joined the group in June and continued with a general eye survey in the field, funded by the PHS and the US Children's Bureau.[54] Fritz later reported that he examined some 400 patients, 127 (32 percent) of whom showed corneal opacities. Later, after examining about 140 patients hospitalized for tuberculosis at Seward and Bethel, he concluded that PKC "is caused by sensitivity to protein, especially that of the staphylococcus and perhaps to that of the tubercle bacillus." He added, however, "there can be little doubt that…pulmonary tuberculosis [and several other conditions] have very little to do with corneal opacities." Instead, he asserted, the problem could be largely prevented by more attention to personal hygiene and better housing.[55]

In a study at Mt. Edgecumbe in the summer of 1949, Fritz, Thygeson, and Durham demonstrated PKC scars in 35 percent of Native children in summer school, in 45 percent of children at the Orthopedic Hospital, and in 25 percent of the sanatorium patients.[56] Using these data and work in the summer of 1950 at Mt. Edgecumbe and Sheldon Jackson College, and with the general population of Angoon and Hydaburg, Fritz and Thygeson concluded that mild attacks tended to clear spontaneously within ten to fifteen days, whereas more severe attacks might last two to three weeks or even several months. When the inflammation diminished, corneal scars remained, most often at the periphery of the cornea but also commonly over the pupil, leaving some children with 20/200 vision or less. The percentage of individuals showing scars ranged from 10.6 percent in the general population of Hydaburg to 45.4 percent in patients, mostly Eskimo, at the Orthopedic Hospital.

The authors could not establish the cause of the disease with certainty, although the evidence strongly pointed to tuberculosis, not staphylococcus, in this population at least. All cases with active PKC had a positive tuberculin reaction and x-ray evidence of tuberculosis. Further, the Eskimo students from northwestern Alaska, where the incidence of tuberculosis was high, had a greater prevalence of scarring than the Indian students from Southeast Alaska, where the tuberculosis rate was relatively low. The most destructive lesions seemed to be in Natives with bone and joint tuberculosis, but badly scarred corneas were found even in children and adults with no evidence of systemic tuberculosis. Experimental treatment with topical cortisone drops gave dramatic results in the active forms of the disease.[57]

From 1958 to 1960, the Arctic Health Research Center studied the epidemiology of PKC as part of its ongoing study of INH prophylaxis of tuberculosis in twenty-four villages of the Yukon-Kuskokwim Delta. Of 4,635 people examined, 40 percent were found to have corneal opacities of varying severity. Of the 1,197 children who were tuberculin tested, 93 percent of those with opacities were tuberculin-positive, compared to only 34 percent of those without scarring. The opacities were found to correlate with tuberculosis infection but not with tuberculous disease, although tuberculin-positive children were still more likely to develop PKC than tuberculin-negative children. The authors concluded that tuberculosis was the major, if not the only, cause of PKC scarring in southwestern Alaska.[58]

PKC has virtually disappeared from the pediatric population of Alaska, but when it does occur it promptly leads the physician to look carefully for evidence of tuberculosis. Many elderly Alaskans still bear the scars of the disease, however— the remnants and reminders of an earlier age. In 1973 an octogenarian Eskimo who had been virtually blind for more than seventy years presented himself at an IHS eye clinic in Nome. The ophthalmologist noted that the old man had severe astigmatism, or irregularity of the spherical shape of the cornea, due to old PKC scars. When he put the appropriate corrective lenses before the patient's eyes, the old man began to bounce violently in the chair, shouting in Siberian Yup'ik. His companion translated: "He says, 'It's wonderful. Don't take it away. Don't take it away!'" When the refraction was completed, the old man was seeing 20/30 and the doctor concocted a temporary pair of glasses for him made out of trial frames.[59]

In the mid-1970s ophthalmologists at the Alaska Native Medical Center began repairing some severe cases of PKC scarring by a procedure known as penetrating keratoplasty. In this operation a section of a full-thickness donor cornea is transplanted to replace the corresponding section of scarred cornea. The results were often quite dramatic, at least initially, in restoring vision in some patients who had been blind since childhood.[60]

Special Role of the Public Health Nurse

The devoted public health nurses working for AHRC and ADH were key to the success of the Ambulatory Chemotherapy Program and both INH prophylaxis studies, but their crucial role in the larger campaign against tuberculosis extended all the way back to the teachers of sanitation employed by the Bureau of Education in the early twentieth century. Some of these women labored for years in the field, flying to and from remote villages in marginal weather, with only brief periods of relief in the larger communities. These were the ones who "sold" the programs to the village councils, and motivated and encouraged the villagers to participate. Besides their tuberculosis duties, they also performed a range of traditional public health nursing skills, such as teaching, giving immunizations, providing prenatal and infant care, treating acute illnesses and injuries, delivering babies, and comforting the dying. They worked at schools, churches, stores, and fish camp tents, as well as in the homes. Their hours were long—often from early morning to well after midnight, or until the last patient was seen or the last record was completed. They slept in the clinic room at the school, in a cramped guest room in the teacher's home, or not infrequently in a sleeping bag on the schoolroom floor.

Some of the AHRC nurses' narrative trip reports chronicle the adventures, hardships, frustrations, and satisfactions they experienced during these critical years in the battle against tuberculosis. The nurse had to prepare for her trip some weeks or even months in advance. She wrote ahead to the BIA teachers, missionaries, and village council presidents of each village she planned to visit, explaining her plans and negotiating a suitable date, balancing her activities with those of the teachers and villagers. Often, because of slow or unreliable mail service, she followed up or confirmed her plans with a radio "sched" from the Bethel hospital. The next task was assembling the records, checking the status of PPDs, sputum tests, x-rays, and admission and discharge records for each village. She then consulted with the doctors at the Bethel hospital to learn of any patients needing follow-up, whether for tuberculosis or other conditions.

She packed her large aluminum trunks with INH, general antibiotics and other drugs, medical supplies, instruments, and records. Her baggage also included motion pictures, filmstrips, posters, pamphlets, and other health education paraphernalia for use in the village. A personal "survival kit" consisted of high-calorie, low-volume foods such as chocolate bars, nuts, and raisins, not to mention a "peace offering" for the local teachers in the form of fresh fruit, bakery bread, or other delicacies not available in the village. Clothing had to be appropriate for a trip by dogsled, a dunking in the river, or even a forced aircraft landing on the windswept tundra. The final essential item was a warm sleeping bag.

Travel to the village was usually by a Cessna 180 or other small single-engine plane on floats in summer and skis in winter. Each nurse had her favorite pilots, knowing who was reliable, who had not been drinking, who carried emergency supplies or equipment, or who especially cared about the villagers. Usually the aircraft took off from the river at about 7:30 a.m., or at first light in the winter. Because of unexpected weather conditions, the aircraft sometimes had to return without landing, or perhaps go on to an unscheduled village. On departure day the weather might be "down," with uncertain prospects for returning home. Ice fog was a particular nuisance, since it could last for days, requiring the nurse to be packed and ready to fly on perhaps fifteen minutes' notice. If the return plane was already loaded, perhaps with a sick patient en route to the hospital, the nurse might have to leave her equipment behind. The ice or mud conditions of freeze-up or break-up could preclude landing for weeks on end.

While in the village, other means of transportation were sometimes necessary. A skiff with a "kicker" might take her across the river to a fish camp or to the next settlement on the slough. In the winter she might travel by dog team or, after the mid-1960s, by snowmobile, or make an edgy trip up or down the frozen Kuskokwim or Yukon by truck or snowplane.[61]

One chemotherapy nurse reported the program activities of a typical week in early 1955 as follows:

1st day: Began home visits to chemotherapy patients; rounded up someone to interpret at meetings. In the evening, presented the aims and purpose of the chemotherapy program at a general meeting of the villagers at the school, using blackboard, posters, slides, and movies. Excellent attendance.

2nd day (Sunday): Oriented individual selected as interpreter and tried to persuade her to serve as Chemotherapy Aide, subject to the decision of the village council. Tuberculin tested 35 children.

3rd day: Visited chemotherapy patients in their homes. Spent the evening orienting the Chemotherapy Aide in the responsibilities of the job. The school teachers were present and offered their assistance, if she felt she needed help.

4th day: In the morning, continued home visits and worked on records. In the afternoon, read tuberculin tests and provided general medical care to sick children and their mothers who came in. In the evening, had a formal meeting with the village council, seeking formal approval of the program.

5th day: Left for neighboring village, then returned a week later for the x-ray survey of the village.[62]

Public health nurses were the foot soldiers of the campaign against tuberculosis, without whom the job could not have been done.

Twilight of the Sanatorium Era

The heady success of the Ambulatory Chemotherapy Program demonstrated within a few years that tuberculosis hospitals, a mainstay of treatment for almost three-quarters of a century, were becoming obsolete. Patients treated in the earlier stages of the disease, at least, were found to be cured as rapidly on home treatment as they were in the sanatorium. Moreover, case finding reached such a level of efficiency that more and more of the cases identified were at a stage when they could be quickly cured. One measure of this trend was the fact that the percentage of far advanced disease among newly reported cases declined by 56 percent between 1952 and 1956. Likewise, between 1952 and 1958 the number of new cases reported annually declined by nearly two-thirds.[63] The length of hospital stay was also declining because of earlier diagnosis at a stage more amenable to effective treatment. Years of searching for cases by x-ray surveys and tuberculin-testing campaigns, not to mention educating physicians and the general public, were finally paying off. Many patients were being started on drug therapy while waiting for a hospital bed, thus getting a head start on treatment. The waiting period for a hospital bed decreased from almost two years in 1953 to about six months a mere two years later, largely because of the opening of the new Anchorage hospital and the availability of beds in Washington State. By mid-1957 home treatment, increased x-ray surveys, and sufficient beds at last allowed a reduction in the need for tuberculosis beds in treatment facilities.[64] The number of hospital beds had reached a maximum of 1,350 at the end of 1955, at which time almost 98 percent were filled, but thereafter the numbers began fall rapidly. By the end of 1959 the total number was 373, all of them in Alaska.[65]

Certainly one important factor was the use of effective drugs. Although streptomycin, PAS, and INH had done much to bring the epidemic under control, they were not always easy to administer, nor were they always acceptable to the patient. Streptomycin remained in injectable form only and was associated with allergies and severe and sometimes permanent side effects, especially deafness or balance disorders due to nerve damage to the inner ear. PAS had to be taken frequently and in large doses, often twenty-four pills a day. The need for new, safer, and more acceptable medications was great, but the first new breakthrough in drug therapy came only in 1968, when ethambutol was introduced on the market. This drug was no more effective than PAS, but it had the distinct advantage of smaller dosages and less-toxic effects. The other major new drug, rifampin, was discovered as early as 1957 but not brought to market for the treatment of tuberculosis until 1972. Shortly thereafter, the combination of rifampin and INH became the standard treatment for the disease. Whereas the classic treatment regimen of streptomycin, PAS, and INH was usually given for eighteen to twenty-four months, with all the problems such a long course entailed, newer studies demonstrated equally good treatment results from a combination of rifampin and INH given for only six to nine months. Several other drugs, including pyrazinamide, were introduced at about this time, but they never caught on as first-line drugs in Alaska, and were used instead for those patients who developed resistance to the older drugs.

Surgery, until the 1950s a critical component of tuberculosis treatment, went into a steep decline once the value of chemotherapy was firmly established. Dr. Robert Moles, the first thoracic surgeon at the Anchorage hospital, arrived in July 1954, but carried out no pulmonary surgery until mid-November, when he performed an apical resection and an upper lobectomy, both for tuberculosis. In January 1955 he carried out his first thoracoplasty, in which he removed the second, third, fourth, and fifth ribs of a patient. By 1957–58 the most common operations for tuberculosis were wedge and segmental resections, in which a relatively small piece of diseased lung was removed. A few lobectomies continued to be performed, but thoracoplasties had been totally discontinued. Occasionally other tuberculosis procedures, such as phrenic nerve crush and the breaking up of pleural adhesions, were carried out.[66]

In the spring of 1956 the number of Alaskans hospitalized for tuberculosis peaked at 1,398. After April 1957 all Native tuberculosis patients were admitted to the Anchorage hospital, leading to the gradual shutdown of the tuberculosis service at Mt. Edgecumbe and the Seward Sanatorium.

By late 1958, the number of Alaskan patients in tuberculosis hospitals was down to 472, including 441 beneficiaries of the ANHS, 22 sponsored by ADH, and 9 by the VA. At the same time, some 1,500 patients were receiving drug treatment at home. Of those funded by the territory, twelve were housed at the new Wesleyan Hospital now at the site of the Seward Sanatorium, which had closed in July of that year.[67] By the end of the year the ADH waiting list for admission had fallen to zero, and by the end of the following year all Native tuberculosis patients were either at Anchorage or Mt. Edgecumbe. The very success of these figures led the ATA to express its concern that funding levels for tuberculosis control would be cut because the disease was receding as a threat to the public.[68]

In the closing years of the tuberculosis epidemic, the Anchorage hospital was led by Dr. Martha R. Wilson, a medical tuberculosis specialist who had previously worked at Mt. Edgecumbe and at the Tacoma Indian Sanatorium. She became the service unit director in 1963 and guided the hospital through eight years, as it gradually transformed from a tuberculosis sanatorium to a general medical and surgical referral hospital for Alaska Natives. In 1965 these changes were reflected in the new name—the Alaska Native Medical Center, which it and its successor hospital have maintained to this day.[69]

By 1963 the Anchorage Hospital still had 161 beds for tuberculosis, including 30 on the pediatric wards, but only 4 percent of the total admissions that year were for tuberculosis. Another dramatic indicator of the decline in tuberculosis was the number of children admitted with primary tuberculosis or its complications. In 1964 the pediatric tuberculosis census averaged about fifty, often including cases of tuberculous meningitis and miliary tuberculosis. In May 1968, only four years later, not a single child with tuberculosis was left in the hospital. The adult tuberculosis unit continued to shrink until February 1973, when the final thirty-one-bed ward was converted to a psychiatric day hospital. Thereafter all those found with active tuberculosis were briefly evaluated on a general medical ward or were begun on treatment on an outpatient basis.[70]

After the last ward was closed, Lillie H. McGarvey, the chair of the Anchorage Service Unit Native Board of Health, hosted a celebration on September 15, 1973, at the Anchorage Westward Hotel to observe the end of the sanatorium era in Alaska. Among the speakers were Drs. Albrecht, Chao, and Comstock. Many Natives attended the event and several spoke movingly of their personal encounters with tuberculosis. The sanatorium era was over in Alaska.

Notes

1. Memorandum from Hugh J. Wade to Arthur J. Altmeyer, November 21, 1947, Governor Correspondence, roll 273.

2. The 22nd session of the territorial legislature in March 1955 formally asked the secretary of Health, Education, and Welfare and the surgeon general to enter into contracts with the territory for the operation, maintenance, and staffing of all hospitals for "Indians" within Alaska. The territory had expressed an interest in this idea in the previous legislature, perhaps spurred by Dr. Albrecht, who had always supported the idea of a unified health program for the Natives. The idea persisted as late as 1957, when territorial officials prepared a detailed plan for the transfer, but nothing further came of the effort. See House Joint Memorial No. 21, *Laws of Alaska 1955* (Juneau: 1955), 493–94; "Bills of Interest to the Health Department by the 22nd Session of the Legislature," ADH, March 28, 1955, Governor Correspondence, roll 350; "Consolidation of All Alaska Native Health Services under the Alaska Department of Health" (Juneau: ADH, 1957).

3. Ruth M. Raup, "The Indian Health Program from 1800 to 1955," DHEW, PHS, March 11, 1959, 22–26.

4. "Not with Answers," editorial, *ADT*, July 22, 1953.

5. "Doctor Blasts Existing Health Program for Alaskan Natives after Survey of Remote Areas," *ADT*, n.d., scrapbook #2, ATA Collection. Dr. Fritz took many opportunities to needle federal and state health officials throughout his long subsequent career in Alaska.

6. Thomas Parran, ed., *Alaska's Health: A Survey Report to the United States Department of the Interior* (Pittsburgh: Graduate School of Public Health, University of Pittsburgh, 1954), i–iv.

7. Parran, *Alaska's Health,* I-2.

8. The Railbelt is that more heavily populated area of south-central Alaska served by the Alaska Railroad, which runs from Seward to Fairbanks.

9. Parran, *Alaska's Health,* III-11 to III-14, III-17.

10. Parran, *Alaska's Health,* VI-34 to VI-48.

11. Letter of Thomas Parran to Douglas McKay, Secretary of the Interior, November 23, 1953.

12. C. Earl Albrecht, "The Alaska Health Plan," *AH* 6, no. 7–8 (July–August 1948); A. B. Colyar, "Arctic Health Research Center, An Introduction," *Alaska Medicine* 1, no. 1 (March 1959), 31–33.

13. Parran, *Alaska's Health,* V-vi.

14. Parran, *Alaska's Health,* VI-34.

15. F. J. Phillips, "A Preliminary Report of Out-Patient Treatment of Pulmonary Tuberculosis," *Alaska Medicine* 3 (March 1961): 1–4; ATA, *Annual Report* (1953–54), 8.

16. The Parran Committee in 1953 took note of the limited outpatient use of antimicrobial drugs by the Alaska Native Service at Bethel. Dr. Beryl Michaelson, the ANS physician there, had begun prescribing outpatient chemotherapy for tuberculosis after reading about its use in a medical journal. According to her account, she provided medication, including streptomycin injections, to anyone with tuberculosis, no matter what the presenting problem was, in order to prevent cross-contamination in the crowded, makeshift Quonset-hut hospital where she worked. When some patients began to improve, they asked to continue their medication at home. She asked for help from the ANS area medical director and the territorial commissioner of health, both of whom refused to support her initiative, presumably because of the cost of the medication and because the care of the patients in the villages could not be adequately supervised. Michaelson claimed that Dr. Parran was so impressed with the results of her work that he went to the ANS medical director and asked why such treatment was not being done elsewhere. Soon afterward she was abruptly transferred to Mt. Edgecumbe, as she thought, for causing embarrassment to ANS. Whatever the full facts of the story, the idea of outpatient therapy was certainly not original with Dr. Michaelson. Her use of it, in fact, might even have been harmful in the long run, since patients seemed to be given drugs almost indiscriminately with little attention to long-term follow-up—a sure formula for the development of drug resistance. See Beryl Michaelson, "Indian Health Service Doc," in *In Her Own Words: Oral Histories of Women Physicians,* ed. Regina Merkel Morantz, Cynthia Stodola Pomereau, and Carol Hansen Fenichel (Westport, CT: Greenwood Press, 1982), 141–44.

17. Merilys E. Porter and George W. Comstock, "Ambulatory Chemotherapy in Alaska," *Public Health Reports* 77, no. 12 (November 1962): 1021–32.

18. Phillips, "Preliminary Report of Out-Patient Treatment."

19. Porter and Comstock. "Ambulatory Chemotherapy in Alaska."

20. "Akiachuk General Information, July 1957," typescript, AHRC Papers, Robert Fortuine Collection, University of Alaska Anchorage Archives.

21. Charles R. Hayman, "Tuberculosis Problem Is Studied from Territorial Standpoint," *AH* 12 (August 1955).

22. Porter and Comstock, "Ambulatory Chemotherapy in Alaska."

23. Louise Lear, "Chemotherapy in Alaska," *American Journal of Nursing* 57 (March 1957): 320–22.

24. Lear, "Chemotherapy in Alaska."

25. Lear, "Chemotherapy in Alaska."

26. See Philip Nice and Walter Johnson, *The Alaska Health Aide Program: A Tradition of Helping Ourselves* (privately published by Philip Nice, 1998).

27. Lear, "Chemotherapy in Alaska."

28. Some aides had their own way of doing things. One insisted on weighing all patients in alphabetical order, because the cards were arranged that way. Thus a patient named Wassillie might have to wait until the end of the day no matter when he presented himself to the clinic. See Lear, "Chemotherapy in Alaska."

29. Lear, "Chemotherapy in Alaska."

30. ATA, *Annual Report* (April 1, 1955 to March 31, 1956).

31. Porter and Comstock, "Ambulatory Chemotherapy in Alaska."

32. Porter and Comstock, "Ambulatory Chemotherapy in Alaska."

33. "First Annual Report of the Aniak Health Council, May 1954–55," Alaska, Territorial Government, Governor, General Correspondence, 1909–1958, RG 80-14, roll 349.

34. Phillips, "Preliminary Report of Out-Patient Treatment."

35. George W. Comstock, "Isoniazid Prophylaxis in an Undeveloped Area," *American Review of Respiratory Disease* 86, no. 6 (December 1962): 810–22.

36. Comstock, "Isoniazid Prophylaxis."

37. C. V. Brown, "Acute Isoniazid Poisoning," *American Review of Respiratory Disease* 105 (1972): 206–16.

38. Comstock, "Isoniazid Prophylaxis."

39. George W. Comstock, Shirley H. Ferebee, and Laurel M. Hammes, "A Controlled Trial of Community-wide Isoniazid Prophylaxis in Alaska," *American Review of Respiratory Disease* 95, no. 6 (June 1967): 935–43.

40. This time Bethel was included, even though a substantial number of non-Native individuals lived there. The author was one of many non-Natives who took INH prophylaxis for a year in Bethel in 1964–65.

41. Mary L. Hanson, G. W. Comstock, and C. E. Haley, "Community Isoniazid Prophylaxis Program in an Underdeveloped Area of Alaska," *Public Health Reports* 82, no. 12 (December 1967): 1045–56.

42. George W. Comstock and Shirley Ferebee Woolpert, "Preventive Treatment of Untreated, Nonactive Tuberculosis in an Eskimo Population," *Archives of Environmental Health* 25, no. 5 (November 1972): 333–37.

43. George W. Comstock and Shirley H. Ferebee, "How Much Isoniazid Is Needed for Prophylaxis?" *American Review of Respiratory Disease* 101 (1970): 780–82.

44. George W. Comstock, Shirley Ferebee Woolpert, and Carol Baum, "Isoniazid Prophylaxis among Alaskan Eskimos: A Progress Report," *American Review of Respiratory Disease* 110, no. 2 (August 1974): 195–97.

45. George W. Comstock, "How Much Isoniazid Is Needed for Prevention of Tuberculosis among Immunocompetent Adults?" *International Journal of Tuberculosis and Lung Diseases* 3, no. 10 (October 1999): 847–50.

46. G. W. Comstock, C. Baum, and Dixie E. Snider, Jr., "Isoniazid Prophylaxis among Alaskan Eskimos: A Final Report on the Bethel Isoniazid Studies," *American Review of Respiratory Disease* 119, no. 5 (May 1979): 827–29.

47. George W. Comstock, Laurel M. Hammes, and Antonio Pio, "Isoniazid Prophylaxis in Alaskan Boarding Schools. A Comparison of Two Doses," *American Review of Respiratory Disease* 100, no. 6 (1969): 773–79.

48. Among the key players who assisted in the fieldwork in Alaska were public health nurses Merilys E. Porter in the Ambulatory Chemotherapy Program and Mary Lou Hansen, Theresa Overfield, and C. E. Haley in the prophylaxis studies. Laurel M. Hammes was the AHRC biostatistician. In the PHS Tuberculosis Program, Drs. Shirley H. Ferebee Woolpert and Dixie E. Snider assisted with the analysis of the data.

49. Myron Yanoff and Jay S. Duker, eds., *Ophthalmology* (St. Louis, MO: Mosby International Ltd., 1999): 5.1.9; Mark H. Beers and Robert Berkow, *The Merck Manual of Diagnosis and Therapy*, 17th ed. (Rahway, NJ: Merck & Co., 1999), sect. 8, chap. 96.

50. Robert White, "Notes on the Physical Condition of the Inhabitants of Alaska," in George W. Bailey, Treasury Department, US Revenue-Cutter Service, *Report upon Alaska and its People*, (Washington, DC: GPO, 1880), 141–49; Irving C. Rosse, "Medical and Anthropological Notes of Alaska," in Treasury Department, US Revenue-Cutter Service, Treasury Document No. 429, *Cruise of the Revenue Steamer* Corwin *in Alaska and the N. W. Arctic Ocean in 1881 . . . Notes and Memoranda* (Washington, DC: GPO, 1883); H. M. W. Edmonds, "The Eskimos of St. Michael and Vicinity, as Related by H. M. W. Edmonds," ed. Dorothy Jean Ray, *Anthropological Papers of the University of Alaska* 13, no. 2 (1966): 30.

51. Ella Higginson, *Alaska: The Great Country* (New York: Macmillan Company, 1908), 383–84.

52. Emil Krulish, "Report on Health Conditions among the Natives of Alaska," in US Department of the Interior, BoE, "Report on the Work of the Bureau of Education for the Natives of Alaska, 1911–12," *Bureau of Education Bulletin*, no. 36, whole no. 546 (Washington, DC: GPO, 1913), 31.

53. N. Berneta Block, "Alaska's Crippled Children," *Alaska Life* 9, no. 12 (December 1946): 10–15.

54. C. Earl Albrecht, "Ophthalmologist Reports," *AH* 5, no. 12 (December 1947).

55. Milo H. Fritz, "Corneal Opacities among Alaska Natives," *AH* 5, no. 12 (December 1947).

56. Milo H. Fritz, Phillips Thygeson, and D. Durham, "Phlyctenular Keratoconjunctivitis among Alaskan Natives," *American Journal of Ophthalmology* 34 (1951): 177–84.

57. Milo H. Fritz and Phillips Thygeson, "Phlyctenular Keratoconjunctivitis among Alaskan Indians and Eskimos," *Public Health Reports* 66, no. 29 (July 20, 1951): 934–39. When I began practicing medicine in southwestern Alaska in 1963, active PKC was still common among the Eskimos. The prompt, dramatic cures with prednisolone drops were most gratifying to both patient and doctor.

58. Robert N. Philip, George W. Comstock, and Joseph H. Shelton, "Phlyctenular Keratoconjunctivitis among Eskimos in Southwestern Alaska. I. Epidemiologic Considerations," *American Review of Respiratory Diseases* 91, no. 2 (February 1965): 171–87. In the second phase of their study, the investigators found that corneal opacities were less frequent among persons who had received INH prophylaxis than among those who had received a placebo. PKC was almost entirely prevented during the actual period of taking INH, but subsequently the drug and placebo groups had an identical incidence of PKC. The authors concluded that "PKC and corneal scarring in this population were usually caused by local implantation of *M. tuberculosis* on or near the sensitized cornea." See Robert N. Philip and George W. Comstock, "Phlyctenular Keratoconjunctivitis among Eskimos in Southwestern Alaska. II. Isoniazid Prophylaxis," *American Review of Respiratory Diseases* 91, no. 2 (February 1965): 188–96.

59. Sandy Wolf, "Don't Take it Away," *Alaska Medicine* 27, no. 1 (January/February/March 1985): 12.

60. R. E. Smith, D. W. Dippé, and S. D. Miller, "Corneal Transplantation in Alaska Natives," *Alaska Medicine* 17, no. 4 (1975): 58–61; R. E. Smith, D. W. Dippé, and S. D. Miller, "Phlyctenular Keratoconjunctivitis: Results of Penetrating Keratoplasty in Alaskan Natives," *Ophthalmological Surgery* 6, no. 3 (1975): 62–66. Dr. Robert Werner, ophthalmologist at the Alaska Native Medical Center, informed me on August 23, 2004, that the long-term results of these surgeries were quite poor.

61. For several stirring accounts of the life of a public health nurse in Alaska, see Effie Graham, Jackie Pflaum, and Elfrida Nord, eds., *With a Dauntless Spirit: Alaska Nursing in Dog-Team Days. Six Personal Accounts* (Fairbanks: University of Alaska Press, 2003). Another good source for the role of the public health nurses in Alaska is Rie Muñoz, *Nursing in the North 1867–1967* (Alaska Nurses'

Association, n.d.). A few other published accounts of individual nurses in Alaska include: Dolores M. Zeis and Edna Foster, "Public Health Nursing in the 49th State by Dog Sled, Boat, and Plane," *American Journal of Nursing* 58, no. 10 (1958): 1376–79; Louise Lear, "Chemotherapy in Alaska," 320–22; Lois M. Jund, "Dog Sled Nurse," *Wellesley Alumnae Magazine* 40, no. 4 (1955): 22–24.

62. "Outline of Program in Akiachuk," typescript, February 19–22, 1955, AHRC Records.

63. ADH, *Alaska TB Report, 1952–57*, April 1958.

64. Charles R. Hayman, "Tuberculosis Problem Is Studied from Territorial Standpoint," *AH* 12 (August 1955); *Alaska TB Report, 1952–57*.

65. An interesting sidelight of the hospitalization program in Alaska was the low rate of discharge against medical advice ("A.M.A."), which in some states reached the level of 50 percent. Overall the rate for Alaskan patients was around 2 percent, ranging from veterans, where the rate was 25 percent, to 0 percent among ADH beneficiaries. ADH, Division of Tuberculosis Control, *Alaska Tuberculosis Report. 1958* (Anchorage: 1959).

66. Surgical logs of the Alaska Native Medical Center, 1954–958.

67. "22 Persons Hospitalized for TB in Territory," *JAE*, October 23, 1958.

68. "Alaska TB Figures Given," *Homer Herald*, November 6, 1958.

69. Dr. Wilson and her husband, Joseph F. Wilson, a thoracic surgeon, arrived in Anchorage in 1961. Martha Wilson maintained her commitment to and enthusiasm for the tuberculosis program throughout her decade at the hospital, both as a clinician and later as its director. She personally oriented all new physicians heading to the field hospitals in tuberculosis awareness, as well as in the diagnosis and management of cases. In his first years at the hospital Joe Wilson performed various thoracic surgery procedures for tuberculosis, but this aspect of his work gradually declined as chemotherapy rendered much of it unnecessary. He led the general surgery service for many years, and later conducted important research in bronchiectasis and alveolar hydatid disease.

70. In its last years the tuberculosis ward was under the direction of Dr. Richard Chao, who had come over from the Seward Sanatorium to PHS in July 1956. Dr. Chao, who was born in China, retired in 1973 and later began a new career in Anchorage as an acupuncturist.

: 7 : A Resilient Foe

The Price of Complacency

Change, Stability, and Longevity: The Fraser Era

Since 1945 the principal responsibility for tuberculosis control had remained with the territorial government, although other agencies sometimes championed their own approach. By 1953, however, nearly everyone acknowledged that a successful effort required a unified command under ADH, an approach that was strongly endorsed by the Parran Report in 1954.[1]

The intensive campaign of the early and mid-1950s had been successful in reducing substantially the number of new active and newly reported far advanced cases. Only one person with primary tuberculosis was reported in 1958. Over the next few years the rates seemed to increase again, although most of the increase, notably, was in patients with minimal disease, demonstrating that case finding was increasingly effective.[2]

The numbers in the case registry also continued to decline steeply. In 1952 there were 5,814 cases listed, including suspects, but by 1960 this number had fallen to 1,903, a decline of two-thirds. In the 1940s and 1950s, the great majority of new cases were first discovered in the far advanced or moderately advanced stages, but by 1960 the majority were classified as primary or minimal. That year 20 percent of new cases hospitalized were reactivations of known treated cases, indicating the need for a more effective follow-up program.[3] Although the number of new cases consistently fell from 1954 through 1958, the number thereafter fluctuated, suggesting that case finding with the available resources had leveled off.[4]

In April 1964 Dr. Robert I. Fraser became the chief of the Unit of Tuberculosis Control in the Alaska Division of Public Health. Following a residency in internal medicine he had served briefly as a tuberculosis consultant to ADH, then took a six-month fellowship in pulmonary diseases at the famous Brompton Hospital in London.[5]

Reporting on his first year as chief, Dr. Fraser acknowledged that the public was becoming increasingly apathetic about tuberculosis now that dramatic cases of disease and death were disappearing from the daily scene. He then set forth the principles by which he proposed to lead the fight against tuberculosis:

- Continue tuberculin skin testing of the school population
- Continue mass x-ray surveys in high-incidence Eskimo and Indian areas for at least another decade
- Continue the x-ray programs involving other high-risk groups, such as prisoners and food handlers
- Orient and motivate the public health nurses and allied staffs in the tuberculosis program
- Develop chemoprophylaxis for specific indications under close direct supervision
- Continue the primary tuberculosis case registry
- Continue to upgrade the state laboratory services, including introduction of new culture media, allowing tuberculosis culture reports to be available in three weeks instead of the eight to ten weeks formerly needed
- Continue to review and report x-rays forwarded by private practitioners and PHS field physicians
- Explore new methods of tuberculosis education directed toward the high-risk and high-incidence groups
- Rely on widespread tuberculin testing in the school and preschool population for early diagnosis rather than on BCG[6]

One of Fraser's special areas of interest was chest clinics in the field, particularly as the need for hospital beds continued to decline. Chest clinics had first been conducted by health department physicians in December 1936, held in conjunction with x-ray surveys.[7] Soon after his arrival, Fraser encouraged the establishment of chest clinics in each of the PHS field hospitals. By 1965 such clinics had been established at Bethel, Kotzebue, Barrow, Tanana, and Kanakanak, and in the referral hospitals at Mt. Edgecumbe and Anchorage.[8] At Bethel, where the needs were greatest, the state funded a tuberculosis coordinator clerk, but her work was limited by the lack of travel funds. At Kotzebue the clinic was especially effective, while in the Kanakanak and Tanana Service Units, work began on only a limited scale.[9] The Tuberculosis Control Unit also enlisted the help of the private sector by providing financial support in Juneau, Anchorage, Fairbanks, Ketchikan, Nome, and Kodiak to physicians interested and knowledgeable in chest diseases and tuberculosis for the diagnosis, treatment, and follow-up of tuberculosis patients in their own clinics.[10]

The development of these services in the PHS hospitals and in the private sector freed up the limited resources of the Tuberculosis Control Unit to focus on more remote areas, such as villages in the Lower Yukon, Nunivak Island, and around Norton Sound. The state budget, however, did not permit transportation of a team on short notice to investigate outbreaks. To address this problem, representatives of the affected state and federal agencies met in 1964 to develop a long-term strategy for dealing with the remote villages. Since these were in a sense still "hot spots" on the tuberculosis map of Alaska, the concept became known as Hot Spot Teams. A rapid-deployment force consisting of a physician, public health nurse, and x-ray technician made up the team, which would go on short notice to a village where there was a concentration of cases. The nurse would administer tuberculin tests to all those eligible, the technician would x-ray the positive reactors, and the physician would evaluate each suspected active case and decide whether immediate hospitalization or home treatment was appropriate. In 1965 a Special Tuberculosis Project Grant from the Tuberculosis Branch of the Centers for Disease Control (CDC) to the Alaska Department of Health and Welfare (ADHW) funded the program.[11] By 1966 a Hot Spot Team was able to descend on short notice on any remote community where new active cases had been detected.[12]

The manner in which the team functioned has been described by Dr. Keith R. Hooker, a CDC itinerant physician based in Anchorage. When in 1967 a new active case turned up in Kalskag, on the Kuskokwim, the team physician first reviewed health records and recent x-ray survey records from the village. The physician and technician then flew to Bethel and by bush plane to Upper Kalskag, where the health aide assisted in rounding up the patient's extended family and friends for tuberculin testing and x-rays. The technician also x-rayed all those children who had recently converted their tuberculin test and their household contacts, and all recent converters were placed on INH prophylaxis. All "old" tuberculosis cases in the village were asked to submit aerosol-induced sputum samples. The team then proceeded by dogsled to Lower Kalskag, where the procedure was repeated.

When the films were read upon the team's return to Anchorage, three new active cases were identified. All were flown to Anchorage for a thorough diagnostic evaluation and treatment as necessary at the Alaska Native Medical Center. Later the sputum from all these patients was reported as positive. The Hot Spot Team physician returned to the Kalskags two months later and skin-tested all remaining children whose tuberculin tests had originally been negative. One additional converter was identified, and one additional active case was found by a positive sputum sample. Members of the Hot Spot Team continued to visit these villages regularly for follow-up.[13]

Another significant outbreak occurred around this time at Noorvik, with a population of 380. In May 1961 five children from the village were hospitalized for tuberculosis in a single month. Tuberculin testing before and after revealed thirty-nine conversions (18 percent) in a school population of 216. An x-ray survey in the village, conducted shortly after, included 90 percent of those over two years of age, exactly half of whom showed evidence of tuberculosis. By July 1961, twenty-five new cases of active tuberculosis had been identified. Many conditions conducive to spread were identified in the community. Fevered spring subsistence activities had caused many of the adults and children to be overtired. An epidemic of mumps had occurred in March, followed shortly by a flu epidemic. Sleeping arrangements in the homes were cramped, and adults and children spent long hours in two crowded village establishments: a pool hall where movies were shown and a local coffee shop.[14]

Although not all outbreaks were as dramatic as these, almost every year new cases were concentrated in one or more communities. In 1963, for example, seven active and an additional seven probably active cases were reported from Kwethluk, on the lower Kuskokwim, and in 1965, eleven active cases were identified in Karluk, on Kodiak Island. Each outbreak was followed up by visits of the public health nurses or by the Hot Spot Teams.

Beginning in 1966 the statistics seemed to show that the cumulative efforts of several agencies and many committed workers were paying off. The new case rate fell a whopping 52 percent over the previous year. Nearly 25 percent of the new cases reported were in persons previously treated, a finding that demonstrated the urgency of providing prolonged follow-up and surveillance of this annually increasing reservoir of individuals who had previously suffered from tuberculosis. Surveillance was carried out through continued x-ray surveys in the smaller communities of the state, while in the larger communities greater reliance was placed on chest clinics and on the cooperation of local private physicians.[15] Another major source of new cases was individuals who were previously tuberculin-positive and whose infection had become progressive. Those most at risk for reinfection were adolescents, young adults, pregnant women, those with debilitating disease, those on steroids, and those with certain specific diseases such as silicosis and diabetes. The best indicator of a developing problem was the annual school and preschool tuberculin-testing program. In 1967 the number of Alaskans with a positive tuberculin test was estimated at 60,000, and this was the group on which DPH began to focus its control efforts.[16]

The following year was the first in recorded history in which there were no deaths attributable to tuberculosis in Alaska. Children entering school showed a tuberculin positivity rate of only 1.6 percent, the lowest ever. The majority of new cases were minimal, a stage at which most were noninfectious and could be easily and effectively treated.[17] In light of these hopeful trends, Fraser suggested in 1968 that "the ultimate disappearance of TB can be projected some time in the future if an adequate surveillance program can be continued."[18]

Thus, as Alaska moved into the 1970s, the priorities of DPH began to be stated in slightly different terms:

- Careful supervision of those with active disease to insure that the medication was taken as prescribed for the necessary length of time
- Identification and supervision of contacts of active cases with a positive sputum
- Careful surveillance of those individuals identified in each community with significant risk of breaking down with active disease

- Tuberculin testing of preschool and school-age population as an early warning system[19]

In 1970 and 1971 the majority of new active cases were again in the category of minimal, primary, or extrapulmonary disease, all categories with little potential for spread. The moderately advanced and far advanced cases in Alaska constituted only 24 percent of the total, in marked contrast to the situation in most other states. Over three-quarters of new cases were in those who were known to be tuberculin-positive, a group that also included individuals previously treated for active disease, or with previous x-ray evidence of healed tuberculosis. Of the ones with a previous tuberculosis history, 57 percent had already received some INH, and an additional 15 percent had been advised to take it but had not done so.

DPH recommended that all those with a positive tuberculin test, whether or not they had had active tuberculosis, have an annual chest x-ray, while those with a prior history of tuberculosis should in addition submit sputum samples every six months. Those newly diagnosed with active disease required only a short period of evaluation in a community hospital for diagnosis and tuberculosis education, with the long-term supervision of the drug treatment left to the public health nurses.[20] These increasingly shorter hospitalizations for active tuberculosis permitted earlier return to economic productivity.

In 1972 the tuberculosis hospital census in Alaska occasionally dropped to one to two patients, a dramatic decline since the 1960s. On the other hand, the shorter hospitalizations, an average of two weeks, put a heavier burden on the public health nurses to motivate patients to continue on drug treatment for their pre-scribed twelve to eighteen months. The job was made more difficult by the fact that severe alcoholism was present in at least 20 percent of the active cases.

The improving tuberculosis situation that year allowed DPH to give more emphasis to the prevention and care of other types of chronic lung disease, a long-standing priority of Dr. Fraser.[21] The section began a program of education for private physicians, hospital nurses, and public health nurses in the use of inhalation therapy in the home and in effective rehabilitation programs for those with chronic pulmonary disease. A contract inhalation therapist held workshops in nearly all of the smaller community and IHS field hospitals. In the larger communities, DPH physicians offered chronic pulmonary disease consultations in addition to their tuberculosis work.[22]

By the end of 1973 the tuberculosis situation in Alaska was stable. Since 1967 the statewide new case rate had hovered between 30.5 and 41.0 per 100,000, with no real evidence of a downward trend. The Native rate in 1973 was 147.5 per 100,000, still over thirteen times the rate for whites. Between 1968 and 1973 only nine deaths had occurred from tuberculosis, and in three of those years (1968, 1971, and 1972), none at all. The tuberculosis case registry at the end of 1973 showed only 520 cases on file, of which 7 were hospitalized and 173 were on drug treatment at home. Only 8 percent of new cases were far advanced, while 81 percent fell into the categories of minimal (47 percent), primary (22 percent), and nonpulmonary (12 percent). The cases by age showed that 44.7 percent were in the young adult group (aged 15–44), and another 17.8 percent in the 0–14 group, with a slight preponderance in males.

Some new cases were being identified by the periodic village x-ray surveys, but increasingly they were recognized by tuberculin test conversions among schoolchildren. Once a child's test converted, it was almost certain that he or she had been in close contact with an "open" case, usually in the household, although occasionally infection could be the result of prolonged contact with another person at school or church. The source case was usually an individual previously treated for tuberculosis, perhaps inadequately by contemporary standards. Several major village outbreaks illustrate the problem.

A large outbreak occurred in 1970 in Tanacross, an Athabascan village of about seventy-five not far from Tok. There were eighteen occupied homes in the village, plus an elementary school, a church, a post office, and a community hall. The village had little health care coverage, in part due to frequent turnover of the public health nurse position responsible for the community. The last x-ray survey had been in 1967 and the last skin testing in 1968. Between August and November 1970, four villagers with active tuberculosis were admitted to the Alaska Native Medical Center. These included an eight-year-old boy with pulmonary tuberculosis, his fifteen-year-old sister with primary tuberculosis and erythema nodosum (an autoimmune skin disease often triggered by tuberculosis), and a seventeen-year-old boy with a pleural effusion. The fourth was a thirty-four-year-old half brother of the first two cases living in the same household. He had already been diagnosed with scrofula in 1966 but was admitted in December 1970 with a seven-month history of sputum-positive far-advanced pulmonary tuberculosis. Two surveys in the region in November by the mobile x-ray team uncovered four more cases of active tuberculosis, thus bringing the total to eight, six of them in adolescents. Another new case was diagnosed in the village in early 1972. One person, a firefighter who was alcoholic, was probably the source case for the entire outbreak. Of the eight members of his household, three were known tuberculin-positive reactors in 1970 and four more developed positive skin tests and active tuberculosis.[23]

Another representative village outbreak of this period was in 1978–79 in Toksook Bay, a Yup'ik village of 373 on the western coast of Alaska. In July 1978 a young man was found to have a positive sputum culture, and an investigation of his family revealed that four out of five siblings had converted their PPD test; two showed active pulmonary tuberculosis. The next month a young woman was identified as a converter and she too was found to have a positive sputum, although she had no contacts with the first family. In November a third young adult from the village developed active tuberculosis in the form of a pleural effusion. Contact follow-up revealed two converters among her in-laws.

In December a DPH team carried out an extensive tuberculin skin-testing survey of the village. All persons known to be tuberculin-negative were skin tested, while those who were known positive were asked to submit an induced sputum specimen and undergo a chest x-ray. These efforts turned up eight recent converters from seven families, although only one with active disease. Again, none had any apparent connections with the earlier cases. A second survey team in January 1979 discovered four new converters, one with positive sputum, from four additional families. In sum, these extensive investigations, which determined the tuberculosis status of 98 percent of the village, revealed a total of twenty new converters, half of whom had active tuberculosis. All were put on preventive therapy or double drug treatment. By January 1979 a total of 37 individuals, or 10 percent of the population, were taking anti-tuberculosis drugs, and 142, or 38 percent, were known to be infected with *M. tuberculosis* and thus at risk for further problems in the future.[24]

The annual school tuberculin-testing program thus remained a basic tool for the identification of new cases of tuberculosis. The extension of this program throughout the state permitted an evaluation of the risk of this population for the development of tuberculosis, the prompt detection of new cases, the evaluation and follow-up of household contacts, and the provision of reliable figures comparing the risk of the youth of Alaska developing tuberculosis with those in other states.[25]

In 1962 the Tuberculosis Control Program had adopted the tine test as its preferred screening method for tuberculin testing. This technique involved the application to the forearm of a small plastic device with four sharp prongs (tines) coated with the tuberculin antigen. The test was read forty-eight to seventy-two hours later and considered positive if there was 2 mm or more of induration around the insertion of one or more of the prongs. This method, which replaced the intradermal method for screening purposes, was much simpler and faster to perform, thus allowing the public health nurses to screen larger numbers of schoolchildren within a shorter time. It was soon clear that more new cases were being found through this method than through the mass x-ray surveys that had been so much a part of the Alaska scene since the 1930s.[26]

During the 1972–73 school year, nurses administered 57,510 tine tests, including 3,941 in preschool children and 10,082 in adults. The positivity rate for adults was 7.7 percent, and 0.4 percent for schoolchildren.[27] The percentage of positive tuberculin tests in children entering school declined during the 1970s, except for 1975–76, when the rate rose unexpectedly to nearly 1 percent. In 1982 ADH began requiring tuberculin testing in kindergarten, first, third, seventh, and eleventh grades, plus pre-elementary students and all those entering an Alaskan school for the first time.[28] The rates remained at a moderate level until 1984, when they reached a peak of 2.07 percent. Likewise, the tuberculin positivity rate for fourteen-year-olds declined until 1976–77, increased steadily to a high of 2.20 percent in 1978–79, and then began to decrease again.[29] These fluctuations suggested that tuberculosis might be making a comeback in the villages.

Although the population of the state was increasing during the early 1980s, the number of new cases kept pace, leading to a fairly stable overall tuberculosis incidence averaging about 19 per 100,000 for the period 1980 through 1986. These figures hit their highest point in 1985, with 110 total cases, 68 of whom were Natives, up from 46 the previous year. Cases were widely distributed in western and northern Alaska, and the increasing numbers were worrisome.

Dr. Fraser retired on May 1, 1987, having served as tuberculosis control officer for twenty-three years, far longer than any other individual. He had presided over the decline and fall of the disease in Alaska, from near the end of the sanatorium era, when tuberculosis was still a frightening prospect, to the late 1980s, when the campaign against tuberculosis had lost its sense of urgency in both Alaska and the nation at large.[30] Moreover, with his retirement at the same time as his longtime associate Peggy Dunsmore the tuberculosis program lost most of its institutional memory.

The Fraser years saw a considerable change in the way tuberculosis was viewed in Alaska. In the 1960s, as a result of the success of the Ambulatory Chemotherapy Program and INH prophylaxis studies, the battleground of tuberculosis changed from the sanatorium to the village. The tuberculosis hospitals rapidly emptied out and were either closed or turned to other uses, and patient follow-up was turned over to field chest clinics. The era of mass screening for tuberculosis was also over, except for the essential annual school tuberculin-testing program, which acted as an indicator of tuberculosis activity in the community. Mobile Hot Spot Teams allowed the DPH staff to respond quickly to village outbreaks.

With the seeming success of the tuberculosis control program on all fronts came a gradual and perhaps inevitable shift of emphasis and funds by all health agencies to other program priorities. Signs of trouble were appearing, however, as shown by a few disturbing village outbreaks and the rising tuberculin sensitivity among schoolchildren. Tuberculosis was making a comeback.

A New Look at Strategy

After Fraser's retirement, the functions of communicable disease control, including tuberculosis, were transferred to the Epidemiology Section of the Division of Public Health. Dr. John Middaugh, chief of the section, assisted by CDC epidemic intelligence officer Dr. Michael Beller, served as the interim tuberculosis control officer pending the recruitment of a new staff physician. Dr. Michael Jones, an infectious disease specialist, arrived on October 1, 1987, to head the tuberculosis program, although he also had other communicable disease responsibilities. Many of the day-to-day functions of the tuberculosis program, as before, were carried out by nurse epidemiologists and public health nurses.[31]

Shortly after taking over in May, Middaugh asked the Division of Tuberculosis Control at CDC to conduct a comprehensive review of the Alaska tuberculosis program, to see if it could be made more responsive to the changing tuberculosis situation in the state. Dr. Alan B. Bloch and Walter Q. Page came to Alaska and made an intensive study of the Alaska program from June 22 to 26, 1987. After consulting with representatives from many agencies, interviewing physicians and others in Anchorage, Fairbanks, and Bethel, and reviewing program management reports and tuberculosis statistics, the team concluded that Dr. Fraser's sudden retirement had led to a crisis of leadership in the tuberculosis program. The team noted further that case finding, diagnosis, treatment, and preventive methods needed to be brought in line with currently accepted practices.

The team recommended that day-to-day management be turned over to a nurse-epidemiologist, to be supervised by a communicable disease physician-epidemiologist. DPH should no longer provide direct clinical services to patients but instead contract with pulmonary specialists in the private sector. Vigorous contact investigation should be the centerpiece of case finding and screening. X-ray screening surveys should be replaced by sputum smear and culture examinations on individuals with chronic chest symptoms. Skin testing should be extended to all school staff, hospital and extended-care-facility workers, and correctional employees before hire, with preventive INH treatment given to all those who tested positive. INH prophylaxis should also be more consistently and widely applied to those already infected. Directly observed therapy (DOT; see below), rarely in use at that time in Alaska, was recommended whenever possible for patients on treatment or on INH prophylaxis. The tuberculosis program was also advised to give increased attention to groups at high risk—the homeless, those infected with HIV/AIDS, and minorities.[32]

In response, the Epidemiology Section in January 1988 prepared a "Strategy for the Elimination of Tuberculosis in Alaska." This document particularly emphasized the following:

- Diagnosis and treatment of all culture-confirmed cases
- Epidemiologic investigation of all close contacts
- Effective skin-test screening programs
- Assistance to insure compliance with drug treatment

The strategy affirmed the major recommendations of the review team regarding laboratory tests, consultations, clinical services, disease reporting, x-ray surveys, and the use of directly observed therapy.[33] Implementing these changes, however, proved difficult because of budget constraints over the next few years. The previous year IHS, then in the midst of contracting with Native health corporations for the management of health facilities, had terminated a long-standing annual grant of $400,000 to DPH in support of tuberculosis control. This period was also one of severe cutbacks in state funding for public health; in fact, under the administration of Governor Walter J. Hickel (1990–1994), the funding for the Epidemiology Section decreased by nearly one-third, including the loss of some $400,000 in tuberculosis control funds, although $200,000 was later restored. Some of the deficit in these years was made up by support from CDC, but funds remained in short supply.

Dr. Jones resigned from the Epidemiology Section in January 1994. The position remained vacant until the arrival, on April 3, 1995, of Dr. Elizabeth A. Funk, who has provided leadership in tuberculosis control until the present time.[34]

Early in 1995 Dr. Middaugh again asked that a CDC team review the Alaska tuberculosis program, especially since the reported cases of the disease were climbing significantly in the Native population. The review was conducted that winter by four individuals from the CDC Tuberculosis Control Division, under the direction of Drs. Carl Schieffelbein and James Creek, the latter an epidemiologist with IHS. Their report was submitted in April.

The report acknowledged that tuberculosis control services in the metropolitan areas were going well, but that the state was being challenged to provide adequate services in isolated Native communities. Many of these problems could be traced to an erosion of the health infrastructure as a consequence of the loss of skilled tuberculosis expertise, the reduction in state funding, a de-emphasis on tuberculosis as a priority, and the loss of IHS funds for prevention. The CDC team was particularly concerned about the striking increase in cases of active disease in the villages. From 1993 to 1994, for example, several village outbreaks (to be discussed below) had sent the statewide incidence rates up 63 percent, to 15.5 per 100,000, the highest since 1985. The overall Native rate was up 60 percent from 1993 to 1994, to 66.6 per 100,000, with the incidence in some villages reaching levels of the pre-chemotherapy era.

The number-one priority, according to the report, was the successful completion of treatment of active cases. To this end, it was suggested that DOT aides be paid on a uniform scale and provided with bonuses for exceptional work. Patients should also be given incentives for full cooperation in treatment. The authors encouraged the state to make better and more extensive use of Native health corporation resources for the prompt reporting and investigation of tuberculosis outbreaks in the villages. Community health aides should be trained in tuberculosis awareness and be encouraged to submit sputum tests for smear and culture on their own in tuberculosis suspects.

All new cases should be treated with an initial four-drug regimen to minimize the development of drug resistance and hasten sputum conversion. To improve the identification of active cases, the team suggested that all providers be urged to use the state laboratory for tuberculosis specimens, that pharmacies be asked to report any rifampin prescriptions as a way of identifying new cases, and that DPH work more closely with hospital infection-control coordinators. The state laboratory should report its mycobacterial findings more promptly to health care providers, with the tuberculosis control officer providing prompt consultation and recommendations for management.[35]

This report has served as the basis for state tuberculosis control policy up to the present time (2004).

The Embers Flare Up: Village Outbreaks

The great tuberculosis epidemic in Alaska in the first half of the twentieth century caused tens of thousands of people to be infected with the tubercle bacillus. Of those who survived, some healed on their own, some developed active disease and were treated in hospitals or on home therapy, and some were given INH prophylaxis. Many of those who were treated with drugs took their medications intermittently or stopped before their course was completed. All who survived, of course, remained tuberculin-positive and subject to subsequent reactivation or progression of their disease, usually as the result of factors such as poor nutrition, general debility, intercurrent infection, or perhaps even severe psychological stress.

From 1987 through 1991 there were some thirteen village outbreaks in western Alaska, with from three to twenty-three active cases in each. In 1990 alone, three large village outbreaks accounted for twenty-three (34 percent) of the sixty-eight cases of tuberculosis reported. Four substantial outbreaks occurred during those years: Holy Cross (twelve cases, 1987), Chevak (nine cases, 1989), the Pribilof Islands (ten cases, 1990–91), and Savoonga (twenty-three cases, 1990–91). In each of these outbreaks, delays in recognition of an active case led to spread to others in the community. A study of the Holy Cross epidemic showed that the estimated cost of evaluating and treating the infected, not including hospitalization, was $521,000.[36]

An especially troublesome outbreak was the one in 1990 in the village of Savoonga, on St. Lawrence Island. A six-year-old child was admitted to the Alaska Native Medical Center in June with symptoms that had lasted over six months. She had converted her tuberculin test since the previous year and also had a lung infiltrate, although no organisms were recovered. The second patient was a twenty-year-old pregnant woman who had converted her skin test in April and after giving birth was reported as sputum-positive. During July and August three more cases were identified by sputum culture, two of whom had been treated for tuberculosis many years before. One of them had highly infectious sputum and had been coughing for two years. As a result of tuberculin testing and chest x-rays in the village, four more cases were identified in October and an additional three in November. A villager then in prison at Nome was found to have infectious sputum and cavitation of the lung. Fourteen additional tuberculin converters were identified and put on preventive INH therapy, along with thirty-seven of their close contacts who had positive skin tests. Altogether, thirteen cases of pulmonary tuberculosis were identified as the result of the investigation, all but one of whom were sputum-positive. All thirteen were put on supervised therapy (DOT).[37]

In 1994 and 1995 there were no fewer than eight village outbreaks, the largest being at Gambell, the other major village on St. Lawrence Island, where thirteen active cases, twenty-nine tuberculin converters, and thirty-five tuberculin reactors were identified. Just under half of all cases reported in 1994 were associated with outbreaks, among them Chevak, Hooper Bay, Scammon Bay, Lower Kalskag, and Mt. Village. In addition, outbreaks continued at Gambell, Savoonga, and St. Paul.

Some idea of the resources expended in the 1994–95 outbreaks may be gathered from the following: the aggregate village population in the eight villages was 5,725, among whom just under 3,000 tuberculin tests were performed, 810 x-rays taken, and 1,369 sputum specimens processed. A total of forty-nine new cases were identified, together with eighty-four tuberculin test converters. More than 200 people were started on DOT either as treatment or as a preventive measure. One of the encouraging features of these investigations was the interagency response: community health aides, public health nurses, physician assistants, x-ray technologists, and physicians from regional health corporations, IHS, and the private sector teamed up with staff from the state Sections of Laboratories, Nursing, and Epidemiology to assist in the investigation of contacts and the treatment of cases.[38] Each of these outbreaks also required several years of careful follow-up to identify new cases by tuberculin screening, x-rays, and sputum examinations, and to ensure that those on treatment continued their regimens faithfully.[39] Other important outbreaks occurred at Circle and Shishmaref in 1995.[40]

In October of the following year, a public health nurse noted two tuberculin test conversions in the village of Levelock, on the Kvichak River near Bristol Bay, but contact investigation revealed no source case. Further probing established that these two had lived together in a Quonset hut at a fishing camp the previous summer. Others using the hut came from the village of Kokhanok, on Lake Iliamna, about seventy-five miles away. The chest x-ray of one of the converters revealed evidence of tuberculosis, and his sputum was strongly positive. Further contact investigation led to five other converters, all of whom had active tuberculosis. The entire village of 150 was then investigated, revealing six additional skin test conversions. Twenty individuals known already to have positive skin tests were asked to submit sputum samples, and among these no fewer than eight showed positive cultures for M. tuberculosis. Epidemiological and laboratory testing revealed that the original case at Kokhanok was responsible for infecting as many as nine of the fourteen cases identified in the outbreak. Thus, 9.3 percent of the population of a village of only 150 had active tuberculosis, and an additional 4 percent were newly infected with the organism.[41]

No new village outbreaks were detected during 1997 or 1998, although screening and follow-up continued, especially in St. Paul and on St. Lawrence Island, where two new cases were identified in Gambell and four more in Savoonga. The late 1990s showed a decline in village outbreaks, except for small ones at Elim and White Mountain on Norton Sound, and at Kwethluk, on the Kuskokwim. Between 1995 and 1998, village outbreaks made up only 17.6 percent of the reported cases of tuberculosis, and the number of cases seemed to be declining each year.

In June 2000, however, another outbreak occurred in the Bristol Bay region, the largest in six years. Some twenty-one new cases were identified initially among the residents of several villages, including nine adults and twelve children, and an additional fifty-six converted their skin tests.[42]

These periodic outbreaks in bush Alaska, representing for the most part the reactivation of old cases and subsequent spread in geographically isolated communities, are a unique phenomenon in tuberculosis control in the United States today. To control them promptly and effectively requires resourcefulness, imagination, and cooperation on the part of both state health officials and local Native health authorities.

Other Outbreaks and New Risks

Several other recent outbreaks represent more conventional problems in modern tuberculosis control. For example, in September 1982 four intensive-care unit workers in a Fairbanks hospital were found to have converted their tuberculin tests, and each had been in contact with a patient with tuberculosis admitted in July 1982. Environmental tests showed that air from the patient's room flowed out to the nurses' station whether or not the door was closed. As a result of this incident, the hospital was urged to place any patient suspected of tuberculosis in a room at negative or at least neutral pressure with respect to the corridor.[43]

The spread of tuberculosis by airline travel is another new and worrisome trend and a particular concern in Alaska, where air travel is often the only means of transportation available for a population with a high incidence of infection. In November 1994 a forty-six-year-old man flew without a mask on a two-and-a-half-hour flight from a rural village to Anchorage, despite the fact that he was known to have had two sputum smears positive for acid-fast bacteria (AFB) in the previous month, and had not been treated. DPH successfully tracked down and evaluated the other twelve people on the plane for tuberculosis, but fortunately none showed evidence of infection.

The tuberculosis control program felt that although the risk of spread of tuberculosis on a commercial flight was "exceedingly small," those with infectious tuberculosis—that is, with a positive smear or other evidence of active disease—should not fly except in emergencies. The policy adopted by DPH was that a person diagnosed with infectious tuberculosis may travel without restriction if he or she has completed fourteen days of adequate anti-tuberculosis treatment, with a favorable treatment response, and has had three consecutive negative sputum smears collected on different days.[44]

Another group requiring special surveillance is the prison population. The setting fosters spread, since many people are living in close confinement for extended periods. Many jails and prisons are old and ventilation is less than ideal. The prison population itself, moreover, is largely made up of the lower socioeconomic strata in which homelessness, alcoholism, and drug abuse are widespread. A further element is that Alaska Natives, who have a relatively high rate of tuberculosis infection, make up nearly 40 percent of the prison population in the state.[45] The Alaska tuberculosis control program recognized as early as 1966 that the prison population deserved special attention in x-ray surveys for tuberculosis.[46]

The July 2001 edition of the state manual *Tuberculosis Control in Alaska* recommends that prison residents, who are at special risk for the development of latent tuberculosis infection, as well as for progression of a latent infection to active disease, receive annual tuberculin testing.[47] In November 2000 four prisoners at the Spring Creek maximum-security prison near Seward were found on routine screening to have converted their tuberculin test. Though none had active tuberculosis, the finding prompted the tuberculosis control program to test every inmate and employee—a total of nearly 700 people—to see whether a source case could be discovered. The whole incident was given little attention in the press, since the state felt that there was no public danger involved.[48] Those who were converters were presumably put on prophylactic DOT.

Special Problems of Urban Tuberculosis in Alaska

Anchorage, the one true urban area of Alaska, has its own special problems of tuberculosis control, since tuberculosis rates among certain groups, such as the homeless, prisoners, Asians/Pacific Islanders, and American Indians/Alaska Natives,[49] are well above the national average there. The staff of the Municipality of Anchorage Department of Health and Human Services handles the day-to-day tuberculosis work of screening, case finding, contact investigation, supervision of DOT, and keeping statistics, within the policies set by DPH.

In the years 1994–95 nearly 80 percent of the forty-four reported cases of tuberculosis in Anchorage were either among Asians/Pacific Islanders or Alaska Natives. The citywide rate was lower than that for the state as a whole and lower than the overall national rate. Those for whites and African Americans were also lower, but rates for American Indians/Alaska Natives and for Asians/Pacific Islanders were 2.1 and 1.7 times, respectively, the national averages. Nineteen (43 percent) of the total cases were foreign-born, all but two from Asia. Of the total cases, thirty-six (82 percent) were pulmonary and six involved the lymph nodes, including five cases of scrofula. Of the two remaining cases, one had pleural involvement and the other miliary tuberculosis.[50]

In 2000 the statewide tuberculosis rate was 17.2 per 100,000, the highest in the nation, due largely to a single major outbreak in Anchorage. In the first four months of the year, twenty Anchorage residents were diagnosed with active tuberculosis, nine of them from one extended family. This outbreak began with an infant whose family had recently moved to Alaska and whose medication had run out. An extensive contact investigation led to four infants, a five-year-old, and three adults with active disease. Twenty-four other family members received treatment for latent tuberculosis infection and eleven others were put on preventive INH treatment.[51] This outbreak demonstrates the essential role of surveillance and intensive contact investigation of a newly recognized case.

In summary, in the period 1999 to 2003, ninety-five Anchorage residents were diagnosed with active tuberculosis, of whom 44 percent were foreign-born. Of the total, 40 percent of cases were Asians/Pacific Islanders and another 34 percent were American Indians/Alaska Natives. Alcohol was used excessively by 32 percent and 17 percent were homeless, both figures at least twice the national rates. One individual was HIV-positive. Of the eighty-two culture-positive cases, 10 percent of strains showed resistance to INH but none was multidrug-resistant. Overall, the tuberculosis rate for Anchorage was 7.2 per 100,000, compared with 10.4 per 100,000 for Alaska and 5.6 per 100,000 for the United States as a whole. Within Anchorage, the rate was 42.9 per 100,000 for Asians/Pacific Islanders and 31.8 per 100,000 for American Indians/Alaska Natives.[52]

Tuberculin Testing Program

Annual tuberculin testing as a major means of case finding became a priority of DPH as early as 1966 and has remained so up to the present. All village school and preschool children were screened annually, together with school personnel and even those with previous BCG vaccination.[53] Over the next three decades, periodic tuberculin testing, especially in the villages, led to most of the cases of active tuberculosis identified in the state.

School tuberculin testing in Alaska has two major purposes: to identify children who would benefit from preventive therapy and to detect cases and outbreaks of tuberculosis disease. All schools are required to administer a tuberculosis skin test to each child in pre-elementary school, kindergarten, grades one, three, seven, and eleven, or when entering a district or private school for the first time. Because of high rates of tuberculosis in rural Alaska, many schools screen children every year regardless of grade. The initial screening is usually a Mono-Vac or tine test, and if the screening test is positive, an intradermal PPD is performed. Those with positive PPDs are referred to a physician.[54]

In the 1994–95 school year, 290 children (0.4 percent) showed newly positive PPD skin tests out of more than 71,000 tested. The rates were highest among schoolchildren from the southwestern region of the state, high school students, and Asians/Pacific Islanders, this last group with a rate of 1.8 percent, by far the highest. Notably, white (0.3 percent) and African American (0.4 percent) children had higher rates of newly positive reactions than Alaska Native children (0.2 percent). Only nine children with newly positive reactions were diagnosed with active tuberculosis. These cases led through contact investigation to two significant village outbreaks in which twenty-four additional cases of tuberculosis and thirty-nine people with tuberculosis infection were discovered, all of whom received either drug treatment or prophylaxis.[55] It was of special interest that children receiving care from private physicians were 1.4 times more likely to receive inadequate preventive therapy than those receiving care through the public health, military, community health center, or IHS/Native health corporation system.[56]

Immigrants: New Fuel for the Fire

The first large wave of immigrants to Alaska at the turn of the nineteenth century came directly from northern Europe (especially Scandinavia), Canada, and even Australia to participate in the gold rushes. Many stayed on to build a family and career in Alaska. Around the same time, many Asian immigrants, particularly from China, the Philippines, and Japan, were being brought to Alaska by major seafood processors to work in the huge canneries of Southeast Alaska, Prince William Sound, the Alaska Peninsula, Kodiak Island, and Bristol Bay. They labored under appalling conditions in the crowded and drafty cannery barracks, working long hours and eating a marginal diet. None of them had any health examinations until FY1926, when the US Public Health Service began to require that all cannery workers be given a physical examination before they could be shipped to Alaska.[57]

The early tuberculosis statistics published by the territorial and state governments are difficult to compare, since ethnic categories were often either lumped together or broken out in varying detail. With these limitations in mind, however, we can look at general trends on how tuberculosis affected races other than "white," "Native," and "black." Beginning with the 1960 federal Census, "blacks" and "Asians" were separated from the "other" category. In the 1970s, the average tuberculosis incidence rate for blacks was 17.7 per 100,000, while the rate for Asians was 87.9 per 100,000, higher than that of Alaska Natives.

Over the next two decades, the five-year average tuberculosis rates were as follows:

Five-Year Average Tuberculosis Rates per 100,000, by Race, 1980–2000[58]

	1980	1985	1990	1995	2000
Total Alaska	21.8	17.6	11.1	13.8	10.5
White	5.4	4.8	1.3	2.4	1.9
Alaska Native	92.4	64.6	52.3	59.0	40.8
Black	13.2	7.8	4.5	6.3	11.9
Asian/Pacific Islander	153.1	125.2	49.7	64.8	49.3
Total US	12.3	9.3	10.3	8.7	9.8

By 1981 DPH was reporting that the highest tuberculosis rates among any segment of the Alaska population were in Asians, particularly the foreign-born.[59] Five years later, seventeen cases of tuberculosis—30 percent of the Alaska total—were in the foreign-born, all but one from western and southern Asia. Nearly two-thirds of these individuals had entered the United States within the previous five years.[60] Follow-up studies for 1994–95 and 1996–97 in Anchorage confirmed these trends.[61] The highest proportion of foreign-born cases ever was in 2002, when nineteen (39 percent) of forty-nine cases of tuberculosis reported statewide were born overseas.[62]

Current federal law requires only that immigrants and refugees have a chest x-ray before admission to the United States, thus excluding examination of those entering legally as tourists, students, workers, or on business.[63] In addition, many individuals enter the United States illegally, especially in the Southwest, and numerous lawful entrants stay beyond the expiration of their visas. In Alaska the problem of tuberculosis in the foreign-born is less that of illegal entrants and more that recent arrivals from Asian countries where tuberculosis is highly endemic are not adequately screened or consistently followed up once they settle in Alaska.

In the last two decades the wave of new immigrants to Alaska, particularly from southern and western Asia, has changed the pattern of tuberculosis in Alaska. As many as 80 percent of the new cases each year in the Municipality of Anchorage and nearly 40 percent of cases statewide are foreign-born. The situation is further complicated in that many of these individuals harbor drug-resistant organisms.

Multidrug-Resistant Tuberculosis

The problem of anti-tuberculosis drug resistance was recognized almost immediately after the development of the first such drug, streptomycin. After a few seemingly dramatic cures of tuberculous meningitis and other severe forms of the disease, clinicians found that some patients rapidly relapsed because streptomycin was no longer effective against the organism. Random genetic mutation of the bacteria is considered to be the cause of this phenomenon. As susceptible bacteria are killed by the drug, the resistant bacteria are permitted to overgrow, and soon become the dominant strain. If a patient is treated with INH alone, for example, the drug will initially kill the sensitive organisms but will leave the resistant organisms to multiply, resulting in a resistant strain.

Multidrug-resistant tuberculosis (MDRTB) became a significant problem in the United States during the early 1990s, with severe outbreaks in New York City, Florida, and Michigan. These were due to strains resulting from inadequate, intermittent drug therapy, often the result of patients not taking their medication in the prescribed manner. Such cases are often rapidly progressive and fatal, despite optimal treatment, especially in those who are in some way immunocompromised. At special risk are those previously inadequately treated with anti-tuberculosis medications and individuals from countries where the incidence of MDRTB is high, particularly South Korea, the Philippines, Vietnam, Russia, and countries of Latin America.[64]

DPH initiated routine drug-sensitivity studies in its Anchorage laboratory in August 1965, and that year the state was sending its "occasional" cases of drug-resistant tuberculosis to National Jewish Hospital in Denver for treatment.[65] A couple of years later, the tuberculosis control officer noted that those patients who reactivated after treatment were commonly drug-resistant, as were those who were infected by them.[66]

Comstock et al. noted in 1967 that resistance was infrequently observed in the INH Community Prophylaxis Program. Moreover, after about six years of follow-up of study patients who developed active disease, those with resistant organisms did as well as those with susceptible organisms, as measured by their average length of hospitalization and subsequent lack of relapse.[67]

A significant increase in drug resistance was recognized in 1977, due in part to the medical community's not ensuring that each patient was taking the appropriate medications for the appropriate length of time.[68] By 1978, physicians at Alaska Native Medical Center reported an increasing number of cases with active disease who harbored drug-resistant organisms, most of these among people with long-standing disease and severe social problems, including alcoholism. Some had openly refused treatment and others had taken treatment only sporadically.[69]

During the 1980s routine sensitivities to INH, rifampin, and streptomycin were performed on all organisms isolated. In 1985, resistant organisms were identified in 7.3 percent of isolates, and the following year in 5.6 percent. In every instance the organism was resistant to only one of three drugs tested. All strains were susceptible to INH, while others showed varying degrees of resistance to rifampin and streptomycin. Eight of the twelve patients with drug-resistant organisms were Alaska Natives, two were of Asian descent, and two were Caucasian. None was known to have been previously treated with the antibiotic to which their organism was resistant. All were treated successfully with a multi-drug regimen.[70]

In 1988–89 a village outbreak of drug-resistant tuberculosis occurred in Chevak, a large Yup'ik village in western Alaska. A thirty-nine-year-old man had been given INH briefly on five occasions between 1956 and 1974, and in 1976 he had been hospitalized for cavitary tuberculosis caused by an organism sensitive to INH, rifampin, and streptomycin. After treatment with INH and rifampin, he was lost to follow-up for a year, but when examined again he had progressive disease fully resistant to INH and partially resistant to rifampin. His son, born in 1974, received prophylactic INH for a year after his father was hospitalized in 1976.

In November 1988 school screening showed five recent converters in the village, but extensive investigation failed to reveal a source case. At the end of December a young teen-center worker and her younger brother developed positive skin tests, and the subsequent investigation identified forty-three additional converters. The original patient's son was identified as the source case because of his cavitary tuberculosis and the skin-test conversion of his closest contacts. He was found to have an organism with total INH resistance and 15 percent resistance to ethambutol. When 350 people originally tuberculin-negative were retested in April 1989, 42 new converters (12 percent) were discovered, with the highest percentage, 64 percent, among those of high school age. Intensive cooperation by health authorities of the state, IHS, and Native health corporations, together with village leaders and community health aides, was evident in this investigation, which ultimately identified thirteen active cases of tuberculosis.[71]

In the period 1988–90, resistant strains of *M. tuberculosis* were cultured from eight individuals, or 4.5 percent of the total positives. Five were resistant to INH alone, two others to streptomycin alone, and the last to rifampin and INH.[72] Only three cultures were drug-resistant in 1991, all in individuals who had been given INH inappropriately as single-drug treatment for unrecognized pulmonary tuberculosis.[73] The following year four isolates (8.7 percent of the total) showed drug resistance, two of them resistant to INH alone, a third to INH and rifampin, and the fourth to INH and pyrazinamide. Two of the patients were Asian immigrants, one of whom had had prior anti-tuberculosis therapy.[74]

Perhaps the most important single factor in diminishing the risk of drug-resistant tuberculosis is to avoid treating active disease with a single drug. In 1993, CDC suggested that four-drug therapy be used in areas of the country where INH resistance exceeded 4.3 percent. Since Alaska's rate at that time was approximately 5 percent, DPH adopted the policy of routinely using initial four-drug regimens for all suspected and confirmed patients in Alaska.[75]

In 1996, four out of thirty-five positive cultures (11 percent) identified in Anchorage showed resistance to INH alone; all four individuals were born in the Philippines.[76] During 1999, only two of fifty-nine isolates of *M. tuberculosis*, again in patients from the Philippines, showed single-drug resistance—the first to strep-tomycin and the second to INH.

Summing up the period from 1995 to 1999, 98 percent of 300 isolates statewide underwent drug susceptibility testing and only twelve (4 percent) showed resis-tance. None was resistant to rifampin, and five were resistant to INH alone. Only one isolate, in a patient from India, was resistant to three drugs, namely INH, ethambutol, and streptomycin. Of the twelve with resistant organisms, five were from the United States, five from the Philippines, one from India, and one from American Samoa.[77]

Multidrug-resistant tuberculosis is a serious and increasing problem in many parts of the world, and the economic costs and personal risks are great. The threat in Alaska comes largely from recent immigrants from parts of the world where the resistant strains are widespread. The problem must be addressed by careful health screening and follow-up of all foreign entrants, determination of drug sensitivity in all cultures of M. tuberculosis, and strict adherence of all physicians to the current recommended guidelines for tuberculosis treatment.

Tuberculosis and the HIV/AIDS Epidemic

AIDS was first defined in 1981, followed shortly thereafter by the identification of HIV, the human immunodeficiency virus, as the causative agent. Since infec-tion with HIV greatly impairs the immune system, the victim is susceptible to many types of infection, especially tuberculosis. Someone who is HIV-positive and infected with the tuberculosis organism is many times more likely to become sick with tuberculosis than someone who is infected but HIV-negative.

Between 1972 and 1992, some 1,746 cases of tuberculosis were reported in Alaska, of which only 6 (0.3 percent) developed AIDS either the same year or in a subsequent year.[78] In 1992 the tuberculosis control officer publicly recommended that all tuberculosis patients be offered counseling and HIV antibody testing and that all those with tuberculosis infection be questioned about HIV risk factors. He further recommended that HIV-infected people be skin tested for evidence of tuberculosis infection and those with a negative reaction, especially from groups in which the prevalence of tuberculosis is high, be considered for INH preventive therapy.[79] Of the seventy-eight cases of tuberculosis identified in Alaska in 1997, thirty-one (40 percent) were known to have been offered HIV testing, and two of them (6.5 percent) were HIV-positive. The most recent figures for Anchorage (2000–2001) showed that twenty-eight cases (58 percent) of tuberculosis had docu-mentation of HIV testing, among whom one was positive.[80] These figures show a need for health authorities to increase HIV testing and counseling in the investiga-tion and treatment of all cases of tuberculosis.

The reporting of AIDS in Alaska has been required since 1985, but the testing at the Fairbanks State Laboratory was done anonymously, except for the availability of some epidemiological information on risk factors. In 1999 Alaska began the mandatory reporting of HIV infection in order to track the risk factors of infection and the progression of the epidemic more effectively. Among its other advantages, the new reporting requirement made it possible to evaluate individuals with HIV infection for risk of tuberculosis and to provide them with suitable educational materials and counseling.

Directly Observed Therapy

One of the most important advances for the treatment of tuberculosis in the past few decades was not a drug, vaccine, or operation, but rather directly observed therapy, or DOT. This approach, pioneered in the late 1960s by Dr. John Sbarbaro of Denver, Colorado, entails twice-weekly therapy, administered in person by a nurse or other health worker, to ensure that the drug is taken as prescribed for the full course of treatment. In the sanatoriums, of course, most patients received their drugs on schedule because the nurse or attendant was there to administer it. Once home therapy became the usual mode of treatment, however, the patient had to assume greater responsibility. The result was that some skipped doses or discontinued the drug altogether because of side effects, rebellion, or simple for-getfulness, thus greatly increasing the risk of drug resistance. The success of DOT in addressing the problem, however, has been demonstrated repeatedly, and this method has become the worldwide standard, including endorsement by the World Health Organization.[81]

As early as 1981, the tuberculosis control program offered its services to any physician treating tuberculosis to set up a direct drug administration program for patients not cooperating with treatment.[82] DOT was first used on a broader scale in about 1987, following the first CDC program review, and since that time has gradually become the standard of treatment in all Alaskan hospitals and clinics. In 1988 DPH adopted DOT as its policy for the administration of drugs for both the prevention and treatment of tuberculosis "whenever possible." It further rec-ognized that sometimes incentives, such as provision of room and board during therapy, might be appropriate for those who resist treatment or whose lifestyles made compliance with treatment regimens difficult.[83]

In 1991, 63 percent of fifty-seven tuberculosis patients were receiving either DOT or weekly supervised therapy.[84] Two years later DPH again affirmed DOT as its policy, warning that individuals with a drug-abuse problem were the most likely to fail to complete therapy.[85] Another difficult group, overlapping with the drug users, were the homeless, but the tuberculosis control program was able to report that six out of nine homeless patients treated in 1992 and 1993 had completed their prescribed therapy, another had taken drugs for five and a half months, and the other two were cooperating with the treatment then under way.[86] In 1994 DPH strongly urged health workers not only to use DOT for treatment but to consider its use for the INH preventive therapy. The tuberculosis control program urged physicians treating tuberculosis patients in hospitals to make preparations for DOT prior to discharge, and offered its assistance in making the necessary arrangements for continuing it subsequently.[87]

In 1994 and 1995, during the continuing investigation and follow-up of the persistent St. Lawrence Island outbreak, DOT was used for those identified as active cases, and also for those on preventive therapy. Special DOT clinics were established in Gambell and Savoonga, and some individuals were visited in their homes to ensure cooperation.[88] Similar arrangements were made during an outbreak at Shishmaref in the winter of 1995–96, and for all tuberculosis patients in Anchorage.[89]

DOT proved practical and effective in both urban areas as well as the most remote areas of Alaska. Between 1990 and 1995 the percentage of tuberculosis patients on DOT increased from 40 to 78 percent, with many living in the villages. The public health nurses were in charge of the program in remote areas. Sometimes they provided the service directly, but more commonly the task was delegated to DOT aides, who received modest compensation for their services. They recorded on a calendar each dose of medication administered, and were often the first to note any side effects. They periodically submitted the calendars and reported any uncooperative individuals to the public health nurse, who in turn passed the information to the tuberculosis control program, where it became part of the patient's clinical record. Incentives, which varied in different regions, were often offered to help ensure the patients' adherence to the requirements of their treatment. DOT has now been accepted by almost all health care providers in Alaska, since there is no cost to the client and no additional resources required from the provider.[90]

Tuberculosis Legislation

Until the 1990s, Alaska public health authorities carried out their anti-tuberculosis activities based either on general laws concerning communicable diseases dating as far back as 1913, or on the tuberculosis laws, originally passed in 1946, that established the tuberculosis control program. These laws were supplemented and implemented by regulations promulgated in the Alaska Administrative Code.

One major gap was how to deal with the recalcitrant tuberculosis patient who refused treatment and was thus a public health threat to the community. As early as 1979, Dr. Robert Fraser, the state tuberculosis control officer, had complained that "our hands are effectively tied" when dealing with such patients. He saw the urgent need for a law that would permit the state to incarcerate temporarily the rare patient with active tuberculosis who rejected treatment and was thus a hazard to the public at large.[91] A 1984 law allowed a state medical officer to order a tuberculosis examination to detect an active case of tuberculosis and then to impose the quarantine of the patient for up to six months "when necessary to preserve and protect public health." Such orders had to be in writing and served personally to the individual in question. In the case of violation, the medical officer reported to the nearest law enforcement agency, and the person, if convicted, became guilty of a class A misdemeanor and subject to imprisonment for not more than a year and a fine not to exceed $5,000, or both.[92] This law was defective in that it did not provide for due process protection and made it a crime for a person to refuse to comply with the law.

On June 8, 1995, DPH finally got the legislation it wanted when Governor Tony Knowles signed into law HB274, which expanded the state's authority to issue quarantine orders and require examinations for tuberculosis. The new law also removed the criminal provision, assured due process protection for any individual unable or unwilling to comply with a tuberculosis order, and allowed the person to request confidentiality of all court proceedings.[93] A state medical officer could require that the individual with tuberculosis be admitted to a health care facility, that he or she complete an appropriate treatment plan and follow required infection control precautions, or even be detained in a treatment facility if "substantial likelihood exists…that the person can not be relied upon to participate in or complete an appropriate treatment plan for tuberculosis." The new provision also allowed the patient to be represented by counsel and to elect whether or not the court review was open to the public. Another provision allowed the state medical officer to request the court to issue an emergency detention order to prevent a threat to the public health.[94]

By 2001 the laws in force for the control of tuberculosis in Alaska included the basic law establishing the program, dating from the 1946 special session of the legislature; the procedures requiring reporting, examination, and enforced isolation when necessary (as outlined above); and the requirement that all school employees be tested annually for tuberculosis. In addition, tuberculosis-control regulations were added to the Alaska Administrative Code, including the provision that each child be required to have a tuberculin test within three months of beginning kindergarten or seventh grade, or entering school for the first time, that all school staff be tested within three months before initial employment, and that all classroom workers and volunteer staff be tested annually. Other sections require testing of health care employees at the time of initial employment and annually thereafter, mandatory reporting of cases of tuberculosis by physicians and laboratories. The Administrative Code also requires annual tuberculin testing for care providers in an assisted living home, school-bus drivers, and pregnant women cared for by a midwife.[95] Although no studies document the effectiveness of these measures, the regulations ensure that those who are most at risk for spread of tuberculosis are periodically tested.

A Tuberculosis Report Card for Alaska at the End of the Century

Overall, the last three decades of the twentieth century have seen a consistent decline in tuberculosis in Alaska, a tribute to the dedicated efforts of the Alaska Division of Public Health, whose staff have often labored under miserly budgets born of public apathy. From 1973, when the state's last tuberculosis ward closed, through 2004, the total number of tuberculosis cases reported annually in Alaska has varied between 112 (1973) and 49 (2002), with fluctuations caused mainly by village outbreaks. Since the population has increased by approximately 50 percent over that period, however, the rates have in fact declined more than these figures would suggest. From 1973 until 1981, the overall rate gradually decreased from 34.3 to 20.7 per 100,000, a decline of nearly 40 percent in the nine-year period. From 1981 to 1985, rates were up again, but then a long-term decline resumed. From 1994 to 2000, the Alaskan rate was elevated once more due to village outbreaks and the high numbers of Asians and Pacific Islanders with the disease.

During the 1990s the median age of people with tuberculosis in Alaska was about forty, and 61 percent were male. Regionally, the highest morbidity rates continued to occur in the northern and southwestern parts of the state, where the Native population predominates. These higher rates vary considerably from year to year because of local outbreaks.

In 1999 Dr. Beth Funk, tuberculosis-control officer for the state, carried out an analysis to determine how the Alaska tuberculosis program measured up to the National Tuberculosis Program Objectives, as set by CDC. These standards and Alaska's "report card" are worth examining in more detail because collectively they show the national state of the art in tuberculosis control and indicate how well Alaska, despite its serious logistical and budgetary problems, is performing. The recommendations can be grouped into those dealing with reporting, contact investigation, and treatment.

Reporting. The CDC electronic reporting system for tuberculosis information from the states requires that 100 percent of newly diagnosed cases and at least 95 percent of specified variables regarding these cases be reported annually. In 1999, all sixty-one cases in Alaska were reported electronically, but only 85 percent of the specified variables were reported. Several, such as "directly observed therapy" and "reason stopped therapy" had low reporting frequencies because some of the cases remained open.

Several reporting standards involved laboratory findings. CDC requires that drug-susceptibility results be reported on at least 90 percent of all new culture-positive cases. Alaska exceeded this goal over the period 1995–99. During 1999 only two of fifty-nine isolates of M. tuberculosis demonstrated single-drug resistance, both from patients who emigrated to the United States from the Philippines.

The standard requires that HIV status be reported for at least 75 percent of new tuberculosis cases in the twenty-five-to-forty-four age group. In the five-year period

1995–99, 50.7 percent of this age group was offered testing, although in the latter two years the figure reached 65.4 percent. In the five-year period four individuals tested positive for HIV and eleven refused testing.

All initial positive cultures for the *M. tuberculosis* complex are to be reported electronically to CDC, and for at least 95 percent of the isolates, all information specified in the *Mycobacterium* module of the Public Health Laboratory Information System is to be provided. The Alaska State Public Health Laboratory reports 100 percent of *M. tuberculosis* cultures, including all information available for each specimen, to CDC using the electronic reporting system.

CDC also requires that at least 80 percent of smears for acid-fast bacteria submitted to the state laboratory be reported back within twenty-four hours, whether positive or negative. The positive smears are reported to the provider and to the tuberculosis-control program by telephone within twenty-four hours. Culture-positive reports of tuberculosis organisms must be reported between two and three weeks from receipt of the specimen. In Alaska in 1999, only 42 percent were reported within three weeks, and 66 percent by the end of four weeks. These delays are at least in part due to the decrease in viability of the specimens because of a long transit time to the laboratory and sometimes repeated freeze-thaw cycles while en route.

According to the CDC, reporting of susceptibility of cultured organisms to first-line drugs should be between fifteen and thirty-five days after the specimen was received. In 1999 in Alaska, less than half of cultures had drug susceptibilities reported within thirty-five days, the overall average being thirty-nine days. The mean time from a positive culture to the reporting of susceptibility was 12.6 days.

Contact Investigation. The CDC requires that at least 90 percent of people with a positive smear have their contacts identified. This standard was met in Alaska in both 1998 and 1999, although in the previous three years the figure had ranged from as low as 61 percent in 1995 to 85 percent in 1997. For those contacts of smear-positive individuals, at least 95 percent should be evaluated for infection and disease. Again, the Alaska program has shown definite progress, especially in 1997 and 1998, when the percentage was 80 percent or above. Prompt follow-up is especially difficult in Alaska, however, because of the great distances, fickle weather conditions, and limited resources of the health department.

Treatment. The CDC standard requires that at least 90 percent of people with newly diagnosed tuberculosis, for whom the course of treatment is one year or less, will have completed treatment within twelve months. Alaska reached this goal on average for the period 1994–98.

The standard for preventive therapy for infected contacts of active cases is that at least 85 percent should complete their course of treatment. Alaska has had some difficulty in meeting this objective, with completion rates ranging from 56 percent to 89 percent in the period 1995–99. The tuberculosis-control program acknowledges that this relatively poor showing requires further study and attention.

For those with a positive tuberculin test found on routine screening, the CDC standard stipulates that 75 percent of people starting preventive therapy will complete the prescribed regimen. For the period 1995–98, an average of 89 percent completed treatment, although the figure for individual years ranged from 73 percent to 94 percent.

The tuberculosis-control program in Alaska has also set some program objectives of its own, to reflect some of the unique aspects of the tuberculosis problem in the state. The first of these objectives is that at least 80 percent of Alaska's reported cases of tuberculosis will complete their recommended course of therapy under DOT. Over the six-year period 1994–99, an average of 77.5 percent of patients completed DOT.

Another Alaska objective is that the incidence of tuberculosis among the homeless in Anchorage will be reduced to no more than 50 cases per 100,000. The number of cases of tuberculosis among the homeless decreased from ten in 1998 to only two in 1999. Over the past five years, however, an annual average of four homeless persons with tuberculosis were identified, for a rate of 50 per 100,000. The statewide tuberculosis-control program provides housing for homeless tuberculosis patients when no other resources can be found, in order to facilitate the administration of DOT.

The majority of new tuberculosis cases in Alaska are found among two specific populations—Asians/Pacific Islanders and Alaska Natives, which together have accounted for over 84 percent of all the cases reported in Alaska between 1993 and 2002. The goal for the Asian/Pacific Islander group is to reduce the annual incidence to no more than 30 per 100,000. This goal has never been reached; in fact, the rate since 1993 has varied between a high of 81.9 per 100,000 (1994) and a low of 41.2 per 100,000 (1998). Through 2002 these figures have shown no tendency to decline, and it is expected that high rates among this group will continue.

Tuberculosis among Alaska Natives continues to be the main focus of the tuberculosis control program. Here the hope is that the rate may be reduced to no more than 35 per 100,000. Over the past ten years, the Alaska Native rate has varied from a high of 78.4 per 100,000 in 1996 to a low of about 21 per 100,000 in 2002, this last perhaps the lowest rate ever. The size of the problem, however, is indicated by the fact that over the past ten years, more than 64 percent of reported tuberculosis cases in Alaska have been among Alaska Natives. The Native rate has remained volatile, resulting largely from village outbreaks. A large number of infected individuals still remain in the villages as a legacy of the great tuberculosis epidemic, and periodic flare-ups with secondary cases are inevitable.

Another objective is to reduce the incidence of tuberculosis in children under fifteen years of age to no more than 2 cases per 100,000. This goal was achieved in 1999, with only two cases reported, giving an incidence rate of 1.2 per 100,000.

Finally, the tuberculosis control program set as a goal that the so-called Alaska TB Committee should meet regularly to direct tuberculosis prevention, control, and elimination activities. In 1999 the committee met on a quarterly basis and addressed issues such as screening of homeless people, targeted tuberculosis testing, the new school tuberculin skin-testing regulations, discharge planning for people with tuberculosis, and the distribution of anti-tuberculosis medications. The group consists of representatives from DPH (including Epidemiology, Public Health Nursing, and Laboratories), the Municipality of Anchorage Department of Health and Human Services, the Alaska Department of Corrections, the Norton Sound Health Corporation, the Alaska Native Medical Center, and the Midnight Sun Chapter of the Association for Professionals of Infection Control and Epidemiology.[96]

Since the 1980s, the face of tuberculosis in Alaska has changed markedly. Before that time, Alaska Natives were the primary population at risk, and efforts of health agencies were directed mainly toward prevention and treatment of tuberculosis in this segment of the population. In the last two decades, however, tuberculosis has posed new threats and has required new approaches. The growing importance of groups at increased risk—those infected with HIV/AIDS, immigrants, the homeless, prisoners—the emergence of multidrug-resistant strains of the organism, and the recrudescence of disease among many Alaska Natives who may have been inadequately treated in the 1940s and 1950s have all contributed to increasing tuberculosis rates in Alaska. Tuberculosis control activities, now firmly anchored and centralized in the Division of Public Health, are built around the following:

- Surveillance, mainly through tuberculin-testing programs in schools and institutions
- Contact investigation and follow-up of newly identified cases
- Modern laboratory methods for the identification, reporting, and sensitivity testing of isolates
- Standardized and up-to-date treatment and prevention protocols of individual cases in the form of DOT

Despite the best efforts of DPH, however, it remains the responsibility of the Alaska state legislature and the Commissioner of the Department of Health and Social Services to ensure that sufficient priority is given this enduring Alaskan problem.

Notes

1. Thomas Parran, ed., *Alaska's Health: A Survey Report to the United States Department of the Interior* (Pittsburgh: Graduate School of Public Health, University of Pittsburgh, 1954), VI-46.

2. *Alaska TB Report 1952–57*, ADH, Division of Tuberculosis Control (Anchorage: ADH, April 1958); *Alaska Tuberculosis Report, 1959*, ADH, Division of Health, Section of Tuberculosis Control (Anchorage: ADH, March 1960).

3. *State of Alaska Tuberculosis Report 1960*, ADHW, Division of Health, Section of Tuberculosis Control (Anchorage: ADHW, March 1961).

4. *State of Alaska Tuberculosis Report 1961*, ADHW, Division of Health, Unit of Tuberculosis Control (Anchorage: ADHW, February 1962).

5. Edwin O. Wicks, "Alaska Department of Health News," *Alaska Medicine* 6 (March 1964): 26–27.

6. *State of Alaska Tuberculosis Report 1964*, ADHW, Division of Public Health, Tuberculosis Control Unit (Anchorage, ADHW, March 1965).

7. J. A. Carswell, "Poverty and Tuberculosis with Particular Reference to the Economic and Social Significance of High Death Rates among Alaskans," *Journal of the National Tuberculosis Association* 34 (1938): 233–46; *Biennial Report of the Office of the Commissioner of Health for the Period July 1, 1938, to June 30, 1940, Inclusive* (Juneau: Territory of Alaska, n.d.).

8. Robert I. Fraser, "The Private Physician in the Modern Treatment of Pulmonary Tuberculosis," *Alaska Medicine* 7 (December 1965): 76–77.

9. Robert I. Fraser, "Tuberculosis in Alaska, 1965, and a Perspective for 1966," typescript, ADHW, January 1966.

10. Fraser, "Private Physician."

11. "New Plans to Combat TB Ready," February 25, 1955, unidentified newspaper clipping, scrapbook #1, ATA Collection; Keith R. Hooker, "A New Approach to Tuberculosis in Alaska," *NTRDA Bulletin* (July–August 1968): 9–12.

12. *Annual Report, 1966*, ADHW; Robert I. Fraser, "Trends in Tuberculosis, Alaska 1965 and a Perspective for the Year" (typescript, presentation for Alaska Tuberculosis Association Meeting, March 26, 1966).

13. Hooker, "New Approach."

14. Lawrence H. Winter, "Increase in Tuberculosis Is Noted," *AH* 18 (October 1961).

15. *State of Alaska Tuberculosis Report 1966*, ADHW, Division of Public Health, Tuberculosis Control Unit (Anchorage: ADHW, April 1967).

16. *State of Alaska Tuberculosis Report 1967*, ADHW, Division of Public Health, Tuberculosis Control Unit (Anchorage: ADHW, April 1968).

17. *State of Alaska Tuberculosis Report 1968*, ADHW, Division of Public Health, Tuberculosis Control Unit (Anchorage: ADHW, April 1969).

18. *State of Alaska Tuberculosis Report 1969*, ADHW, Division of Public Health, Section of Tuberculosis Control and Chest Diseases (Anchorage: ADHW, April 1970).

19. *State of Alaska Tuberculosis Report 1970*, ADHW, Division of Public Health, Section of Tuberculosis Control and Chest Diseases (Anchorage: ADHW, April 1971).

20. *State of Alaska Tuberculosis Report 1971*, ADHSS, Unit of Tuberculosis Control and Chest Diseases (Anchorage: ADHSS, June 1972).

21. As early as 1969 the name of the tuberculosis control program had been changed to Section of Tuberculosis Control and Chest Diseases.

22. *State of Alaska Tuberculosis Report 1972*, ADHSS, Section of Tuberculosis Control and Chest Diseases (Anchorage: ADHSS, June 1973); *State of Alaska Tuberculosis Report 1973*, ADHSS, Section of Disease Control (Anchorage: June 1974).

23. Clarice Dukeminier, "Description of an Outbreak of Tuberculosis in an Alaskan Village, 1970–71," unpublished report, ADHSS, DPH, n.d. This report discusses in some detail some reasons why the Tuberculosis Control Unit could have done a better job.

24. Elfrida H. Nord, "Tuberculosis in Toksook Bay," *Alaska Medicine* 21, no. 4 (July 1979): 53–56.

25. *State of Alaska Tuberculosis Report 1965*, ADHW, Division of Public Health, Tuberculosis Control Unit (Anchorage: ADHW, March 1966).

26. Another reason the use of the tine test was appropriate was that in Alaska there is almost a total lack of tuberculin sensitivity to any *Mycobacterium* except *M. tuberculosis*. See Lydia B. Edwards, George W. Comstock, and Carroll E. Palmer, "Contributions of Northern Popula-tions to the Understanding of Tuberculin Sensitivity," *Archives of Environmental Health* 17, no. 10 (October 1968): 507–12.

27. *Tuberculosis Report 1973*.

28. "Students Must Have TB Test," *Alaska Education Weekly* (January 1982): 6.

29. *State of Alaska Tuberculosis Report 1977*, ADHSS, Section of Communicable Disease Control (Anchorage: ADHSS, June 1978); *State of Alaska Tuberculosis Report 1984*, ADHSS, Division of Public Health, Section of Communicable Disease Control (Anchorage: ADHSS, June 1985).

30. E. W. Piper, "The Nemesis of TB. Architect of Search and Destroy War on Tuberculosis Says It's Not Over Yet," *Anchorage Daily News*, September 29, 1987, E1.

31. John P. Middaugh, personal communication, October 7, 2003.

32. Alan B. Bloch and Walter Q. Page, "Alaska Tuberculosis Program Review, June 22–26, 1987" (typescript, 1987).

33. "Strategy for the Elimination of Tuberculosis in Alaska, Division of Public Health, Section of Epidemiology, January 1988." *Alaska Medicine* 31, no. 1 (January/February 1989): 17–19.

34. John P. Middaugh, personal communication, October 7, 2003.

35. Carl W. Schieffelbein and James Creek, "Alaska Program Review" (typescript, February 13–17, 1995).

36. Michael E. Jones, "Tuberculosis Update," *EB*, no. 10 (May 26, 1992); Michael E. Jones and John P. Middaugh, "The Epidemiology of Tuberculosis in Alaska. 1987," *Alaska Medicine* 31, no. 1 (January/February 1989): 9–16.

37. Michael Jones, "Tuberculosis Outbreak in Savoonga," *EB*, no. 21 (November 26, 1990).

38. "Village Tuberculosis Outbreaks—Update," *EB*, no. 8 (March 9, 1995).

39. Sue Anne Jenkerson, "Public Health Partners Bring Village TB Outbreaks under Control," *EB*, no. 27 (October 25, 1995).

40. Beth Funk, "Shishmaref Teams up to Fight Tuberculosis," *EB*, no. 11 (February 22, 1996).

41. E. A. Funk, "Tuberculosis Control among Alaska Native People," *International Journal of Tuberculosis and Lung Disease* 2, no. 9 (1998): S26–S31.

42. "State Battles New Tuberculosis Outbreaks,"Associated Press State & Local Wire, June 13, 2000; Maureen Clark, "Alaska Tops Nation with Highest TB Rate," Associated Press, June 12, 2001.

43. "Tuberculin Conversions among Staff of an Intensive Care Unit," *EB*, no. 10 (May 20, 1983).

44. "Tuberculosis and Air Travel," *EB*, no. 27 (November 4, 1996).

45. "Finance Subcommittee on Corrections Will Review Native Prison Overcrowding In Alas-ka's Prisons," Alaska State Legislature News Release, Juneau, Alaska, March 17, 1997.

46. *State of Alaska Tuberculosis Report 1964*, ADHW, Division of Public Health, Tuberculosis Control Unit (Anchorage: ADHW, March 1965).

47. *Tuberculosis Control in Alaska, "To Eliminate Tuberculosis in Alaska,"* ADHSS, Division of Public Health (Anchorage: ADHSS, July 2001), 25, 74.

48. Jon Little, "State Screens Prison for TB," *ADN*, November 29, 2000.

49. These categories are used by DPH for their official tuberculosis statistics.

50. Bruce Chandler, "Tuberculosis in Anchorage, 1994–1995," *EB*, no. 16 (March 26, 1996).

51. Bruce Chandler, "Update—Tuberculosis in Anchorage," *EB*, no. 9 (May 15, 2000).

52. Bruce Chandler, "Tuberculosis in Anchorage, Alaska, 1999–2003," *EB*, no. 22 (October 20, 2004).

53. *Manual for the Control of Tuberculosis in Alaska* (Anchorage: Alaska Department of Health and Welfare, Division of Public Health, Unit of Tuberculosis Control, 1966), 8.

54. An incident in October 1991 demonstrated the importance of constant vigilance in the school testing program. Routine testing in the Seward schools led to the identification of twenty-four positives, including ten among the staff. Investigation revealed the probable source case to be a member of the staff, who was promptly put on anti-tuberculosis medication and given sick leave. In January 1992 it was reported that an additional thirty-nine children and one staffer in Seward had converted their tuberculin skin tests. Since the positives were about equally divided among elementary school and high school students, Dr. Michael Jones, the state tuberculosis control officer, expressed skepticism about the results, especially the lack of "clustering" of cases that might suggest a common source. Repeat testing with tuberculin from another manufacturer a few days later revealed that only three of the forty persons were in fact PPD positive. The culprit seemed to be a tuberculin product named Aplisol, for when 60 to 85 percent of these same individuals were tested with a product from a different company they showed no reaction. In light of these findings the tuberculosis control program discontinued use of Aplisol. See Nancy Erickson, "TB Tests Find Bug in Seward: 14 Students, 10 Staffers Infected; Just One Gets Sick," *ADN*, November 22, 1991; Dwayne D. Atwood, "TB Tests Puzzle Officials: 40 More Cases Turn up During Seward Retest," *ADN*, January 23, 1992; "New Tests Contradict Seward TB Report," *ADN*, January 31, 1992; Michael Jones, "False-Positive Aplisol® PPD Reactions," *EB*, no. 9 (May 12, 1992).

55. Michael G. Landen, "Alaska School Tuberculosis Screening, 1994–1995," *EB*, no. 25 (May 27, 1997).

56. Michael G. Landen, "The Risk of Inadequate Tuberculosis Preventive Therapy among Alaska Schoolchildren," *EB*, no. 26 (May 28, 1997).

57. George A. Parks, *Report of the Governor of Alaska to the Secretary of the Interior, 1926* (Washington, DC: GPO, 1926).

58. These figures were calculated as the mean of the five-year period centered on the reported year, using official state morbidity figures and race-specific population figures from the US Census.

59. Jones and Middaugh, "Epidemiology of Tuberculosis."

60. "Alaska's TB Morbidity Drops—but the Battle Is Far from Over," *EB*, no. 19 (June 2, 1993).

61. Chandler, "Tuberculosis in Anchorage, 1994–1995"; Chandler and Funk, "Tuberculosis in Anchorage, 1996–1997."

62. Beth Funk, personal communication, March 14, 2003.

63. *MMWR* 44, no. 38 (September 29, 1995): 703–7.

64. Michael E. Jones, "Drug-Resistant Tuberculosis," *EB*, no. 11 (March 27, 1992). See also World Health Organization, *Anti-Tuberculosis Drug Resistance in the World*, WHO Publication WHO/TB/97.229, chapter 3.

65. *State of Alaska Tuberculosis Report, 1965*, ADHW, DPH, Tuberculosis Control Unit (Anchorage: ADHW, March 1966); Robert I. Fraser, "The Private Physician in the Modern Treatment of Pulmonary Tuberculosis," *Alaska Medicine* 7 (December 1965): 76–77.

66. *Manual for Tuberculosis, 1966*, 51; *State of Alaska Tuberculosis Report, 1967*, ADHW, Division of Public Health, Tuberculosis Control Unit (Anchorage: ADHW, April 1968).

67. George W. Comstock, Shirley H. Ferebee, and Laurel M. Hammes, "A Controlled Trial of Community-Wide Isoniazid Prophylaxis in Alaska," *American Review of Respiratory Diseases 95*, no. 6 (June 1967): 935–43.

68. *Tuberculosis Annual Report, 1977*, ADHSS, Division of Public Health (Anchorage: ADHSS, June 1978).

69. David Templin and Martha Wilson, "The Resurgence of TB in Alaska?" (issue paper, typescript, Alaska Native Medical Center, January 1978).

70. Jones and Middaugh, "Epidemiology of Tuberculosis."

71. J. R. Krevans, "An Unusual Epidemic of Isoniazid Resistant Tuberculosis in a Western Alaska Eskimo Village—Portents for the Future?" *Circumpolar Health 90: Proceedings of the 8th International Congress on Circumpolar Health,* ed. Brian D. Postl, Penny Gilbert, Jean Goodwill, et al. (Winnipeg: University of Manitoba Press, 1991), 339–40.

72. "Tuberculosis in Alaska, 1988–90," *EB,* no. 11 (June 3, 1991).

73. Jones, "Tuberculosis Update."

74. "Alaska's TB Morbidity Drops."

75. "Tuberculosis Treatment Update: Did the Patient Really Swallow All Those Pills?" *EB,* no. 13 (June 23, 1995); Funk, "Tuberculosis in Alaska, 1995."

76. Chandler, "Tuberculosis in Anchorage, 1994–1995."

77. Elizabeth Funk, "Tuberculosis in Alaska 1999," *Epidemiology Bulletin, Recommendations and Reports* 4, no. 4 (July 12, 2000).

78. Michael Jones, "Tuberculosis Update," *EB,* no. 10 (May 26, 1992).

79. In 1999 the Division of Public Health concluded that routine anergy testing was unreliable and did not recommend it further, since even in the face of a negative tuberculin test and evidence of anergy, an individual could still have either latent tuberculosis infection or full-blown tuberculosis. Beth Funk, "Latent Tuberculosis Infection (LTBI)," *EB,* no. 10 (June 26, 2000); Jones, "HIV Infection, Tuberculosis (TB), and Anergy Testing," *EB,* no. 20 (September 2, 1992).

80. "Tuberculosis in Alaska, 1992," typescript, ADHSS, DPH; "Recent Trends in Alaska," typescript (n.d.), ADHSS, DPH; Jones, "HIV Infection and Anergy Testing"; Chandler, "Tuberculosis in Anchorage, 2000–2001."

81. Michael D. Iseman, *A Clinician's Guide to Tuberculosis* (Philadelphia: Lippincott Williams and Wilkins, 2000), 306–7.

82. Robert I. Fraser, "Tuberculosis," *EB,* no. 1 (January 16, 1981).

83. "Strategy for the Elimination of Tuberculosis in Alaska," *Alaska Medicine* 31, no. 1 (1989): 17–19.

84. "Tuberculosis in Alaska, 1988–90."

85. "Alaska's TB Morbidity Drops."

86. "Tuberculosis in Alaska, 1992."

87. "Tuberculosis Threatens Rural Alaskans," *EB,* no. 25 (October 25, 1994).

88. Jenkerson, "Public Health Partners."

89. Funk, "Shishmaref Teams up"; Chandler, "Tuberculosis in Anchorage, 1994–1995."

90. Salynn Boyles and Sandra W. Key, "DOT Possible Even in Remote Areas of Alaska," *TB Weekly,* December 23, 1996; Funk, "Tuberculosis in Alaska, 1995."

91. *State of Alaska Tuberculosis Report, 1979,* ADHSS, Division of Public Health, Tuberculosis Control Unit (Anchorage: ADHSS, August 1980).

92. *Alaska Statutes* 18.15.135–138.

93. Sarah Boyles and Ken Kimsey, "New Alaska TB Law Restores Due Process, Court Confidentiality," *TB Weekly,* August 14–21, 1995: 11.

94. *Alaska Statutes* 18.15.136, 137, 139, 143.

95. The text of these regulations may be found in *Tuberculosis Control in Alaska, July 2001,* ADHSS, Division of Public Health, 84–96.

96. Beth Funk, Personal communication, March 14, 2003; Funk, "Tuberculosis in Alaska 1999."

:: Epilogue

An Uncertain Peace

Why Did Tuberculosis Spread So Rapidly in Alaska?

In concluding this story of tuberculosis in Alaska, it is appropriate to look backwards one more time to explore why this disease, which was probably endemic and sporadic in Alaska prior to 1741, spread so rapidly and destructively through the Alaska Native population over the course of the next two centuries. By the end of World War II, tuberculosis was truly the scourge of Alaska. It permeated every Native village and nearly every Native household, causing suffering, mental and physical pain, crippling, and despair.

There can be of course no definitive or scientific answer to this question. Four main hypotheses can help explain the facts:

1) Before the arrival of Euro-Americans, the Native population had no prior contact with the tuberculosis organism and hence no natural immunity to it.
2) Alaska Natives had some natural immunity to tuberculosis because of their long association with it. A new, possibly more virulent tuberculosis organism, however, was introduced into Alaska by Euro-Americans and selectively affected the Natives more severely.
3) Changing physical and environmental factors in the Alaska Natives' lifestyle promoted the rapid spread of tuberculosis.
4) Psychosocial and cultural stress caused by confrontation with the dominant Euro-American culture reduced immunity to tuberculosis and hastened its progression in affected individuals.[1]

In my opinion, the latter three items each probably played a part in the rapid and extensive spread of tuberculosis in Alaska between about 1800 and 1950. Tuberculosis is likely to have been present as a sporadic disease in Alaska prior to 1741. Due to their previous exposure to an indigenous organism, Alaska Natives presumably had some natural immunity to the strain of the organism that was reintroduced by Europeans. This new strain, which had been very destructive in Europe throughout the eighteenth and nineteenth centuries, could have been more virulent for Natives than for whites, since the latter by long association were beginning to show a reduced susceptibility to it. The paleopathological evidence, if the indigenous organism in question really was *M. tuberculosis*, seems to demonstrate such resistance, as evidenced by a significant healing response in the form of the calcified granulomas and a calcified lymph node in the pre-contact body from Barrow, as well as the concentric layers of fibrosis and calcification in the lymph node from the body from St. Lawrence Island.

A number of physicians and scientists over the years have suggested that Alaska Natives have mounted a good immune response to tuberculous infection. In 1942 Marcia Hayes questioned the popular notion that Natives were genetically more susceptible to tuberculosis and argued instead that the high rates were simply the result of poor economic conditions, malnutrition, excessive exposure to the disease, and lack of facilities for isolation and treatment.[2] Dr. Philip Moore, director of the Mt. Edgecumbe Orthopedic Hospital, observed that Alaska Native patients responded just as well and as quickly to treatment as non-Natives, "once given a clean environment, a proper place to live, good food, adequate medication and surgery when indicated." He thus felt that where there was a lower resistance to the disease, it was attributable to the poor environment in which they lived, not to any race-based lack of immunity.[3] The authors of the Parran Report (1954) also gave particular attention to this topic:

> There is excessive mortality in native infants from miliary, bone and meningeal tuberculosis and a declining rate in adolescents followed by progressively increasing rates with advancing age. These facts led to the tentative conclusion early in this survey that the native has a relatively high degree of natural resistance to tuberculosis, and that the excessive mortality he suffers is due primarily to overwhelmingly wide spread of infection enhanced by crowding and filth.
>
> During this survey we had the opportunity to examine clinical records and serial x-ray films, and consult with experienced physicians concerning the resistance of the native. All evidence that we have obtained supports the conclusion that the native now has as much "natural resistance" to tuberculosis as does the white resident of the States.

The report concluded that the high mortality rate in Alaska Natives was instead due to a high prevalence of tuberculous infection and to living conditions highly conducive to the spread of the disease.[4]

In the 1962 report of the Ambulatory Chemotherapy Program, Porter and Comstock noted that "many patients improved even without treatment and under unfavorable home conditions. This must indicate appreciable resistance against tuberculosis among Alaskan natives, a conclusion in keeping with the clinical impression that exudative tuberculosis is unusually uncommon among them."[5]

Another factor was that as Native communities became more and more influenced by Euro-American society, the environmental conditions under which the

Natives lived generally changed for the worse. Some small villages were consoli-
dated into larger artificial units by the government to facilitate the administration
of schools and other official agencies, or because of die-offs of the population in
epidemics. Occasionally the government established new Native communities, laid
out and designed for its own purposes. These communities brought with them a
more densely massed population, leading to new problems. Sanitation became
worse, especially in permafrost regions, because solid and biological waste simply piled up as village populations increased. New types of frame housing were
established as part of the effort to "civilize" the Natives, but these homes were
difficult and expensive to heat. Because of the shortage of lumber and high costs
of construction, most houses were small and intended for a single family. Instead,
they often became home to a large extended family or to several families, with the
result that tuberculosis and other infectious diseases could easily spread from an
infected person to other family members. People gathered more frequently and in
larger numbers in public places as well, since village life revolved around school
and church activities. The use of store-bought clothing also became widespread.
Although these articles had the benefit of being washable, they were in most cases
less appropriate for the climate than the traditional parkas, mukluks, and other
homemade items.

Many Natives adopted a more sedentary lifestyle as they settled into larger
communities, attended school, and participated in the cash economy. Their diets
also changed for the worse, with greater consumption of refined carbohydrates
and preserved foods instead of high-nutritional-value foods such as fish, caribou,
and sea mammals, supplemented with local plants, especially berries. Occasionally there were periods of hunger or even starvation, resulting either from natural
cycles or, more likely, from wasteful overhunting and overfishing caused by the use
of newer technologies.

Another important factor was the spread of acute infectious diseases that periodically swept through Native communities, sometimes with a gross mortality of
30 percent or more within a few weeks' time. Smallpox, influenza, measles, and
syphilis caused the greatest devastation, although diphtheria, whooping cough,
typhoid fever, mumps, streptococcal disease, and poliomyelitis could also decimate
a population with little or no prior exposure. These diseases had long ago become
endemic in the Western world, affecting primarily children, most of whom had
received at least some immunological protection from their parents. As a consequence, the diseases tended to be milder among Europeans, while in the Native
population they attacked all ages and commonly resulted in a high case-fatality
rate. Those who recovered from such diseases were often left vulnerable to the
development or progression of a tuberculous infection.

Finally, the introduction of tobacco and alcohol had far-reaching effects on
the health of Alaska Natives and their susceptibility to tuberculosis. Tobacco use

undoubtedly contributed to chronic diseases of the lung, which in turn became a fertile field for tuberculosis and other respiratory infections. Alcohol abuse also had many adverse effects, including simple debility, nutritional deficiency, and a manner of living that made its victims vulnerable to tuberculosis.

The earliest, most rapid, and perhaps most radical changes occurred among the Aleut and Alutiiq peoples, who first confronted the Russian adventurers and fur traders in the eighteenth century. Many Natives were killed outright in armed encounters, while many others were abducted from their villages and virtually enslaved, with the men forced to hunt at sea or otherwise work according to Russian priorities, while the women were compelled to make clothing and cook for the invaders, and sometimes satisfy their sexual appetites. Some were forcibly and permanently relocated to faraway Prince William Sound and Southeast Alaska, where they were made to live in Russian barracks and eat Russian food. Most ultimately adopted the Russian Orthodox Church and discovered that their traditional beliefs were incompatible with the new faith. They necessarily learned at least some of the Russian language in order to survive. Their traditional diet, well suited to their needs, progressively deteriorated.

For other Native groups, the forced acculturation was slower but no less inexorable. Although there was little armed conflict between Natives and whites after the Americans arrived in force after 1867, there was a constant struggle, if not for the land, then for the values, attitudes, and even the souls of the Natives. Sometimes the pressures for change were purposeful and explicit, as in the schools and missions; in other situations the pressure for change was more subtle and the result of Alaska Natives' curiosity about and exposure to new technology and goods, such as guns, knives, boats, clothing, new foods and drinks, and new methods of building, lighting, and heating houses. Chapter 2 has already described the stern efforts of teachers, nurses, and doctors to change how Natives thought and lived in order to avoid the ravages of tuberculosis. Their efforts were well meaning and based on good "science," as science was practiced in their time, yet some Alaska Natives must have felt that these authority figures did not value their viewpoints or their cultural practices.

The epidemics that periodically swept through their communities also caused the breakup of families, orphaning of children, and loss of subsistence providers. The epidemics also left survivors with a feeling of hopelessness and loss, not only the physical loss of those they loved but also the loss of something more intangible—a sense of control. That their own traditional methods of healing were ineffective, while most Europeans survived these epidemic diseases, only heightened their sense of powerlessness. Such an experience could destroy their faith in the way of life of their ancestors, leaving them with few spiritual anchors to which their lives could be moored.[6]

Harold Napoleon, in his penetrating essay *"Yuuyaraq,* 'The Way of the Human Being,'"* calls the survivors of these epidemics "listless, confused, bewildered, heart-broken and afraid." Writing specifically of the Yup'ik, Napoleon felt that the people were traumatized by the enormity of their gruesome experience and turned their sorrow inward. They became fatalists, and silently began to abandon the old beliefs by which their lives had always been governed. Much of the joy of their traditional life went out of them. Teachers and missionaries encouraged them to turn away from their old cultures once and for all and become "good, civilized Americans" who would contribute to the economic welfare of their nation. Parents no longer passed on the old values to their children, and even seemed to be ashamed of their beliefs.[7]

Another especially insightful view of this process is that of Ann Fienup-Riordan, an anthropologist who has described the long-term relationship between Euro-Americans and Alaska Natives in terms of seven overlapping stages: resistance, coexistence, population disruption, attempted assimilation, global incorporation, dependency, and finally empowerment.[8] The spread of tuberculosis among the Natives, as discussed here, is primarily related to the stages of population disruption, attempted assimilation, global incorporation, and dependency. Each of these stages involved severe cultural pressures on the Natives—pressures to change from a traditional way of life to that of "mainstream" America. "Old" values were systematically devalued, initially by teachers, missionaries, and officials, and later to a greater or lesser extent by the Natives themselves, who wanted the benefits of the new culture. The process, in some sense at least, was successful, although the stress of such changes may have been greater than we shall ever know.

It is worth pointing out here that from about 1750 to 1900 a similar process of severe sociocultural change took place in Western Europe and contributed greatly to the rise of tuberculosis. During this era the disease, which had been sporadic in earlier times, became the principal cause of death, particularly among the lower socioeconomic classes. Most authorities relate this great increase in the disease to the effects of the Industrial Revolution, when countless rural people were uprooted from their traditional open-air agricultural way of life, thrust into wretched urban tenements, and made to work long hours in poorly ventilated and crowded shops and factories. Others worked long hours in stifling mines and dark offices. All suffered major changes in diet, often leading to malnutrition.[9]

Although tuberculosis is now far less prevalent than it was 100 years ago, as general industrial and social conditions, not to mention control and treatment measures, have improved, hotbeds of tuberculosis in the United States are still to be found mainly among clusters of recent immigrants, migrant workers, refugee groups, drug abusers, and people living in homeless shelters, long-term care facilities, and prisons.[10]

Recent research indicates that cultural, physical, and psychological stresses increase susceptibility to infection or aggravate disease in individuals. The new field of psychoneuroimmunology has been defined as "the study of the intricate interaction of consciousness (psycho), brain and central nervous system (neuro) and the body's defense against external infection and aberrant cell division (immunology)."[11] Both animal and human studies are demonstrating increasingly that many environmental stressors can modify the basic immune competence of the host and lead to suppression of the immune response. Among the forms of stress that have been studied are trauma, natural disasters, change of residence, prolonged rumination, malnutrition, crowding, drug and alcohol usage, bereavement, and feelings of "burnout," depression, loneliness, and hopelessness. These studies have shown, to various levels of scientific persuasion, that psychological stress is an important factor contributing to the development of several infections, including HIV/AIDS, herpes simplex, and the common cold, and may influence their onset, course, and outcome.[12] It has long been known to clinicians that the tubercular patient's state of mind is crucial to his or her clinical progress. One older study showed that stressful life events among tuberculosis patients extended back fourteen years from their admission to the hospital and sharply increased approximately two years before admission. Others have reported that alcohol abuse, dietary deficiencies, and homelessness can influence the progression of tuberculosis, probably through a mechanism of immune suppression.[13] The fundamental and long-lasting stresses of acculturation among the Alaska Natives as they adjusted to (or resisted) modern Euro-American culture over the past two centuries may well have contributed to their susceptibility to the ravages of tuberculosis.

I believe that the rapid and destructive spread of tuberculosis among the Alaska Native population between 1800 and 1950 was caused by a combination of factors. It began with the reintroduction of the new strain of *M. tuberculosis* then widespread in Europe and North America. The epidemic gained momentum as Natives confronted major physical and environmental changes brought on by cultural pressures from the Euro-American society. These changes also bred severe psychological and social stresses which themselves promoted the acquisition and progression of the disease.

The Alaska Tuberculosis Epidemic in Perspective

The tuberculosis epidemic in Alaska was one of the crucial events in the history of Alaska, and especially for the Alaska Native people. For a century—from approximately 1860 to 1960—the disease literally decimated the population. Although reliable figures bearing out this statement are only available for the last decade or so of this era, both the white and the Native population perceived tuberculosis to be the major killer of Alaska Natives for over a century. The disease was a constant force in Native villages, flaring up especially in the months and years after major epidemics of influenza and measles.

It has been widely reported, even in the scientific literature, that Alaska, during its great epidemic, had the highest known rates of tuberculosis of any place in the world. This was probably true, at least by one important measure. The 1953 paper by Weiss cited several times in this book stated, "No available report, not even that based on tests of 'Chinese children of the poorest classes,' shows levels of [tuberculin] sensitivity exceeding those observed among the [Yukon-Kuskokwim] delta Eskimos."[14] In the context of this statement, the author was referring to the finding that in the Yukon-Kuskokwim Delta in the years 1948–51, 89 percent of children five to eight years old had a positive tuberculin test. The highest recorded annual mortality from tuberculosis in Alaska Natives was 1,011 per 100,000, in 1932, at a time when reporting figures for tuberculosis were untrustworthy. If true, this rate would mean that a Native village of 300 people would have about three tuberculosis deaths a year, although the rates in local areas were known to be much higher. The highest mortality rate in the modern era of reporting was 765 per 100,000, in 1945. The highest incidence rate for tuberculosis reported for all Alaska Natives in a single year was 1,823 per 100,000, in 1952. Again, in more understandable terms, a village of 300 persons might show five or six new cases of active tuberculosis each year. Although these figures may seem small, consider that over a ten-year period, about fifty-five people in the village would develop the disease, many of them children or young adults in the prime of life. Another figure showing the impact of the disease on the Alaska Native people is that a peak of 1,311 Alaskans were hospitalized for tuberculosis in December 1955. Although the figure for Alaska Natives hospitalized is not available, 88.5 percent of new cases that year were Native. Thus an estimated 1,160, or approximately 3.04 percent, of the total Native population were hospitalized that year for tuberculosis, or, stated another way, about one out of every thirty-two Alaska Natives was living in a tuberculosis hospital on December 31, 1955.

The Inuit (Eskimos) of Canada also had a devastating experience with tuberculosis. In 1950, the Inuit mortality rate from tuberculosis, according to the Canadian Department of National Health and Welfare, was 718 per 100,000, while in 1958 the tuberculosis morbidity rate reached a peak of 2,143 cases per 100,000. The hospitalization figures in Canada, however, were even more impressive. At the end of 1956, for instance, 703 Inuit, or about 7 percent of the entire population, were in the hospital for tuberculosis, more than twice the rate in Alaska.[15] Moreover, the epidemic lasted longer in Canada, with tuberculosis mortality rates still about 14 per 100,000 in 1969, a time when virtually no deaths were occurring in Alaska.[16]

Perhaps the highest tuberculosis mortality figure ever reported was 9,000 per 100,000, among the Indians of the Qu'Appelle Valley Reserve in western Canada in the late nineteenth century. This meant that 9 percent of the population was dying of tuberculosis *each year*, barely three decades after they had been forced to move to a reserve.[17]

Nor were such high rates limited to indigenous peoples in the twentieth century. A report from London set the death rate from tuberculosis at 1,121 per 100,000 in the years 1771–80, and another study from that era found the cause of death in 36 percent of nearly 700 autopsies almost certainly due to consumption.[18] During the mid-nineteenth century, tuberculosis mortality in many industrialized cities of Europe and the United States hovered from 400 to as high as 800 per 100,000, with a natural decline beginning in most areas about 1870.[19] In selected neighborhoods these figures could be much higher; for example, a New York City study in 1894 found the tuberculosis mortality for the Upper West Side to be 49 per 100,000, while in the tenements of lower Manhattan it reached 776 per 100,000.[20]

Seeking Peace: The Mausoleum of Japonski Island

This history of tuberculosis in Alaska might be fittingly concluded by retelling a recent story that has had not only wide coverage in Alaskan newspapers, magazines, and on television, but which has been circulated throughout the nation. This episode has once again brought to the mind of Alaskans the heartache of the great tuberculosis epidemic, and what it meant to some of the families who suffered its ravages. The story came to light at a time when many still had bitter personal memories about their own experiences with tuberculosis.

In the fall of 1998 the Alaska Department of Transportation began planning for a proposed multimillion-dollar expansion of the Sitka Airport, located on Japonski Island. Plans called for the removal of a concrete ammunition storage bunker, dating from World War II, which stood in the way of extending the taxiway. Robert Sam, a Tlingit of the Sitka tribe with a long-standing commitment to the local cemeteries of Sitka, pointed out to the authorities that this bunker housed the remains of well over 100 tuberculosis victims who had died between 1947 and 1966 at the Alice Island Sanatorium, the Orthopedic Hospital, and the new Mt. Edgecumbe Sanatorium. The remains had been placed in wooden caskets stacked up in the bunkers, encased in cement, with each crypt identified only by a number. An additional eighteen to twenty victims, he reminded them, were interred in another bunker on Coast Guard property not far away.[21]

During the period in which the bodies were placed in the bunkers, neither the Bureau of Indian Affairs, nor, after 1955, the Public Health Service, had budgetary provision for the return of the remains of the deceased, although individual families could personally pay the costs of having a body shipped home. The distances involved and the cost of air freight precluded almost all families in northern and western Alaska from being able to afford this alternative.

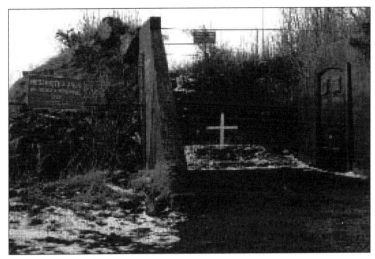

:: Tuberculosis mausoleum on Japonski Island. ::
(Photo by Matthew Hunter)

Bob Sam took on the responsibility of righting this injustice. Working closely with the state Department of Transportation, Mt. Edgecumbe Hospital, the Alaska Federation of Natives, various regional Native organizations, and other state and federal agencies, he was determined to identify the remains of each victim through hospital records, and to try to match the names with living relatives—not an easy task, since some of the villages listed for the patients no longer exist. By December 1998 he had identified thirty families; in one poignant case he located the widow of a victim just a few days before she died.[22] By July 2000, relatives of all the victims except two had been identified. Approximately thirty-eight were ultimately reburied in Sitka, including the remains of three children from the Kuskokwim whose families decided that Sitka was their last "village."

On the weekend of July 7–9, 2000, a public memorial service was held in Sitka, at which time some 300 family members, friends, and visitors—some coming great distances—were given a chance to hear the whole story, to try to understand, and to grieve. Many took the opportunity to meet with and thank some of the surviving doctors, nurses, and other caregivers who were also attending the gathering. Several clergymen, representatives of the state agencies, and Bob Sam were among the speakers, followed by storytelling, gift-giving, and a reception and buffet dinner sponsored by the Sitka tribe and the Alaska Native Brotherhood and Sisterhood. On Sunday various Sitka churches held special remembrances, including "A Journey Back Home" service at St. Michael Russian Orthodox Cathedral. That afternoon at Mermaid Cove on Charcoal Island, there were prayers, sharing, storytelling, and a ceremonial reopening of the crypt.[23]

The actual transfers began that month, and over the following month or so Alaska Airlines flew out approximately four sealed caskets a day, each with a small chunk of concrete from the bunkers as a reminder of this sad story. The state of Alaska paid all shipping and reburial costs.[24] The remains were ultimately laid to rest in some sixty-seven Alaskan communities from Barrow to Metlakatla.[25]

The story of the Sitka Mausoleum and its aftermath is a symbol of the entire story of tuberculosis in Alaska. On the starkest level, it reminds us how a strange and deadly disease attacked the lives of many Natives and how the victims, often in the prime of life, were snatched from their homes and taken to a distant and unfamiliar place where many suffered in loneliness and died. It tells of the worried families left at home and the hardships they underwent to cope without a spouse or child or parent. It tells us that Alaska is an enormous place and that transportation and communication fifty years ago were expensive, unreliable, and often simply nonexistent. It tells us that bureaucracies then (as now) were always underfunded and sometimes unfeeling. But, as readers of this book should appreciate, this story also recounts the constant and tireless efforts of the health leaders of the territory to obtain funds to put a system in place to find, prevent, and treat tuberculosis despite huge fiscal and bureaucratic obstacles. The story also reminds us that fiscal and administrative rules made in Washington, D.C., may appear totally irrelevant in faraway Alaska. The administrators at Mt. Edgecumbe simply had no authority to spend money to transport bodies home. At all the hospitals, however, they made every effort to notify relatives of the death of loved ones. That this effort failed at times because of language barriers, distance, lost messages, or human error is regrettable, but it should not be attributed to indifference.

The use of the ammunition bunkers for burial seems now—a half century later—rather cold-blooded and disrespectful, yet I suspect that at the time the Alaska Native Service saw it as a reasonable solution to a difficult problem. The simple wooden caskets were treated respectfully and placed in a safe and relatively inaccessible place. All Alaskan tuberculosis hospitals had chaplains, and whenever possible interment services were held in keeping with the deceased's religious preference. When no information was available, the local Presbyterian minister led the service.[26]

This story should also remind us that countless nurses, physicians, technicians, and support personnel worked in Alaska for minimal pay, sometimes under dangerous and appalling physical conditions, to provide care and preventive tuberculosis services in the villages as well as in the hospitals. These were generally idealistic people of strong commitment who loved their work and deeply respected and cared for the Native people. In addition, scores of committed volunteers worked at all the hospitals and made regular contact with families one of their major priorities. Employees and volunteers alike worked very hard to brighten the lives of those committed to their care, especially the children. Sometimes they may have had lapses in cultural sensitivity, but this was through ignorance, not ill will or prejudice.

This tale, of course, had a positive ending. Once the state of affairs was fully recognized, it was at last set right. True, fifty years and more had passed and the world had already moved on, perhaps in an attempt to forget an uncomfortable period in Alaskan history. People, in any case, are usually most reluctant to disturb the remains of those who have died. When the situation demanded action, however, a chain of events led to the ultimate identification of all the remains and repatriation of the majority. Many individuals were able to find some peace, after decades of uncertainty, when the bones of their family members at last came home again. The whole process was set in motion by the leadership of a single Alaska Native, Robert Sam, who felt deeply about the task before him. He was helped by many others, especially Diane DeRoux and Frank Mielke of the Alaska Department of Transportation, but also by Alaska Native organizations, some twenty-eight state and federal agencies, the airlines, and many volunteers. The present-day outpouring of leadership, cooperation, selfless effort, and good will that this incident has evoked should remind us all that these were some of the very qualities that have characterized the course of Alaska's enduring struggle with tuberculosis.

Notes

1. Dr. George W. Comstock, in a personal communication on September 19, 2003, suggests a fifth hypothesis. He was struck by the fact that although he had read over 10,000 chest x-rays of Alaska Natives in the 1950s, he rarely or ever saw a case of exudative tuberculosis (tuberculous pneumonia), whereas this type of tuberculosis was far more common among poor blacks in Georgia and Alabama. Some experimental evidence exists suggesting that people on a high-protein diet, such as the traditional Eskimo diet, tend to have fibrotic tuberculosis, while those on a protein-deficient diet, like the poor blacks, have more of the exudative type.

2. Marcia Hayes, "Some Problems of Health in Alaska," *Proceedings of the 6th Pacific Science Conference* (1942): 465–72.

3. Philip H. Moore, "Tuberculosis of the Bones and Joints as Found in the Alaskan Native," typescript (n.d. [1954?]), 3. Copy in the files of the Alaska Department of Health and Social Services, Division of Public Health, Epidemiology Section.

4. Thomas Parran, ed., *Alaska's Health: A Survey Report* (Pittsburgh: University of Pittsburgh Graduate School of Public Health, 1954), VI-33.

5. Merilys E. Porter and George W. Comstock, "Ambulatory Chemotherapy in Alaska," *Public Health Reports* 77, no. 12 (December 1962): 1021–32. "Exudative tuberculosis" refers to the rapidly progressive forms of tuberculosis characterized by an intense inflammatory reaction and tissue destruction.

6. For further discussion and examples, see Robert Fortuine, *Chills and Fever: Health and Disease in the Early History of Alaska* (Fairbanks: University of Alaska Press, 1989), 225, 230, 232, 237.

7. Harold Napoleon, *Yuuyaraq: The Way of the Human Being* (Fairbanks: Alaska Native Knowledge Network, 1996). I have drawn heavily on Napoleon's work in this section. Although his analysis of the effects of epidemic disease and forced acculturation focuses on the later development of alcoholism and other self-destructive behaviors, I think that many of his insights also support my theme here: that the severe cultural disruption and destruction caused by the epidemics and their aftermath also contributed to the susceptibility of the survivors to chronic diseases such as tuberculosis.

8. Ann Fienup-Riordan, *Culture Change and Identity among Alaska Natives: Retaining Control* (Anchorage: Henry M. Jackson Foundation, 1992), 1–6.

9. René and Jean Dubos, *The White Plague: Tuberculosis, Man and Society* (Boston: Little, Brown and Company, 1952), 65–66, 197–208; Thomas Dormandy, *The White Death: A History of Tuberculosis* (New York: New York University Press, 2000), 73–84.

10. Lawrence Geiter, ed., *Ending Neglect: The Elimination of Tuberculosis in the United States* (Washington, DC: National Academy Press, 2000), 31–33.

11. K. R. Pelletier and D. L. Herzing, quoted in Lawrence T. Vollhardt, "Psychoneuroimmunology: A Literature Review," *American Journal of Orthopsychiatry* 61, no. 1 (January 1991): 35–47.

12. Vollhardt, "Psychoneuroimmunology"; Janice K. Kiecolt-Glaser, Lynanne McGuire, Theodore F. Robles, and Ronald Glaser, "Psychoneuroimmunology: Psychological Influences on Immune Function and Health," *Journal of Consulting and Clinical Psychology* 70, no. 3 (2000): 537–47.

13. Massimo Biondi and Luca-Gionata Zannino, "Psychological Stress, Neuroimmodulation, and Susceptibility to Infectious Diseases in Animals and Man: A Review," *Psychotherapy and Psychosomatics* 66 (1997): 3–26.

14. Edward S. Weiss, "Tuberculin Sensitivity in Alaska," *Public Health Reports* 68, no. 1 (1953): 23–27.

15. Pat Sandiford Grygier, *A Long Way from Home: The Tuberculosis Epidemic Among the Inuit* (Montreal and Kingston: McGill-Queen's University Press, 1994), 71, 83–85. It must be pointed out, however, that the Eskimo patients in Canada tended to stay in hospital longer because of the great distances to and extreme isolation of some of their communities. For further insights into the Canadian experience, see also "Life as a TB Patient in the South," *Inukitut* no. 71 (1990), 20–29, and Frank James Tester, Paule McNicoll, and Peter Irniq, "Writing for our Lives: The Language of Homesickness, Self-Esteem and the Inuit TB 'Epidemic,'" *Etudes/Inuit/Studies* 25, no. 1–2 (2001): 121–40.

16. S. Grzybowski and K. Styblo, "The Relevance of Studies of Tuberculosis in Eskimos to Antituberculous Program Planning," in *Circumpolar Health*, Proceedings of the Third International Symposium, Yellowknife, NWT, ed. Roy J. Shephard and S. Itoh (Toronto: University of Toronto Press, n.d.), 334–41.

17. Dubos and Dubos, *White Plague*, 191.

18. Michael E. Teller, *The Tuberculosis Movement: A Public Health Campaign in the Progressive Era* (New York: Greenwood Press, 1988), 6.

19. Geiter, *Ending Neglect*, 23; Selman A. Waksman, *The Conquest of Tuberculosis* (Berkeley: University of California Press, 1966), 20–21.

20. Sheila M. Rothman, "Seek and Hide: Public Health Departments and Persons with Tuberculosis, 1890–1940," *Journal of Law, Medicine, & Ethics* 21, no. 3–4 (Fall–Winter 1993): 289–95.

21. The Coast Guard had been using the site for tool storage until Sam brought the situation to light, after which it allowed members of the Sitka tribe full access and made a formal apology to the tribe. See James MacPherson, "Bitter History: Bodies of Tuberculosis Victims Found in Forgotten Mausoleum," *Alaska* (April 1999): 14.

22. "Entombed and Forgotten. Now's Time to Make It Right," Dispatch Alaska, *ADN*, December 13, 1998, B7.

23. Mark Boesser, "The Journey Home," *Alaskan Epiphany* 22, no. 2 (August 2000): 6, 28.

24. Liz Ruskin, "A Better Place," *ADN*, July 9, 2000, A1.

25. Will Swagel, "The Journey Back Home," *Alaskan Southeaster* 11, no. 2 (February 2001): 28–31; Ruskin, "Better Place"; Amanda Bohman, "Victims of 50-year Old TB Epidemic Returned to Families," *ADN*, July 29, 2000, B9.

26. Liz Ruskin, "TB's Harsh Toll," *ADN*, July 30, 2000, A1.

Appendix :A:

A Look at Sanatorium Life in Alaska

EXPERIENCES OF TUBERCULOSIS differed, depending on culture, environmental conditions, and socioeconomic status. Even within Alaska, a tubercular white man with independent means might travel to Seattle, Denver, or San Francisco and pay for private care, while his poorer counterpart might receive his care, funded through the territorial Department of Welfare, in a state sanatorium in Seattle. A veteran might be sent to a veterans' hospital in the continental United States, where he would receive adequate but no-frills care at no personal cost, while a child with orthopedic problems might spend as long as three years away from family. The focus of this book is on Alaska Natives, who had by far the most serious tuberculosis problem in Alaska, and who experienced the greatest disruption and turmoil. This section will examine some of the features of hospital life for an Alaska Native with tuberculosis.

In the 1940s, when tuberculosis beds in Alaska were in critically short supply, an Alaska Native might be diagnosed in the village through an x-ray survey, then wait two years or more before being called to the hospital. In such cases the public health nurse would attempt to create optimal conditions in the home, both for the patient's comfort and the family's safety. Poverty, a crowded household, and the stark reality of village life, however, often rendered these arrangements irrelevant. Many patients became sicker, some died, and others in the household were nearly always infected.

Sooner or later, a person who survived long enough would be notified by the nurse, or by a telegram, that a bed had become available at a sanatorium. The message would indicate that an airplane would be arriving in the village, perhaps within days, to take them to a hospital in a faraway location, such as Skagway, Sitka, Seward, or even Tacoma, Washington, for treatment. Most had little concept of where these places were.

The individual had no real choice in the matter: the decision had been made by distant health officials on the basis of a positive x-ray or sputum test. A few flatly refused to go to the hospital, or agreed to go only if they could be assured that they could go to a certain hospital, or be accompanied by a friend or relative from the village. The nurse, in good faith, might promise to do her best to comply with these wishes, but when the exigencies of the program thwarted the plan, the patients felt betrayed and angry.[1]

Those who had been summoned to the hospital were taken away with only enough time to grab a few essentials before boarding a plane, often for the first time in their lives. They were permitted a single small suitcase, and specifically advised to bring only a few toiletry articles, pajamas, a bathrobe, slippers, and a sweater. Optional articles that were permitted included writing materials, photographs, and materials used in crafts and handiwork.[2] They were required to put on a cloth mask covering the nose and mouth and to wear it until they reached the hospital ward.

Robert Mayokok, the noted Eskimo Inupiat artist and writer, wrote of his experience when he left his village for the hospital in 1947:

> When a single-motored plane came for me, I did the worst thing any father would have done. . . . I did not see my children to say good-by to them. They were in school when I left. I thought it was for the best, but I have never ceased to regret that ever since. My only thought was that it was better that way, in a short time I might be dead anyway. . . . If you are compelled by circumstances to leave your children, be sure to give them an affectionate farewell. I thought of my children every day, and how circumstances denied me their companionship. I am still hoping for the best. But, may God's will be done.[3]

Some indeed assumed that they were going away to die, and their fears were augmented by the rumor—not far from the truth, as events showed—that the doctors threw away the bodies of those who died at the hospital if the family could not pay for transportation home.[4] Even those lucky ones who survived sometimes did not return for two or even three years. By then they had discovered that they would no longer be able to hunt, fish, trap, or carry out their household chores as before.

The first stop was usually a regional center, such as Bethel, Kotzebue, or Barrow, where the patient was transferred, still with mask and single suitcase, to a larger two-engine plane for the trip to Fairbanks or Anchorage. This aircraft might include several other tuberculosis patients who had been brought in from other villages for transport to the sanatorium.

Most of the patients destined for the sanatoriums came from the villages of northwestern and western Alaska, although some were sent from Bristol Bay, the Aleutians, and the Interior. Few had ever spoken on a telephone, seen a television set, or eaten at a restaurant. They discovered paved streets, traffic lights, supermarkets, multistory buildings, elevators, and escalators for the first time. For those from the tundra of northern and western Alaska, or from the Aleutians, even trees were a novelty, particularly the massive Sitka spruce of Southeast Alaska.

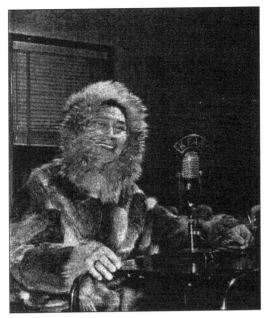

:: Studio photo of Robert Mayokok. ::
(Courtesy of University of Alaska Fairbanks, Rasmuson Library,
Alaska and Polar Regions Department, Robert O. C. Steiner
Collection, Box Z, Folder 53, 91-164-123)

On arriving in Seattle, Mayokok described his feelings:

The houses looking like pictures in a picture book seemed to be catapulting toward us a few inches below the belly of our plane. Suddenly there was a slight bump. We knew that we had landed. Simultaneously 40 or 50 of us Natives sighed with relief. The big plane stopped moving. The stewardess opened the door and we found that there was a stairway already placed from the plane to the ground. We filed out, stepping on the new soil, far from Alaska.

We saw trees, trees, trees everywhere. In the barren coasts of Alaska none of my people have ever seen trees, except those who live in the Interior. We saw enormous buildings, as high as the skies. What was inside we could not even imagine. We saw cement walks and endless paved roads. We saw wonders we have never seen before in the Eskimo land. We saw swarms of people.[5]

At their final destination, they were loaded into an ambulance or van and driven to the hospital, where their own clothes were taken away. They were bathed, given scanty lightweight pajamas, and unceremoniously put to bed either in a single room, if very sick, or with one to three roommates. If their disease was active, they were not even allowed out of bed to the bathroom.

A few were lucky enough to find someone from their village, or at least some-one who spoke their language. Sometimes it was a nursing assistant, housekeeper, kitchen worker, or other employee who could help communicate with the doctors and nurses. Finding other patients in the same circumstances was a comfort to some. As Mayokok wrote. "At the sanatorium, I met men and women from all over the territory. I admired their pluck and courage. Each one was determined to lick the TB." But it was hard to bear the sadness all around. "Some of the patients were brought in too late...too far gone...and they last only a few days. I believe many of them died of loneliness and homesickness. Only those who panted to live, because of their love for their families, turned for the better."[6]

Being in the hospital for a long period left both physical and psychological scars. As the patient lay for months in bed, he or she would think of the family at home and the responsibilities not being faced. There was always concern about money, and whether the house was warm and the children and spouse were getting enough to eat. Still others had marital or other relationships that were aggravated by the separation.

Mayokok noted that it was especially difficult for Eskimos to adjust to the hospital routine, since they had never been used to being confined. At home they moved about wherever and whenever they wanted to. He found it especially irksome to wait for a wheelchair or stretcher to go for an x-ray: "I always feel like a bird in a cage with no where [sic] to fly."[7]

According to a study carried out in the Seattle hospitals, it was the older patients who found hospitalization especially hard. Most spoke little English and thus were dependent on other Natives to express even their basic needs. They found themselves isolated not only from staff but from Natives who did not speak their language. Those who did better in the hospital setting were individuals with healthy family ties, and who before getting sick were self-sufficient, stable, and well adjusted. Similarly, those who could speak English, had lived in towns, had had positive past relationships with whites, and had completed more classroom education generally made a good adjustment. Some, on the other hand, adapted reasonably well to their new surroundings and made the best of what they came to understand as a necessary evil. Younger people, especially if they knew some English and were willing to try to speak it, were even more flexible and receptive to new ideas and new surroundings. They had a smaller investment in the "old life," not to mention fewer family responsibilities back in the village. Most of them learned quickly and readily took advantage of classes and training opportunities.[8]

In the era of chemotherapy there were dozens of pills to be swallowed each day. After 1951 nearly every hospital patient was on PAS as well as twice-weekly streptomycin injections. PAS was dispensed in large tablets and the standard daily dose was about twenty-four pills, divided into four doses. Many patients had serious difficulty swallowing such a large number of large pills several times a day for months on end. INH tablets, in use after 1952, were distinctly smaller as well as less frequently taken, but they too added to the burden, along with vitamins and other prescribed medications. Some drugs had serious, or at least bothersome, side effects.

Many patients with pulmonary tuberculosis required surgery, either because of the extent of their disease or as a means for shortening their treatment. The extent of surgery varied from the removal of an entire diseased lung to simply injecting air into the peritoneal cavity. All these procedures were unpleasant for the patient, several were not without considerable risk, and a few led to long-term disabilities. The major thoracic surgical procedures used in Alaska included pneumonectomy, lobectomy, segmental resection, thoracoplasty, and pneumonolysis, all of which are described in the introduction to this book. All these operations were thoracotomies, in which the chest wall was opened, and all required extended periods of general anesthesia. The "minor" surgical procedures, also described earlier, included thoracocentesis, pneumothorax, pneumoperitoneum, phrenic crush, and phrenicectomy. Each of these procedures, though generally less dangerous, could be quite painful.[9]

A few Natives were terrified at the prospect of surgery. One Seattle hospital wisely scheduled young cases with a good prognosis first, in order to increase the confidence of the other patients, but another took the opposite approach and operated first on those who were sickest (and thus in greatest need). Several of the earlier patients died, causing even greater anxiety and reluctance to cooperate.[10]

The hallmark of sanatorium life everywhere was routine. Most tuberculosis specialists of that era believed that patients required a strict daily discipline to get well, one justification being that a routine would take away much of the worry of everyday decision making. The typical daily schedule in 1954 at the Seward Sanatorium, handed out to patients, looked something like this (slightly abbreviated):

6:15   Awakened to use bedpan, wash and brush teeth. Before you wash in the morning, put your sputum cup in your paper bag and fold over the top of the bag, so that the contents will not spill out. Now wash your hands and face and brush your teeth. Every patient is expected to brush his teeth twice daily, morning and afternoon.

8:00   Breakfast. It is important that you eat all the food offered you. Meals are planned so that you may have as balanced and nourishing a diet as possible. Even though you may not like some of the food served, you should learn to eat all of it.

8:45   Morning care begins. You will receive a full bath once a week, with a complete change of linen, and will have a shampoo once a month if your condition permits.

9:00–10:30	This period is used by those who have occupational therapy time, for the amount of time allotted you by the doctor. Those whose condition does not permit occupational therapy activity will continue their bed rest treatment.
8:45–11:00	This is the time needed by the nurses to do morning care. Work will be done so that your basic treatment, bed rest, will be interfered with as little as possible. Those not receiving care will try to relax and rest. Nourishment will be passed out during this period and also bedpans to those who need them.
11:30	Lunch.
12:30	Bedpans will be passed out.
1:00–3:00	This is your afternoon sleeping period and is not broken for any except unusual reasons. All patients are encouraged to sleep. If this is not possible, try to relax and lie as still as possible. There will be no talking, reading, or any other activity during this period.
3:00	Temperature time, patients are encouraged to read their own thermometers.
3:30–4:00	Wash basins will be passed out. Everyone will brush his teeth and wash his face and hands.
3:00–4:00	is also visiting hour. Instruct your visitor to talk quietly. They should not sit on the beds, neither should there be any kissing or petting. All visitors should wear masks.
4:30–5:00	Dinner. Eat all that is served you.
5:00–9:00	Your rest treatment still continues but to help divert your mind and relax you, movies will be shown for one hour twice a week on each ward. On Sundays there will be visiting among the patients. If you are in Class II or higher, you may visit by wheelchair. If you are in Class I, you will have to go by stretcher and remain on the stretcher during the entire visiting hour. This is to protect you from becoming too tired. Visiting permits will be issued by the nurses. Please do not visit without a pass. Each patient is allowed two visitors only.
	There will be nourishment passed every night at this time also. We do not encourage you to drink coffee other than at meal-time. Milk is the ideal food especially for you.
9:15	Lights out. You need a great deal of sleep, that is why we ask that you put your lights out early and promptly.
10:00	All radios off.
10:00–6:15	There will be a night attendant to attend to your needs. Remember, though, that they are governed by the orders of the doctors and may give you nothing for which they have no written order.[11]

The meals were also served on a rigid and unfamiliar schedule, with the food itself often strange and unappetizing. All the ANS hospitals made at least an attempt to accommodate the tastes of the Natives, but in practice this boiled down to providing reindeer meat and salmon occasionally, although seal meat, tongue, and moose (usually from roadkill) were also sometimes served. In the early sanatorium years, war surplus military rations, including powdered milk and powdered eggs, were unwelcome staple foods. The fruits and vegetables that were served were unfamiliar to most patients. Food or drink could not be brought in from outside the hospital by the rare family or friends who visited.

Meals, baths, long rest periods, and pills punctuated the day. Until sputum tests were negative (sometimes months), patients had to wear masks whenever they were outside the room or seeing visitors. No one could leave the floor without the permission of the nurse, and to leave the hospital was out of the question until the late stages of the hospital stay, when the patient was no longer infectious to others.

Boredom became a deadening and insidious disease in its own right. Many were unable to read or write and had no means to communicate with their loved ones at home, except when a volunteer was willing to help. Most tuberculosis patients stayed in the hospital for six to nine months at a minimum, and in the pre-drug era often as long as two or three years. The second patient to be admitted to the new Alaska Native Hospital in Anchorage, in November 1953, stayed 660 days. A few children suffering from chronic lung disease or more serious orthopedic disabilities stayed so long that they even lost their ability to speak their own language.

ADH tried to ease the transition to the hospital by making available several articles and pamphlets that described what a Native patient should expect in the hospital, but these also largely missed their mark. One purports to be written by a Native at the Skagway Sanatorium, but reflects more the viewpoint and issues of the nurses and doctors than those of the Natives.[12] Another pamphlet takes the point of view of a Native woman who was discharged from the hospital telling a new patient what to expect.[13] Quite aside from the inappropriateness of some of these efforts, many of the older Natives did not read English.

Patients were categorized into different groups depending on their clinical response as they gradually progressed through various stages of treatment. Each category had its own restrictions and incentives. At the Seward Sanatorium during the 1950s, all patients were classified as follows:

Class I. Patients must remain in bed throughout the 24 hours, they should be lying flat in bed all the time except at meal times when they may sit up on a back rest. Writing is permitted only for 1/2 hour daily, no handiwork is allowed. Reading is to be limited to 2 hours.

Class II. Patients may go to bathroom once daily. They may sit up on a back rest for meals and for 30 minutes daily to do their writing; at all other times they should be flat in bed. Reading allowed. Baths will be taken in bed and usual rest periods taken.

Class III. Patients may go to bathroom three times daily, bathe or shave themselves in the morning. They may sit up on a back rest for meals and from 3–5 p.m. and do their writing during that period. At all other times they are to remain flat in bed.

Class IV. Patients may eat lunch and supper out of bed and remain up for 1/2 hour after meals. Reading and writing are allowed at any time except rest period. They are to make their beds daily and give aid to nurses as required.

Class V. In addition to the above, patients are allowed walking exercises for a certain length of time specified by the physician. They are to make their own beds in the morning and to remain in bed during rest period.

All patients began in Class I, and only slowly progressed through the other stages depending on their temperature chart, body weight, and x-ray findings, but most of all on the basis of their sputum smears and cultures. Except for those in Class V, patients spent nearly all their time in bed, usually flat on their backs gazing at the ceiling. Most of the time they could neither read, nor write, nor talk to friends, nor listen to the radio. When in the presence of staff or visitors, or whenever they were out of their room, they had to wear a cloth mask covering the nose and mouth.

The "rule book" from the Seward Sanatorium reminded the new patient at the outset that the sanatorium was a "training school." By carrying out the prescribed tasks faithfully, it went on, "you will learn to discipline your emotions." The pamphlet then intoned:

[C]heerfulness and the determination to get well, you must provide. . . . You will also learn how to live with others without being in danger to their health. And, when you leave the hospital you will be, we hope, a messenger of health and a teacher of others. For these reasons, it is expected that you will enter wholeheartedly into the spirit of our hospital. Be helpful and encouraging to others. Taking the cure depends on you. The doctors and nurses only guide you to do the right things.

It then went on to list thirty-four regulations. The first instructed patients not to sneeze or cough without covering their mouth and nose with a paper tissue, and the last bluntly reminded patients that the territory had a law requiring isolation of patients with contagious diseases. In between were many other prohibitions, of which the following are a sample:

- Patients cannot show visitors through the hospital.
- Women patients are allowed only in the women's division and men patients are allowed only in the men's division.
- Patients are not permitted to visit each other at any time without permission of the nurse in charge.
- Men and women patients are not to visit each other within the hospital or while out on exercise, without permission from the doctor.
- No patient is allowed to associate with an employee, or to have deals of any sort.
- Patients must not exchange wearing apparel.

- Patients should not discuss their illnesses with one another.
- Patients must not congregate in rooms, lavatories, or halls.
- Patients' personal belongings are to be reduced to such proportions as can be kept on the bedside table and these are to be kept neat and orderly at all times.
- The use of the telephone by patients is forbidden.
- All windows, doors controlling ventilation in all rooms and wards are to be operated only by direction of the nurse or doctor.
- Non-cooperation on the part of the patient is cause for disciplinary action.

Despite these rigid pronouncements, the pamphlet breezily suggested that "the regulations provided are not arbitrary, disciplinary rules, but safeguards devised entirely for your benefit."[14]

A similar rule book survives from the Anchorage hospital. The rules were much the same, although there were some additional restrictions imposed. For example:

- All notes, packages, letters, etc., must go through the hospital post office. Only short, open notes may be handled by the ward worker of the nursing department and that only within the ward she works.
- Do not use chair seat as a storage shelf.
- Do not float emesis basin in wash basin.
- At meal time place any leftover food on your tray in one receptacle. Papers and liquids are kept separate. All dishes must go out to be sterilized for next meal.
- Keep belongings in your storage space or on the bed. Anything which drops to the floor is contaminated and is placed in a box in the linen room for proper decontamination.

At the end of these rules and prohibitions, a list of "contraband articles" was appended. These included private radios or TV sets, firearms or other articles considered dangerous, personal drugs, and alcohol. Curiously, smoking was discouraged only because it increased coughing and dulled the appetite. Bed patients were not permitted to smoke, but "up" patients could smoke except while in bed.[15]

Most of these regulations and routines may have been necessary for the function of an orderly institution, although one must wonder whether words like "contraband, "nourishment," or "emesis" were lost on most readers. Many of the regulations seem unnecessarily harsh, and even an impediment to recovery from a serious illness, but they were common in sanatoriums of the era and by no means unique to Alaska.[16] For Alaska Natives, however, such rules flew in the face of their daily habits of living.

The regulations provided that patients be segregated by sex and age, even when more than one member of a single family was admitted to the hospital. By the rules, however, even couples had to be separated, with the men on one ward, women on another, and the children on yet a third. Visiting was possible only at brief times and then only in the central area of the hospital, with everyone wearing a mask. Mothers could not visit their infant children unless the latter were on the seriously ill list. If a tubercular mother delivered a baby in the hospital, the child was taken away at birth and put in a foster home until the mother was released from the hospital. Even when an older child and his or her mother were admitted to the same hospital, they were able to visit each other only once a week.[17]

Although most patients were quite cooperative and well behaved, boredom and frustration sometimes broke through and led to disciplinary problems. Stir-crazy patients on occasion were known to sneak out of the hospital and even run away in their pajamas, only to be brought back by the police. Sometimes they brought back alcoholic beverages from the bars or stores while on pass, but more commonly alcohol was smuggled in by visitors. Noninfectious patients were occasionally given permission to leave the hospital for a day or even for a weekend to visit friends or relatives, but all too often they returned not only intoxicated themselves but armed with bottles for their friends on the ward as well. Bottles, full or empty, were discovered by nurses or doctors hidden under pillows, in jigsaw puzzle boxes, and in a variety of other ingenious caches. Occasionally the situation got completely out of hand, with patients passing out from excessive drinking or getting into brawls on the ward. One patient at Anchorage was arrested for striking a nurse, and on another occasion the medical officer of the day had to engage in hand-to-hand battle in the tuberculosis ward with a drunk patient brandishing a knife.[18]

Despite all the restrictions and regimentation, the hospital staff did what they could to make life easier for the patients. The social service department and local volunteers actively tried to keep families in touch by writing letters or arranging for radio messages to be sent to the village. Local or traveling entertainers often came to the hospital to present a show. At the time of major holidays, the volunteers decorated the wards, piped in appropriate music, and arranged small gifts for everyone.

Christian chaplains and other church representatives visited the sanatorium at least twice a week and usually held Sunday services. They talked with the patients, comforted them, prayed with them, and sometimes wrote letters for them. For some patients, these visits offered new hope and encouraged them to persevere with the long course of treatment.

The patients themselves tried to keep up each others' spirits. News accounts from the individual wards in the various sanatorium newspapers, edited by the patients, brimmed with words of encouragement, funny stories, gossip, praise, good cheer, and optimism. The patients loved to celebrate birthdays, a going-away party, and especially to give recognition to those who were making progress in their struggle against the common enemy. Particularly prominent were the accolades patients

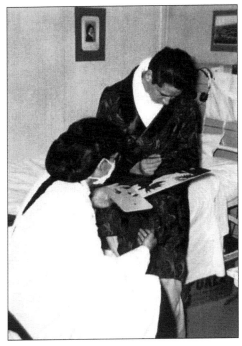

:: Tuberculosis patient receiving art instruction ::
at Seward Sanatorium, 1950s.
(Courtesy of Margery Albrecht)

bestowed on each other for reaching coveted milestones, such as being allowed out of bed for one hour or graduating from one hour to two or three, especially if accompanied by "BRP" ("bathroom privileges").[19]

The occupational therapy department organized many manual activities, including drawing, painting, sewing, weaving, beadwork, ivory carving, leather work, woodwork, and other crafts for the patients. Live radio, recordings, movies, and later television were available to help fill up the long hours. Some patients played musical instruments, such as guitars or harmonicas. Despite these respites—and the best intentions of the staff—life in the sanatorium was dull, restrictive, burdensome, vexatious, and seemingly endless. Keeping busy helped occupy the hands and mind, but it was no substitute for freedom and for the familiar faraway life that they had known with family and friends.

Children who were hospitalized for tuberculosis had their own set of problems and issues, and those with tuberculosis of the bones and joints had a particularly difficult time. Some were as young as five or six years old, although most were older. When first sent to the hospital, many had at least one painful, swollen joint, sometimes with a draining sinus. Those with tuberculosis of the spine often had a hunchback appearance, sometimes with urinary incontinence or paralysis of the lower extremities. These children usually required at least two years in the hospital, much of that time immobilized in plaster casts that greatly restricted activity, a particular hardship for a growing, active child. Wearing restrictive casts for long periods caused atrophy of the major muscles of the body, not to mention almost intolerable itching of the skin underneath the plaster. Surgical procedures requiring bone grafting and the fusion of major joints were commonplace, and despite improvements, many were left permanently disabled and disfigured even after a long and difficult recovery period. Family rarely visited because parents were unable to afford the cost of air travel from the village.

Going home from the sanatorium was in many ways a happy time, but it had its dark side. Patients returning from the sanatorium were given detailed rules for convalescence, including rest periods, and in later years a supply of medication. They were admonished to live a structured life with a nonstrenuous regular daily routine. Yet prolonged absence sometimes led to marital difficulties or family adjustment problems. Children, some of whom had physical deformities that set them apart, found village life and even foods unfamiliar and their friends either gone or moved on to other friends. Adults commonly had residual disabilities that prevented them from taking up the tasks of village life as before. Excessive drinking claimed not a few victims.[20]

Were there any redeeming aspects to the months or years spent in the sanatorium? At least some of the victims of tuberculosis in Alaska came away from the experience stronger and even better able than before to cope with the world around them.

Those who spent months or even years in a sanatorium made new friends— often for life. For many it was the first chance to meet Alaska Natives of other cultures. Because they shared rooms and the total sanatorium experience, an Athabascan might get to know a Yup'ik, a Tlingit an Alutiit, or an Aleut an Inupiat, perhaps for the first time. These unplanned and unforeseen contacts often began in young adulthood, and may even have contributed in a small way to the emerging pan-Native movement, which culminated in the formation of the Alaska Federation of Natives in 1966.

The very success of the tuberculosis control program in Alaska, especially after effective drugs became available, fostered a certain level of confidence in the value of modern health care among Alaska Natives. Many of those who initially distrusted or avoided the government's health care program were thankful to see those with tuberculosis coming home from the hospital alive and well. It is reasonable to suggest that the confidence engendered by the tuberculosis program spilled over into other health programs.

It was probably tuberculosis more than any other health problem that focused the attention of the territorial and federal governments on the plight of the Alaska Natives and thus assured a great increase in the level of public consciousness regarding Native health problems. The massive buildup of facilities and personnel addressed the specific problem, to be sure, but it also precipitated a wider interest in their general health status. Moreover, the new resources available for tuberculosis rather rapidly outpaced the need, especially after the mid-1950s, freeing up many hospital beds and health workers for a more comprehensive health program addressing other significant but hitherto neglected health problems. The Alaska Native Medical Center became a tertiary care general hospital for all Alaska Natives as a direct result of the declining tuberculosis epidemic.

Finally, many Natives learned new skills while in the hospital, which allowed them to flourish in fields they had not even dreamed of. For some the sanatorium made possible their first real opportunity to learn English, a skill that was to serve them well throughout their lives. Others learned a new trade or vocation, permitting them to earn a living commensurate with their physical limitations both in the villages and in larger communities. With their intimate and forced familiarity with the hospital environment, some went on to find jobs in the health field, not just as janitors, maintenance men, and cooks, but also as nurses, practical nurses, technicians, and dental assistants. A few became members of the earliest generation of community health aides.

Of particular interest is that some tuberculosis patients first discovered—or at least first developed—their talent in music, carving, drawing, or sewing while in the sanatorium, and later derived their livelihood from their newly found skills. The rehabilitation programs, especially the one at the Seward Sanatorium, also prepared many Natives for new jobs as storekeepers, clerks, bookkeepers, barbers, village airline agents, and nursing assistants, to name a few of the training programs. Occasionally Alaska Natives who spent time in a tuberculosis hospital went on to notable careers. A few representative examples demonstrate the breadth of talents these individuals developed, in some cases, at least, as a result of their hospital stay.

Robert Mayokok, quoted above, wrote at length about his life and in particular his experiences as a tuberculosis patient at Seward, the Anchorage Native Hospital, and at a sanatorium in Seattle. He had an amazing career, even before his sickness, as a reindeer herder, crew member on the ship carrying the famous explorer Knud Rasmussen to the Siberian coast, and on other voyages to Wrangell Island, Herschel Island, and the Aleutians. He later took a long journey to Boston, New York, and Philadelphia, exhibiting reindeer and lecturing on Eskimo life, including an interview by Lowell Thomas, Sr. In 1947, at the age of forty-four, he learned he had tuberculosis and entered the Seward Sanatorium, where he remained for three years. While there he underwent major chest surgery, and while recovering, started to write stories of his experiences. He also began to draw with India ink on paper, skins, and ivory, and later worked with color as well, talents he had not discovered in himself before his time in the hospital. After discharge Mayokok became a full-time artist and writer—in fact one of the best-known artists of his time in Alaska.[21]

Another well-known Alaska Native whose career was influenced by tuberculosis was the great sprint-musher George Attla, the "Huslia Hustler." Attla developed tuberculosis of the right knee when he was eleven years old and spent most of the next six years in hospitals, including the Mt. Edgecumbe Orthopedic Hospital. There he underwent a surgical fusion of the knee joint, which left him with a permanently stiff knee and his characteristic "kick." When Attla finally returned home to his village, he recalled, "It was a big shock.... After being in the hospital that long and then going home, I found out that I had forgotten a lot of the things I had learned as a kid. And I was a man when I got home. I really didn't know how to make a living out there." Sprint mushing was one thing he could do as well as—and ultimately better than—anyone else. His competitive spirit was legendary among other mushers. Charlie Champaine, a well-known musher in his own right, said of him, "He's a driven guy. He's the ultimate dog racer. He has that blood lust. George is always the last one to give up; he doesn't trade for second place."[22]

A few others, among the many other veterans of the tuberculosis sanatoriums, might be briefly mentioned. Sidney Huntington was an Athabascan whose portrait of Native life, *Shadows on the Koyukuk: An Alaskan Native's Life along the River,* is well known. As a youngster Huntington spent six months under treatment for tuberculosis at the Eklutna Indian School, where he was a student.[23] Walter Austin, known as "Uncle Walter," is a Tlingit musician and counselor who spent two years in the sanatorium at Mt. Edgecumbe. While there he learned many traditional songs from patients of other cultures, and later became very active in the Spirit Days celebrations and in Native musical groups.[24] Melvin Olanna was an Inupiat from Shishmaref who became an exceptional ivory, wood, and whalebone carver. He took up sculpture as a young man because he had a bad limp secondary to tuberculosis of the bone, and knew he would never make it as a hunter.[25] Agnes Kunnuk, one of the original King Island Dancers group, had problems with tuberculosis most of her life, but it didn't keep her from touring with the dance group throughout the United States and even to Tokyo.[26] Two of many who worked in the health field were Alex Marks and Phil Tutiakoff. Marks, a former patient, was trained during the late 1940s to manufacture braces for the Mt. Edgecumbe Orthopedic Hospital. ACCA purchased most of the equipment for the brace shop, but Alex operated the shop and established himself as a skilled worker providing an essential service to the territory and to the Native people.[27] Phil Tutiakoff, a prominent Aleut leader in the health field and longtime community health aide at Unalaska, suffered from severe Pott's disease since childhood.

These are only a sampling of the many Alaska Natives who were all afflicted by tuberculosis but were able to rise above it, and even use their experience with the disease to help them excel in their chosen fields.

Despite these positive influences and successes, however, the sanatorium experience of most tuberculosis patients would not be a fond memory. The patients were physically sick, lonely, and probably anxious, and they and their families faced an uncertain future. The tedious months or years they spent in bed in an alien and unfamiliar environment were frustrating and unhappy. That so many made the best of their enforced idleness shows the strength and adaptability of the human spirit.

Notes

1. W. H. Oswalt, *Napaskiak, An Eskimo Village in Western Alaska*, technical report 57-23, Alaskan Air Command (Fort Wainwright: Arctic Aeromedical Laboratory, January 1961), 94.

2. *Dear Lucy* (pamphlet given to tuberculosis patients, Juneau, ADH and ATA, 1955).

3. Robert Mayokok, "A Marked Man: My Battle with Tuberculosis," *Alaska Journal* 13, no. 4 (1983): 21–26.

4. Oswalt, *Napaskiak*, 94.

5. Mayokok, "Marked Man."

6. Mayokok, "Marked Man."

7. Mayokok, "Marked Man."

8. Margaret L. Lantis and Evelyn B. Hadaway, "How Three Seattle Tuberculosis Hospitals Have Met the Needs of Their Eskimo Patients" (typescript, paper presented to the Nursing Section of the National Tuberculosis Association in Kansas City, MO, 1957), 5.

9. One patient described the sensation of the pleura being punctured as "being kicked by a mule." He went on, "there was a crunch, a stab, and a prayer, O God, let me die quickly." Quoted in Thomas Dormandy, *The White Death: A History of Tuberculosis* (New York: New York University Press, 2000), 261.

10. Lantis and Hadaway, "Three Seattle Tuberculosis Hospitals," 9.

11. "Seward Sanatorium, Bartlett, Alaska," mimeographed pamphlet (1954), Alaska State Historical Library, Juneau, MS 113-1-79.

12. Elsie Bruce, "How Can I Cure Tuberculosis?" *AH* 4, no. 10 (October 1946).

13. *Dear Lucy*.

14. "To the Patient in Seward Sanitorium," printed pamphlet (n.d.), Albrecht Collection, UAA Archives.

15. "To the Patient," typescript (n.d.), National Archives, Pacific Alaska Region. RG 513, box 3, file 56.13.

16. See, for example, Betty MacDonald, *The Plague and I* (1948; repr., Pleasantville, NY: The Akadine Press, 1997).

17. Nancy Olsen, "Ward Five News," *San Chat*, Seward Sanatorium (1954).

18. For a further discussion of these issues, see Robert Fortuine, *Alaska Native Medical Center: A History 1953–1983* (Anchorage: Alaska Native Medical Center, 1986), chapter 13.

19. See, for example, Rena James, "Ward Two News," *San Chat*, Seward Sanatorium (1954).

20. James W. VanStone, *Point Hope, An Eskimo Community in Northwest Alaska*, technical report 57-22, Alaskan Air Command (Fort Wainwright: Arctic Aeromedical Laboratory, March 1961), 127.

21. Yvonne Mozee, "Robert Mayokok," *Alaska Journal* 6, no. 4 (1976): 242–49; Mayokok, "Marked Man."

22. Tim McDonald, "A Legend in His Own Time," *ADT,* December 15, 1988, N6. Another Native athlete whose life was marred by tuberculosis was Ephraim Kalmakoff, a fourteen-year-old boy at the Jesse Lee Home in Seward. Ephraim stunned the spectators of the Mt. Marathon race in 1928 by beating the existing record by two minutes. His own record stood for the next

thirty years. In 1931, just after the race that year, Ephraim was diagnosed with pulmonary tuber-culosis, and died in 1935 without reaching his twenty-first birthday. See Mike Dunham, *ADN*, July 1, 2002.

23. Sidney Huntington, *Shadows on the Koyukuk: An Alaskan Native's Life along the River*, with Jim Rearden (Anchorage: Alaska Northwest Books, 1993).

24. Mike Dunham, "Uncle Walter Drums and Heals the Nations," *ADN*, July 14, 2000, H15.

25. Jan Ingram, "Melvin Olanna's Death Leaves Void in Artistic Landscape," *ADN*, November 3, 1991, H4.

26. Caroline Cremo, "Native Dancer Dies at 74," *ADN*, January 27, 1988.

27. Moore, "ACCA Lends Great Aid."

Appendix :B:

Tuberculosis Mortality and Morbidity Reports

T UBERCULOSIS mortality figures for Alaska were incomplete and definitely suspect during the earliest years. Many diagnoses of tuberculosis, especially in the western and northern parts of the territory, were not made by health professionals but rather by teachers, missionaries, and magistrates, usually on the basis of cough, long-standing illness, and perhaps spitting blood. Some deaths in the more remote villages were probably not reported at all. Certainly, x-rays and sputum tests were not done. These earlier reports are included below, however, because the figures, whatever the source, were the basis for policy and action.

The earliest figures in the table, from 1926 to 1929, were taken from a 1934 report by F. S. Fellows, published in *Public Health Reports* vol. 49, no. 9, pp. 284–98. Mortality figures from 1930 to 1936 are extracted from a paper by J. A. Carswell, published in 1938 in the *Journal of the National Tuberculosis Association* vol. 34, pp. 233–46. Figures from 1937 to 1946 were compiled from official records by Frederick Swanson in 1949, in his unpublished detailed study of tuberculosis in Alaska titled *Alaska's Tuberculosis Problem*. The figures listed from 1945 to 1951 are largely taken from an unpublished 1956 paper by Margaret L. Lantis and Evelyn Hardaway, "How Three Seattle Hospitals Have Met the Needs of their Eskimo Patients." Unfortunately, only rates are given, and thus the numbers of deaths are estimates only. A few annual death reports are given in the *Governor's Reports*. It is unfortunate that this very period of uncertainty in statistics represents the height of the tuberculosis epidemic in Alaska.

Reliable standardized morbidity reports are available only since 1952, and the tables and graphs since that date are taken from official DPH reports.

All rates have been recalculated using prorated annual population figures based on decennial US Census figures.

Table B-1. Tuberculosis Deaths and Mortality Rates, Alaska, 1926–1951

Year	White Deaths from TB	Native Deaths from TB	Total Alaska Deaths from TB	White TB Mortality Rate per 100,000	Native TB Mortality Rate per 100,000	Total TB Mortality Rate per 100,000	U.S. TB Mortality Rate per 100,000
1926	22	193	215	77	644	371	~85
1927	17	177	194	59	590	333	
1928	14	180	194	49	600	330	
1929	13	208	221	45	694	373	
1930	11	224	235	37.0	740.9	392.0	71.1
1931	18	281	299	58.5	921.9	491.5	
1932	25	303	328	78.6	986.0	524.5	
1933	13	238	251	39.6	768.2	393.2	
1934	21	213	234	61.9	682.0	359.2	
1935	12	276	288	34.3	876.7	433.5	55.1
1936	18	238	256	50.0	750.1	377.9	55.9
1937	26	220	246	70.1	688.0	356.3	
1938	21	225	246	55.1	698.2	349.7	
1939	15	306	321	38.3	942.7	448.1	
1940	17	257	274	38.6	788.7	357.5	45.9
1941	19	256	275	38.8	782.5	336.8	44.5
1942	14	243	257	26.0	739.9	296.6	43.1
1943	22	279	301	37.5	846.2	328.4	42.5
1944	30	216	246	47.2	652.6	254.5	41.2
1945	21	257	278	30.7	773.5	273.5	39.9
1946	29	215	295	39.6	644.6	228.8	36.4
1947	28*	201*	245	35.8*	594.0	205.6	33.5
1948	24*	213	237*	28.9*	633.9	203.3	30.0
1949	12*	206	218*	13.6*	611.3	179.2	26.3
1950	n.a.	227*	n.a.	228*	672.6	177.4	22.5
1951	n.a	223	n.a.	n.a.	630.1	145.3	20.1

* Estimate based on rates

n.a. Unable to make reasonable estimate from available information

Table B-2. Tuberculosis Mortality, Alaska, 1952–1972
(Rates expressed as deaths per 100,000 per year)

Year	TB Deaths, Whites	TB Deaths, Alaska Natives	TB Deaths, All Races	TB Death Rate, Whites	TB Death Rate, Natives	TB Death Rate, All Races	TB Death Rates, US.
1952	19	171	191	18.3	480.4	128.9	15.8
1953	10	120	130	8.5	329.1	82.3	12.4
1954	14	82	97	12.0	219.7	57.9	10.2
1955	8	45	54	6.7	117.8	30.4	9.1
1956	9	41	50	6.3	105.0	26.7	8.4
1957	13	40	53	8.7	100.2	26.9	7.8
1958	8	15	23	5.1	36.8	11.1	7.1
1959	3	21	24	1.8	50.4	11.1	6.5
1960	3	11	14	1.7	25.9	6.2	6.0
1961	1	11	12	0.6	25.4	5.1	5.4
1962	7	8	15	3.7	18.1	6.2	5.1
1963	4	14	18	2.1	31.1	7.2	4.9
1964	1	4	5	0.5	8.7	2.0	4.3
1965	3	3	6	1.5	6.4	2.3	4.1
1966	2	5	7	0.9	10.5	2.6	3.9
1967	3	2	5	1.4	4.1	1.8	3.5
1968	0	0	0	0.0	0.0	0.0	3.1
1969	3	2	5	1.3	4.0	1.7	2.8
1970	0	0	1	0.0	0.0	0.3	2.6
1971	0	0	0	0.0	0.0	0.0	2.2
1972	0	0	0	0.0	0.0	0.0	2.1

Table B-3. Tuberculosis Cases and Incidence, Alaska, 1952–1972
(Rates expressed as cases per 100,000 per year)

Year	TB Cases, Native	TB Cases, White	TB Cases, Black	TB Cases, Other	Total TB Cases	Native Rate	White Rate	Black Rate	Other Rate	Total Alaska Rate	US Rate
1952	649*	92	—	—	743	1823.3	84.3	—	—	501.5	—
1953	533*	87	—	—	622	1461.8	74.1	—	—	393.9	53.0
1954	651*	109	—	—	760	1744.0	86.8	—	—	453.3	49.3
1955	585*	76	—	—	661	1531.7	56.9	—	—	372.6	46.9
1956	500*	92	—	—	595	1280.1	64.9	—	—	317.9	41.6
1957	369*	62	—	—	431	924.2	41.3	—	—	218.9	39.2
1958	212	40	—	4	256	519.7	25.3	—	80.0	123.9	36.5
1959	299	49	—	8	356	719.3	29.5	—	160.0	164.5	32.5
1960	188	28	—	8	224	442.1	16.0	—	133.3	99.0	30.8
1961	193	56	—	6	255	445.2	31.0	—	70.2	109.2	29.4
1962	260	57	—	6	323	588.3	30.5	—	70.2	134.0	28.7
1963	230	43	—	6	279	511.0	22.3	—	62.5	112.3	28.7
1964	271	61	—	6	338	591.3	30.6	0.0	203.0	132.1	26.6
1965	238	63	—	1	302	510.1	30.6	0.0	32.1	114.7	25.3
1966	119	27	1	0	147	250.6	12.7	12.4	0.0	54.3	24.4
1967	87	21	—	2	110	180.1	9.6	0.0	58.4	39.5	23.1
1968	88	20	—	4	112	179.1	8.9	0.0	111.6	39.2	21.3
1969	67	15	—	7	89	134.1	6.5	0.0	187.1	30.4	19.4
1970	82	16	2	5	105	161.4	6.8	22.4	128.1	35.0	18.3
1971	104	17	1	2	124	200.5	7.0	10.7	40.4	41.0	17.1
1972	79	14	1	3	97	152.3	5.6	10.1	50.0	32.1	15.8

* Category is "Non-White."

Table B-4. Tuberculosis Cases and Incidence, Alaska, 1973–2002

Year	TB Cases, Native	TB Cases, White	TB Cases, Black	TB Cases, Asian	Total TB Cases	Native Rate	White Rate	Black Rate	Asian Rate	Total Alaska Rate	US Rate
1973	81	28	2	1	112	147.5	10.8	19.4	14.2	34.3	14.8
1974	83	15	5	7	110	151.2	5.6	44.3	87.3	33.7	14.2
1975	56	13	4	0	74	102.0	4.8	35.5	0.0	22.6	15.9
1976	51	29	1	4	88	92.9	10.3	8.5	39.3	27.0	15.0
1977	66	13	2	11	92	120.2	4.5	16.4	97.9	23.2	13.9
1978	63	25	2	4	94	114.8	8.5	15.8	32.6	22.9	13.1
1979	68	12	0	10	90	123.9	4.0	0.0	75.0	21.6	12.6
1980	49	11	2	14	76	76.5	3.6	14.7	173.8	19.0	12.3
1981	56	15	1	11	83	87.4	4.7	6.9	119.3	20.7	11.9
1982	60	20	4	12	96	93.7	6.0	26.9	115.5	23.9	11.0
1983	62	23	1	12	98	78.5	6.7	6.14	103.9	24.5	10.2
1984	46	19	0	14	79	55.1	5.4	0.0	110.0	15.4	9.4
1985	68	22	1	19	110	79.0	6.1	5.5	136.8	21.0	9.3
1986	35	12	2	23	72	40.1	3.2	10.6	152.8	13.3	9.4
1987	34	10	3	14	61	42.9	2.6	15.1	141.8	12.1	9.3
1988	35	10	0	6	51	43.0	2.5	0.0	34.5	9.8	9.1
1989	50	2	0	7	59	59.9	0.5	0.0	37.7	11.0	9.5
1990	52	6	1	9	68	60.7	1.4	4.5	45.6	12.4	9.6
1991	56	4	2	8	70	64.4	1.0	8.9	38.8	12.6	10.4
1992	29	6	2	20	57	32.9	1.4	9.0	93.2	10.1	10.5
1993	37	8	0	12	57	41.4	1.9	0.0	53.7	9.9	9.8
1994	65	8	0	19	92	71.7	1.9	0.0	81.9	15.8	9.4
1995	57	8	2	15	82	62.0	1.9	9.0	62.3	13.9	8.7
1996	73	10	0	14	97	78.4	2.3	0.0	56.1	16.3	8.0
1997	39	16	5	18	78	41.3	3.7	22.7	69.7	12.9	7.4
1998	30	11	3	11	55	31.4	2.6	13.7	41.2	9.0	6.8
1999	43	5	0	13	61	44.4	1.2	0.0	47.2	9.9	6.4
2000	72	11	9	17	109	73.4	2.5	41.3	59.8	17.4	9.8
2001*	34	8	0	12	54	34.7*	1.8*	0.0	42.2*	8.5*	5.6*
2002*	21	7	1	17	49	21.4*	1.6*	4.6*	59.8*	7.7*	—

* Morbidity rates for 2001 and 2002 based on 2000 Census figures.

Appendix :C:

Glossary

This glossary briefly defines a collection of technical terms in tuberculosis for the benefit of those not trained in science or medicine.

Acid-fast: Staining characteristic of certain bacteria, including the tubercle bacillus and other mycobacteria, in which the organism is not decolorized by acid and alcohol after having been stained by dyes such as basic fuchsin. Acid-fast bacteria (AFB) stain red under the microscope.

Aerophilic, aerobic: A type of microorganism that requires air for growth.

Aerosol: Liquid or tiny particles dispersed in air in the form of a fine mist for therapeutic or other purposes.

AFB: Acid-fast bacteria. *See* **acid-fast**.

Alveolus, alveoli (pl., as pulmonary alveoli): The thin-walled, saclike dilatations in the lung tissue at the very ends of the respiratory passages, across which oxygen and carbon dioxide pass to and from the pulmonary capillaries.

Ambulatory, ambulant: Describes a patient who is able to walk about; often applied to outpatient care.

Apex of lung, apical: The rounded, uppermost part of each lung. It is a common site for tuberculosis infection.

Artificial pneumothorax. *See* **pneumothorax**.

BCG vaccine: A suspension of a weakened strain (Bacillus Calmette-Guérin) of the bovine type of *Mycobacterium tuberculosis* that is injected into the skin to prevent tuberculosis.

Bifurcation: A forking, or division into two branches, as with the trachea dividing into the two main bronchi.

Blepharoconjunctivitis: An inflammation of the eyelids and conjunctivae, the thin membrane that lines the inside of the lids and covers the "white" of the eyeball.

Bronchiectasis: A chronic lung disease in which there is dilatation of the bronchi, coughing, and large amounts of foul sputum. The condition is usually associated with long-standing bronchitis and sometimes with tuberculosis.

Bronchopleural fistula: An abnormal passage or communication between a bronchus and the pleural cavity, usually the result of a surgical complication, but sometimes due to chronic inflammation, as in tuberculosis.

Bronchus, bronchi (pl.): One of the two main divisions of the trachea which conveys air to and from the lungs. The main bronchi then subdivide into progressively smaller airways.

Bovine tuberculosis: Tuberculosis of cattle, generally caused by the organism *M. bovis*. The organism may also infect humans.

Cachexia: A general weight loss and wasting of the body tissues occurring in the later course of tuberculosis and other chronic diseases.

Calcification: The deposition of lime or other insoluble calcium salts in scarred tissues in the later stages of the healing process.

Cardiac tamponade: Compression and interference with the function of the heart due to fluid in the pericardial sac, sometimes secondary to a stiffening of the pericardium from tuberculosis scarring.

Case fatality rate: The proportion of individuals contracting a disease that die of that disease.

Caseous necrosis: The death of tissue resulting from tuberculosis (and a few other diseases), characterized by loss of identifiable structures of the various cells; the affected tissue has a crumbly consistency and dull, opaque quality similar to some types of cheese.

Catarrh, catarrhal: An old-fashioned word describing the increased flow of mucus or other discharge due to inflammation of a membrane.

Cavity: A hollow space, applied particularly to an advanced tuberculous lesion of the lung. A tuberculous cavity has a lining of thickened inflamed tissue and is usually teeming with bacteria.

Cell-mediated immunity (CMI), cellular immunity: A type of immune response that is initiated by the so-called T-lymphocytes and carried out by T-lymphocytes and other tissue cells. It is the type of immunity that causes skin redness and swelling that results from a positive reaction to tuberculin or PPD.

Chemoprophylaxis: Prevention of disease by the use of chemicals or drugs. The term is particularly applied to the use of INH to prevent tuberculosis.

Chemotherapy: Treatment of disease by means of chemical substances or drugs; usually used in reference to neoplastic disease, but also used to describe the long-term drug treatment of tuberculosis.

Cold abscess: An abscess without heat or the other usual signs of inflammation, such as pain; the word is most often applied to an abscess caused by *M. tuberculosis*.

Conjunctivae (pl.): Delicate membranes that line the inside of the eyelids and cover the exposed surface of the whites of the eyes.

Consumption: Obsolete term for a wasting disease of the body. It usually referred to what we now know as pulmonary tuberculosis.

Converter: A person who has converted the tuberculin skin test from negative to positive.

Cyanosis: A bluish or purplish coloration of the skin and mucous membrane due to insufficient oxygen being carried in the blood. It may occur as the result of severe lung disease, such as tuberculosis.

Death rate (mortality rate): The proportion of the population that dies during a specified period, usually a year. In tuberculosis statistics, the rate is usually expressed as the number of annual deaths from tuberculosis per 100,000 persons in the population.

Decortication: A surgical procedure in which an inflammatory membrane around a lung is removed in order to permit reexpansion of the lung.

Delayed hypersensitivity. *See* **cell-mediated immunity**.

Diaphragm: The muscular partition between the chest and abdominal cavities.

Diathesis: The constitutional state that predisposes a person to acquire a particular disease. The idea of a "tubercular diathesis" was very popular in the nineteenth century.

Dihydrostreptomycin: An antibiotic with some effectiveness against tuberculosis, but its use carries a risk of causing permanent hearing loss.

Droplet nuclei: Particles 1 to 10 microns in diameter, implicated in the spread of tuberculosis and other respiratory diseases. It consists of the dried residue formed by evaporation of droplets coughed or sneezed into the atmosphere.

Dyspnea: Shortness of breath, a subjective distress in breathing, usually associated with disease of the heart or lungs.

Emphysema: A condition of the lung in which the size of the air spaces is increased, either because of dilatation of the alveoli themselves or from destruction of their walls. Smoking is a major causative factor.

Endemic: Present in a community or among a group of people; used to describe a disease prevailing continually in a region.

Epithelioid cells: Cells resembling or having some of the characteristics of epithelium. They are often found in the microscopic structure of a tubercle.

Ethambutol hydrochloride: An anti-tuberculosis drug that inhibits the growth of tubercle bacilli, and is often effective against organisms resistant to other such drugs; the drug may sometimes cause temporary visual impairment.

Ethionimide: A drug used in the treatment of pulmonary tuberculosis; it is always given with other agents because bacterial resistance develops when it is administered alone.

Expectorate: To spit; to cough up sputum from the chest.

Extrapulmonary tuberculosis: Tuberculosis of organs other than the lungs.

Exudative tuberculosis: Forms of tuberculosis in which inflammation causes the escape of fluid, cells, and cellular debris from blood vessels and their deposit in tissue. Examples would include tuberculous pneumonia and pleural effusion.

Far advanced: A classification of tuberculosis according to x-ray appearance established by the National Tuberculosis Association in 1955. Far advanced refers to disease in both lungs more extensive than moderately advanced.

Fallopian tubes: Uterine tubes. The tubes leading from the upper or outer extremity of the ovary to the fundus of the uterus, and which conduct the egg to the uterus. Occasionally these structures may be infected with tuberculosis.

Fibrosis: Formation of fibrous tissue as part of the process of repair or reaction to a stimulus. Fibrosis is an important part of the healing process of tuberculosis, especially in the lungs.

Galloping consumption: An obsolete term for very rapidly progressive pulmonary tuberculosis, usually with tuberculous pneumonia.

Ghon's tubercle (complex): Calcifications seen on x-ray, usually the mid-lung area and the lymph nodes of the root of the lung, resulting from childhood primary tuberculosis.

Giant cells: A cell with many nuclei, often seen in the microscopic structure of a tubercle.

Gibbus: Sharply angulated hunchback deformity of the spine, usually due to the destruction of thoracic vertebrae resulting from tuberculosis. *See* **tuberculous spondylitis.**

Granuloma: A well-circumscribed chronic inflammatory lesion, which is usually small, granular, and firm; granulomas are characteristic of tuberculosis and other chronic infections.

Hectic fever: A type of recurrent or continuous fever typically associated with tuberculosis, with flushed cheeks and hot, dry skin.

Hemoptysis: Spitting of blood resulting from an erosion of a blood vessel of the lungs or bronchial passages, usually the result of tuberculosis or cancer.

Hilum, hilar: A depression on the middle surface of each lung, where the bronchus, blood vessels, nerves, and lymphatics enter or leave the lung.

Histoplasmin: An extract of the fungus *Histoplasma capsulatum*, used in the diagnosis of the fungus disease histoplasmosis; it is also used in skin test surveys of populations to determine the geographic distribution of the fungus.

Histoplasmosis: A disease caused by the fungus *Histoplasma capsulatum* and occurring frequently in some regions, usually acquired by breathing in spores of the fungus in soil and dust; it characteristically affects the lungs and is often similar to a mild form of primary tuberculosis. Occasionally, the disease progresses to produce chronic localized lesions in the lung, such as pulmonary cavitation, with fever and emaciation.

Incidence rate: The number of specified new events—for example, the number of new cases of tuberculosis—during a specified period in a specified population. It is often expressed by the number of new cases per 100,000 population per year.

Induration: The localized hardening of the skin and subcutaneous tissues which may occur at the site of a PPD injection. Typically, a positive reaction is an area of induration of at least 10 mm forty-eight to seventy-two hours after injection.

INH. *See* **isoniazid.**

Intrapleural pneumonolysis: A surgical operation designed to break up scar tissue between the two layers of the pleurae, in order to allow the lung to collapse partially. It was usually performed through two small chest wall incisions, into one of which a "thoracoscope" was inserted to provide visualization. The scar tissue was either cut or cauterized through the other hole.

Isoniazid, INH: Isonicotinic acid hydrazide; an important drug effective in the treatment and prevention of tuberculosis.

Keratitis: Inflammation of the cornea.

King's evil: Historical term for tuberculous lymph glands of the neck (scrofula); it was once thought to be curable by the touch of royalty.

Kyphosis: Hunchback deformity of the upper spine, which may be due to tuberculosis of the vertebral column.

Latent tuberculosis infection (LTBI): Infection by *M. tuberculosis*, with no manifestation of active tuberculous disease.

Lesion: A local pathologic change in the tissues; in tuberculosis, the primary lesion is the tubercle.

Lupus vulgaris: Tuberculosis of the skin, usually manifested by nodules on the face, particularly about the nose and ears.

Lymphadenitis: Inflammation of a lymph node or lymph nodes.

Macrophage: A type of cell deriving from the bone marrow that is widely distributed in the body; these cells are part of the immune system and have the capacity to ingest bacteria.

Malaise: A feeling of general discomfort or unwellness, often the first sign of an infection or other disease.

Mantoux test. *See* **tuberculin test**.

Miliary tuberculosis: A rapidly progressive form of tuberculosis characterized by a general dissemination of tubercle bacilli through the bloodstream, causing the production of countless tiny tubercles in various organs and tissues. It is usually fatal unless recognized early and treated vigorously.

Minimal tuberculosis: A classification of tuberculosis according to x-ray appearance established by the National Tuberculosis Association in 1955. Minimal tuberculosis is defined as lesions confined to a small part of one or both lungs, and without cavitation.

Moderately advanced tuberculosis: A classification of tuberculosis according to x-ray appearance established by the National Tuberculosis Association in 1955. In moderately advanced tuberculosis, one or both lungs may be involved, but the total involvement should not exceed the volume of one lung (or the equivalent in both lungs), and in addition, dense and confluent lesions should not exceed one third the volume of one lung. Moreover, the diameter of a cavity should not exceed 4 cm.

Morbidity rate. *See* **incidence rate**.

Mortality rate. *See* **death rate.**

Multidrug-resistant tuberculosis (MDRTB): Tuberculosis caused by organisms resistant to more than one anti-tuberculosis drug.

***Mycobacterium bovis*:** A species of bacteria that is the cause of tuberculosis in cattle; transmissible to humans and other animals, causing tuberculosis.

***Mycobacterium tuberculosis*:** The species of bacteria that causes tuberculosis in man. Also called tubercle bacillus.

Nasogastric tube: A rubber or plastic tube inserted through a nostril past the back of the throat and into the stomach. In the sanatorium, it was primarily used in children to collect specimens of gastric juice to examine for tubercle bacilli, since sputum specimens were difficult to collect in that age group.

Necrosis: Pathologic death of one or more cells, or of a portion of tissue or organ, resulting from irreversible damage.

Old tuberculin (OT): A heat-concentrated filtrate of a culture of tubercle bacilli grown on a special medium. It has now largely been supplanted by PPD (purified protein derivative), except in the tine test.

Paleopathology: The science of disease in prehistoric times, as revealed in bones, mummies, and archeologic artifacts.

Para-aminosalicylic acid (PAS, PASA): A drug inhibiting the growth of tubercle bacilli, used particularly as an adjunct to streptomycin.

Paracentesis: The passage into a cavity of a needle or other hollow instrument for the purpose of removing fluid such as pus or blood.

Paroxysmal: Sudden recurrence or intensification of symptoms, usually applied to severe coughing spells.

PCR. *See* **polymerase chain reaction amplification technique.**

Peribronchial: Surrounding a bronchus.

Phlebolith: A deposit of calcium in a venous wall or a thrombus.

Phlyctenular keratoconjunctivits. *See* **PKC.**

Phlyctenule: A small blister or ulcerated nodule on the cornea or on the conjunctiva.

Photofluorography: Miniature x-rays made by contact photography of a fluoroscopic screen, formerly used in mass radiographic surveys of the lungs.

Phrenic nerve: A major nerve that supplies motor (movement) function to the diaphragm, and thus in part controls the act of breathing.

Phrenic crush: An operation in which part of the phrenic nerve supplying half the diaphragm is crushed in the neck region in order to reduce the excursions of the lung on that side and thus promote healing of a tuberculous lesion. The effect usually lasted from four to eight months.

Phrenicectomy: An operation in which the phrenic nerve supplying half the diaphragm is cut, in order to reduce the excursions of the lung on that side permanently.

Phthisis, phthisic: An obsolete term for a wasting disease, specifically used for consumption or tuberculosis of the lungs.

Phthisis pulmonale: An obsolete term for pulmonary tuberculosis.

Pleura, pleurae (pl.): The membranes enveloping the lungs and lining the walls of the pleural cavity.

Pleural cavity: The potential space between the parietal and visceral layers of the pleurae, which normally glide over each other as the lung expands and contracts. This space sometimes fills with fluid, such as pus or blood.

Pleural effusion: Increased amounts of fluid within the pleural cavity, often found in tuberculosis.

Pleurisy: Inflammation of the pleurae. Pleurisy is often the first sign of tuberculosis.

Plombage: Formerly, the use of an inert substance inside the rib cage and outside the pleura to maintain collapse of the lung. Materials used included paraffin wax and Lucite balls.

Pneumonectomy: An operation to remove an entire lung.

Pneumoperitoneum: A procedure often used before the chemotherapy era in which air or nitrogen was periodically injected into the peritoneal cavity of the abdomen. The air temporarily restricted the movement of the diaphragm, thereby resting a lung infected with tuberculosis.

Pneumothorax: The presence of air or gas in the pleural cavity. The word also refers to the artificial injection of air, or a more slowly absorbed gas such as nitrogen, into the pleural space to collapse and thereby rest a lung infected with tuberculosis.

Polymerase chain reaction amplification technique (PCR): A diagnostic test for the tubercle bacillus that involves the amplification of characteristic DNA fragments. It is used to confirm the presence of the organism on smear-positive sputum specimens or to identify which species are growing in culture.

Pott's disease. *See* **tuberculous spondylitis**.

PPD (Purified Protein Derivative): A purified form of tuberculin containing the active protein fraction; used in the diagnosis of infection with the tubercle bacillus.

Primary tuberculosis: Infection by *M. tuberculosis*, typically seen in children but also in adults, characterized by a small peripheral pulmonary focus of the disease with spread to hilar nodes; the disease may heal with scarring, lead to cavitation, or may progress to more typical forms of pulmonary tuberculosis.

Psoas abscess: An abscess, usually tuberculous, that usually originates in spinal tuberculosis, and extends through the iliopsoas muscle to the groin region.

Reinfection: A second infection by the same microorganism, after recovery from or during the course of a primary infection.

Rifampin, rifampicin: An antibiotic antibacterial agent used in the treatment of tuberculosis.

Sanatorium: An institution for the treatment and recuperation of chronic disorders, usually tuberculosis, under medical supervision.

Sanitarium: A health resort. *See also* **sanatorium**.

Scrofula: An obsolete term for tuberculous infection of the lymph glands of the neck. This form of tuberculosis was once common among adolescents and accompanied by swelling, draining sinuses, and scarring.

Segmental resection: An operation to remove a diseased section of lung called a segment, which is the largest subdivision of a lobe of the lung.

Sepsis: The presence of bacteria or their toxins in the blood or other tissues; causing severe illness.

Sinus: A drainage tract leading to a pus-filled cavity.

Solarium: A place where a person may take advantage of natural sunlight. Many tuberculosis sanatoriums had a glassed-in solarium, where the patient could absorb ultraviolet rays from the sun.

Spes phthisicorum, spes phthisica: An older concept describing the false sense of hope and optimism found in some individuals dying of tuberculosis. Literally, "hope of the consumptives."

Sputum: Mucous, purulent, or bloody material coughed up from the air passages.

Streptomycin: An antibiotic agent obtained from the natural fungus *Streptomyces griseus* that is active against the tubercle bacillus. It is now used almost exclusively in the treatment of tuberculosis; toxicity includes eighth cranial nerve damage leading to deafness or a disorder of balance.

Surveillance: The collection, analysis, and dissemination of data, principally to monitor disease occurrence within a population.

Thoracentesis: A procedure by which a needle or hollow tube is inserted through the chest wall to draw off fluid from the pleural cavity.

Thoracoplasty: A major surgical procedure that involved reshaping the upper thoracic wall by removing one or more ribs, for the purpose of collapsing part of a lung infected by tuberculosis.

Thoracotomy: Any surgical operation that involves cutting through the chest wall.

Tine test. *See* **tuberculin test**.

Trachoma: A chronic infectious disease of the conjunctiva and cornea of the eye, which produces redness, pain, tearing, and sensitivity to light. Untreated cases may cause blindness.

Trocar: A sharp-pointed instrument equipped with a tube and generally used to puncture the chest or abdominal wall to withdraw fluid.

Tubercle: The basic pathologic lesion caused by *M. tuberculosis*. Although variable in size and detail, tubercles tend to be fairly well-circumscribed, spheroidal, firm lesions consisting of three irregularly outlined zones: 1) an inner focus of necrosis, often becoming caseous; 2) a middle zone that consists of a fairly dense accumulation of large macrophages and multinucleated giant cells; 3) an outer zone of predominately lymphocytes. Where healing has begun, a fourth zone of fibrous tissue may form at the periphery.

Tubercle bacillus: Generally refers to the organism *M. tuberculosis*, but may also refer to the related species *M. bovis*, which can also cause tuberculosis in humans.

Tuberculin test: Application of the skin test to the diagnosis of infection by *Mycobacterium tuberculosis* in which tuberculin or its purified protein derivative (PPD) serves as an antigen. The test is performed by injection of tuberculin or of PPD into the outer layer of the skin, either by a small needle (Mantoux test) or by "tines" (tine test), or by application of test material by means of a "patch." The test is read in forty-eight to seventy-two hours on the basis of swelling, firmness, and erythema, the former being considered the more diagnostic of infection with the tubercle bacillus (*M. tuberculosis*).

Tuberculoma: A rounded tumorlike mass, usually in the lungs or brain, due to localized tuberculous infection.

Tuberculous meningitis: Infection of the coverings of the brain and spinal cord, or meninges, by the tubercle bacillus. The disease usually occurs in children and is almost always fatal without prompt diagnosis and treatment.

Tuberculous pericarditis: Tuberculous infection of the pericardium, the membranes enclosing the heart. The disease often causes scar tissue, which restricts the function of the heart.

Tuberculous peritonitis: Tuberculous infection of the peritoneum, the membrane that lines the outside of the intestinal tract and the inner surface of the abdominal wall.

Tuberculous pneumonia: A consolidation of lung tissue secondary to infection with the tubercle bacillus. Such infections spread rapidly and often lead to galloping consumption.

Tuberculous spondylitis: Tuberculous infection of one or more vertebrae or the joints between them. The disease is often associated with a sharp angulation of the spine at the point of disease. Syn: Pott's disease.

Ziehl-Neelson stain: A stain used for staining acid-fast bacteria, followed by decolorization in acid alcohol and counterstaining with methylene blue; acid-fast organisms appear red, other tissue elements light blue.

Appendix :D:

Alaska Tuberculosis Time Line

Boldface items describe general Alaskan historical events.
Fiscal years run from July 1 of the previous year to June 30 of the year in question.

AD 400	::	Frozen body of St. Lawrence Island woman with possible evidence of tuberculosis
1500s	::	Frozen body of Point Barrow woman with possible evidence of tuberculosis
1741	::	**Bering voyage to Alaska**
1770	::	Two Aleuts said to have died of tuberculosis while crossing Siberia
1778	::	Dr. Anderson, surgeon of Cook Expedition, dies of tuberculosis while in Alaskan waters
1779	::	Captain Clerke, who replaced Cook as commander, dies of tuberculosis in Alaskan waters
1783	::	**First permanent Russian settlement at Three Saints Bay (Kodiak Island)**
1799	::	**Russian-American Company established**
1820	::	Dr. Volkov is first physician assigned permanently to Russian America, at Sitka
1820s	::	Father Veniaminov, missionary in the Aleutians, mentions consumptives and traditional Aleut remedies for consumption
1830s	::	Dr. Blaschke describes "phthisis" as common disease at Sitka, especially among Creoles and Aleuts
1830s–40s	::	Father Netsvetov mentions consumptives in Atka and on lower Yukon
1840s	::	Dr. Frankenhaeuser reports that 20 to 30 percent of all deaths in Sitka are due to tuberculosis, particularly affecting Creole women

1851–52 ::	Eskimo child reported with consumption at Port Clarence
1860s ::	Dr. Govorlivyi at Sitka reports that 60 percent of Tlingit adults have suffered hemoptysis
1867 ::	**The United States purchases Alaska from Russia**
1875 ::	U.S. Army Surgeon Brooke states that phthisis is "not uncommon" and makes up majority of Indian deaths
1879 ::	Dr. Robert White reports on voyage of USRC *Rush* and finds pulmonary phthisis and scrofula in SE Alaska, Aleutians, and Pribilofs
1880 ::	Petroff, in first Alaska Census, lists tuberculosis as "the disease that destroys the greatest number throughout Alaska"
1881 ::	Dr. Irving Rosse on USRC *Corwin* finds tuberculosis and scrofula among whaling crews, as well as among the Natives
1884 ::	**Congress passes First Alaska Organic Act and establishes civil government**
1885 ::	**Sheldon Jackson becomes first general agent for education in Alaska**
1900 ::	Severe epidemic of influenza and measles spreads through western Alaska; many survivors die of tuberculosis
1901 ::	Carroll Fox of USPHS suggests government hospital for tuberculosis
1907 ::	**Harlan Updegraff becomes head of the Alaska Division, Bureau of Education (BoE)**
::	Teachers provided with medical kit and textbooks
1908 ::	BoE appoints first full-time medical officers
1909 ::	BoE's budget has allocation for Sanitation and Medical Relief for first time
1910 ::	First "teachers of sanitation" appointed by BoE
::	*Summer*: Dr. H. E. Hasseltine reports on voyage of *Rush*
::	*November*: BoE opens first Native hospital in rented building in Juneau
1911 ::	*Summer*: Dr. M. H. Foster conducts health survey in southern Alaska
1912 ::	*March*: BoE appoints Dr. Emil Krulish as medical director; he visits southern Alaska
::	*August*: **Congress passes Second Alaska Organic Act**
::	*FY1913*: BoE establishes hospitals in school buildings at Nulato and Kotzebue

	::	BoE contracts with Children's Orthopedic Hospital in Seattle for care of bone and joint tuberculosis
1913	::	Drs. Krulish and Neuman publish *Medical Handbook* to assist teachers
	::	*March*: First territorial legislature provides for governor as health commissioner and passes communicable disease law
	::	*Summer*: Dr. Krulish accompanies *Bear* on its northern cruise
	::	Dr. J. A. Watkins, medical officer on *Bear,* reports on health conditions in the North
1915	::	*March*: Appropriation by legislature in support of communicable disease law
	::	Legislature asks Congress for $125,000 annually for medical relief and for tuberculosis sanatorium
	::	*FY1916*: First specific appropriation for health for BoE
1916	::	*May 9*: New 20-bed Juneau Hospital for Natives opens
1917	::	*FY1918*: "Tubercular camps" are established at Akiak and Nulato
1918	::	*Fall*: **Spanish influenza hits Pacific Rim communities**
	::	BoE sanatorium opens in leased Presbyterian Mission hospital at Haines
1919	::	*Spring*: Influenza reaches Kodiak, Unalaska, Bristol Bay, and Nome
	::	*March 26*: Legislature strengthens communicable disease laws in light of influenza epidemic
	::	*May 1*: Legislature provides for physician as part-time commissioner of health, local boards of health, and health districts
1922	::	Quarantine rules and regulations are promulgated to all physicians
	::	BoE teachers are required to report communicable diseases
1925	::	*FY1926*: USPHS begins examining cannery workers en route to Alaska
1927	::	BoE hospital, with beds for tuberculosis, opens at Fort Gibbon Army post at Tanana
1930	::	*FY 1931*: Office of Indian Affairs (OIA) builds 26-bed tuberculosis annex at Juneau Hospital; x-ray unit is added
1931	::	*March*: Legislature asks that funds for TB be increased
	::	*March 16*: BoE Alaska functions are transferred to OIA
1932	::	328 tuberculosis deaths are reported, the highest number ever
	::	*FY1933*: American Legion asks for TB funding for OIA
1934	::	Fellows publishes first tuberculosis mortality figures for Alaska, covering 1926–30

:: Alaska Tuberculosis Association is founded in Juneau as affiliate of National Tuberculosis Association

:: *Nov. 15*: First appeal for funds by sale of Christmas Seals in Alaska

1935 :: *March*: Legislature sends joint memorial to Congress about tuberculosis problem

1936 :: *March*: **Congress passes Social Security Act**

:: *September*: TDH establishes Communicable Disease Control Division (including tuberculosis)

:: *December*: X-ray surveys for tuberculosis begin

:: TDH holds first itinerant tuberculosis clinics with physician

1937 :: *June*: Communicable Disease Division completes x-ray survey of 11 communities

:: *December*: Aronson begins BCG vaccinations in SE Alaska

1938 :: J. A. Carswell reports on Alaska TB mortality for 1930–36

:: *FY1939*: Tuberculosis teaching units are added to curriculum of all schools in Alaska

:: ATA hires executive director

:: Alaska Native Service (ANS) joins ADH in coordinated tuberculin testing and x-ray surveys

1939 :: *March*: Legislature asks Congress to convert ANS buildings at White Mountain to a Native tuberculosis sanatorium

1940 :: TDH adds tuberculosis clinician to staff

1941 :: *Dec. 7*: **Pearl Harbor attacked**

:: 53 percent of all crippling conditions of children known to ADH in Alaska are due to tuberculosis; among Alaska Natives the figure is 67 percent

:: *FY1942*: Congress appropriates funds for Native sanatorium at Saxman, but it is never built

1942 :: *June 4–5*: **Dutch Harbor bombed by the Japanese**

:: Over 800 Aleuts forcibly evacuated to camps in SE Alaska

1943 :: *Spring*: Legislature cuts to $25,000 a request for $250,000 for tuberculosis control

:: *June*: *Alaska's Health*, TDH newsletter, is inaugurated

1944 :: *June 28*: Congress authorizes transfer of Skagway Army Hospital to ANS for use as tuberculosis sanatorium

:: TDH acquires army surplus ship M/V *Hygiene*

:: *Dec. 9*: Army authorizes transfer of Fort Raymond Hospital at Seward to territory for use as tuberculosis sanatorium

---

1945 :: Tuberculosis causes 20 percent of all deaths; five tuberculosis deaths each week; 60 percent of cases first reported on death certificate

:: *March 21*: ADH is given official status by legislature; Board of Health is established

:: *March 24*: Legislature authorizes negotiations with army for Fort Raymond Hospital and appropriates $14,500 for purchase

:: *April*: Dr. Rudolph Haas drafts tuberculosis control program for territory

:: *April 4*: M/V *Hygiene* leaves Juneau on maiden voyage to SE Alaska

:: *April 14*: First patients are admitted to Skagway Sanatorium

:: *July 1*: Dr. C. Earl Albrecht becomes Alaska's first full-time commissioner of health

:: *August 15*: **VJ Day, end of World War II**

:: *September*: Alaska Board of Health meets for first time

1946 :: *January*: ADH purchases M/S *Hygiene*

:: Alaska Crippled Children's Association is founded and sponsors territorial Crippled Children's Program

:: *February*: Division of Tuberculosis Control is established in ADH

:: ANS officials request funding for 200-bed sanatorium in SE Alaska

:: Lois Jund arrives as tuberculosis education consultant

:: *March*: Dr. Leo Gehrig arrives as tuberculosis consultant

:: Special session of legislature appropriates $250,000 for tuberculosis control and passes comprehensive tuberculosis bill

:: *May*: Health Education Unit is established in ADH

:: *May 10*: War Assets Administration transfers Fort Raymond Hospital to Territory

:: *May/June*: First large survey in bush to identify crippled children

:: *June*: Mass x-ray surveys begin

:: *June 3*: M/S *Hygiene* leaves on maiden voyage

:: *June 28*: Congress authorizes transfer of naval air station and Fort Ray on Japonski Island to ANS

:: *July*: Comprehensive survey of orthopedic needs in territory

:: *July 6*: Seward Sanatorium admits first patients

:: *Summer*: ADH purchases army surplus plane to transport patients and x-ray equipment

:: *August 16*: Alice Island facility on Japonski Island is transferred to ANS

:: *October*: Army small-arms repair truck acquired by TDH begins operation for use as highway mobile health unit

---

1947 :: *Home Care of the Tuberculous* is published

:: Pneumothorax refill clinic established at Juneau

:: ADH establishes Medical Social Service Department

:: *Early*: Mass x-ray survey carried out (by Highway Unit and *Hygiene*)

:: Streptomycin is first used in Alaska

:: Tuberculosis Case Registry becomes functional

:: "Mt. Edgecumbe" becomes official name of ANS complex on Japonski Island

:: *February 6*: Patients are transferred from Skagway to Alice Island Sanatorium

:: Orthopedic Unit is opened at Mt. Edgecumbe; Dr. Philip Moore arrives in Sitka

:: *May*: Photofluorographic x-ray unit is delivered for use in larger towns

:: *May–June*: Dr. Moore organizes orthopedic survey to bush

:: *June–August*: Dr. Milo Fritz carries out ophthalmological survey, showing PKC

:: *July 19*: AMA survey team arrives

:: *August*: Supplemental appropriation for ANS lost in Senate, causing sanatorium crisis

:: *October*: Seward Sanatorium threatens to close because of ANS's failure to pay bills

1948   :: Last general x-ray survey in Alaska (until 1954)

:: Congress provides Special Alaska Public Health Grant

:: Pneumothorax refill clinics are established at Sitka and Seward

:: Plans are made for transfer of ANS PHNs to ADH

:: Twenty-four-bed isolation unit is completed at Kotzebue

:: Moore performs orthopedic surgery at Bethel and Kotzebue

:: Arctic Health Research Station is opened in Anchorage under Dr. Jack C. Haldeman

:: *January*: Tuberculosis patients at Mt. Edgecumbe begin publishing *Island Breezes*

:: *Spring*: Bureau of Budget gives authorization to draw up plans for Anchorage hospital

:: *April*: CCS children are sent to Chicago with funds from American Junior Red Cross

:: *May*: Construction begins on Mt. Edgecumbe Hospital

:: *Summer*: Aronson and ADH begin BCG vaccination in Barrow

:: *July*: First use of streptomycin at Sitka and Seward and later Kotzebue

:: *August*: Capacity of Orthopedic Hospital is raised from 50 to 65 beds

:: *August 8–28*: AMA survey team returns for follow-up

:: *September*: ADH establishes and trains BCG team

:: *October*: Thirty beds are added to Seward Sanatorium

:: University of Alaska Regents donates land for Arctic Health Research Center

1949
:: 5,914 cases in register; 439 beds available
:: *March*: Dr. Coddington, thoracic surgeon, arrives at Mt. Edgecumbe
:: *Spring*: TDH acquires two railway cars for Mobile Railway Health Unit
:: *April*: First patients at Orthopedic Hospital are given streptomycin under research grant from National Research Council
:: Construction bids for new Anchorage hospital are let
:: M/S *Yukon Health* leaves Juneau on first voyage to Yukon
:: Bess Winn, executive secretary of ATA, dies of brain tumor; replaced by Frances Paul
:: *April 19*: M/V *Health* is commissioned
:: *Summer*: Vital Statistics Bureau is established in Health Department
:: *August*: Chest Clinic of Anchorage Health Center begun
:: *August 9*: Ground-breaking for 400-bed Anchorage Hospital
:: *Fall*: Truck Health Unit is permanently discontinued
:: *September*: M/V *Yukon Health* begins operations
:: *November*: Mobile Railway Health Unit begins operation
:: *FY1950*: Twenty-four-bed tuberculosis units added at Bethel, Kanakanak, Kotzebue
:: Annual infection rate of 25 percent in Bethel area

1950
:: Last year that tuberculosis is number one cause of death in Alaska
:: Thirty ACCA chapters in territory
:: *January*: BCG program cut back because of budgetary constraints
:: *February 1*: Case register at 5,279; 3,134 cases considered active or questionably active not hospitalized
:: *March 1*: New Mt. Edgecumbe Hospital opens
:: *April 15*: Division of Tuberculosis Control is transferred to Section of Communicable and Preventable Diseases
:: *May*: Mobile Railway Health Unit ceases operations: staff joins M/S *Yukon Health*
:: *June*: Dr. Francis Phillips named medical director of Seward Sanatorium
:: *June 30*: 439 beds available for tuberculosis in Alaska
:: Dr. Grace E. Field becomes acting director of Tuberculosis Control
:: *August*: Thoracoplasties begin at Seward

1951
:: Tuberculosis drops to second place behind accidents as leading cause of death in Alaska
:: PAS first used in Alaska
:: *February 26*: First "deposit" in bone bank at Orthopedic Hospital
:: *May*: New Anchorage Health Center opens with expanded Chest Clinic
:: *June*: Dr. Moore gives paper at national meeting on streptomycin treatment

:: *September*: First meeting at Juneau of interagency board to set admission priorities for tuberculosis hospitals

:: *December*: BCG program is suspended

1952   :: Accidents again chief cause of death, with tuberculosis in third place with 172 deaths

:: *February*: Territorial Office of Vocational Rehabilitation is reactivated

:: *March*: BCG program is reactivated

:: *April 14*: Additional beds opened at Alice Island

:: *April 15*: 568 tuberculosis patients hospitalized

:: *June*: INH is in use at both Seward and Mt. Edgecumbe

:: *September*: Vocational rehabilitation program begins at Mt. Edgecumbe Hospital

:: *October*: First dentist is stationed at Seward Sanatorium

:: *October 1*: All Mobile Health Units inactivated because of federal budget cuts

---

1953   :: ACCA Treatment Center opens in Anchorage

:: Dr. Beryl Michaelson uses streptomycin on outpatients at Bethel

:: *January*: 602 Alaskan patients hospitalized for tuberculosis; 501 beds available in Alaska

:: *March*: Dr. Coddington, thoracic surgeon at Mt. Edgecumbe, resigns and leaves Alaska

:: *March 15*: 5,774 cases in TB register; 2,400 known active or probably active cases of tuberculosis among Alaska Natives

:: *July 21*: First group from Parran team arrives in Juneau

:: *November 7–8*: Tuberculosis conference on ambulatory chemotherapy in Pittsburgh

:: *November 29*: Ambulatory Chemotherapy Program (ACP) authorized

:: *December 1*: Anchorage Hospital opens officially

1954   :: Dr. Moore uses two-drug treatment at Orthopedic Hospital

:: Tuberculosis drops to 4th place in Alaska as cause of death, at 60.5 / 100,000

:: 1,000 hospital admissions for tuberculosis, compared with 431 the previous year

:: *January 1*: 820 tuberculosis beds are available in Alaska

:: *March 15*: 2,363 known active or probably active in Alaska; Native rate is 6,474 / 100,000

:: *June 1*: Large x-ray truck unit begins operations in Haines

:: *July 1*: Dr. Robert Moles arrives at Anchorage Hospital as thoracic surgeon and medical officer-in-charge

:: *July 1* : $100,000 made available for ACP

:: *Summer*: Congress appropriates $1.18 million to treat 400 Alaskan tuberculosis patients in Washington sanatoriums during 1955

    :: *July–August*: Main Parran team travels in Alaska

    :: *August*: M/S *Hygiene* is reactivated for Alaska service

    :: *October*: Parran Report is published

    :: *October 14*: First Alaskan patients are transferred to Seattle-area sanatoriums

1955   :: Tuberculosis deaths down to 50 (from 240 in 1950), but 955 new cases are identified

    :: The wait for tuberculosis hospital bed is now six months, compared with two years in 1953

    :: ACP begins successively in Bethel, Barrow, Tanana, and Kotzebue Service Units

    :: *May*: 1,205 Alaskans hospitalized for tuberculosis, including 484 in the States; estimated 1,000 patients still requiring hospital treatment

    :: *July 1*: ANS health functions are transferred to PHS

    :: *December 31*: 1,311 Alaskans hospitalized for tuberculosis; 1,350 beds available

1956   :: Dr. Phillips leaves Seward Sanatorium and moves to Anchorage

    :: Use of BCG is gradually phased out

    :: Dr. Moore resigns from Orthopedic Hospital and sets up private practice in Sitka

    :: Tuberculosis bed supply meets demand

    :: *January*: Dr. Albrecht resigns as commissioner of health; Dr. Hayman named acting commissioner

    :: *Spring*: 1,398 Alaskans are hospitalized for tuberculosis

    :: *Spring*: Dr. Aronson makes final follow-up of nineteen-year BCG study

    :: *April*: Unified tuberculosis control field office is set up in Anchorage under Dr. Robert Gardner, and with participation of ADH and DIH

    :: *July*: ACP operating in seventy villages, with 1,625 patients on treatment

    :: *September*: ADH takes over ACP program except in Bethel area

    :: Rose Galaida hired as first medical social worker in tuberculosis program

    :: *October*: M/S *Hygiene* out of service

1957   :: 3,705 tuberculosis patients are under home care and observation by PHNs; of these 2,176 are taking anti-tuberculosis drugs

    :: *April*: All new tuberculosis cases will be treated within the territory

    :: *Summer*: Frances L. Paul retires after twenty-three years of leadership with the Alaska Tuberculosis Association and nine years as executive secretary

    :: ANHS Area Office moves from Juneau to Anchorage

    :: *December*: INH prophylaxis study begins in Bethel area

    :: *December 1*: No more Alaskan patients at Firland, Laurel Beach, or Riverton sanatoriums, Seattle

1958   :: *July 1*: Seward Sanatorium closes

1959	::	Routine annual tuberculin testing of preschool and schoolchildren is begun by PHNs
	::	*January 3*: **Alaska becomes the forty-ninth state**
	::	*Early*: Waiting list for beds finally eliminated
	::	*End*: All tuberculosis patients are returned to Alaska; 373 tuberculosis beds available
1960	::	1,903 cases in Tuberculosis Case Registry
	::	Native death rate from tuberculosis is 27.5 / 100,000
	::	For the first time, majority of new cases of tuberculosis are primary or minimal
	::	Average annual infection rate of 1 percent in children under 3 in Bethel area
	::	*February*: 1,200 x-ray films from northern villages lost in fire in Kotzebue
1961	::	*May*: Large tuberculosis outbreak in Noorvik
	::	*July 1*: Drs. Martha and Joseph Wilson arrive at the Anchorage Hospital
1962	::	New cases of tuberculosis up from 255 in 1961 to 353
	::	Dr. Karola Reitlinger, longtime radiologist at ADH, resigns
	::	ADHW officially adopts tine test for tuberculin sensitivity screening
1963	::	*October*: First villages begun on community-wide INH prophylaxis in Bethel area
1964	::	*April*: Dr. Robert I. Fraser becomes chief, Unit of Tuberculosis Control
1965	::	Service Unit Hospitals develop local chest clinics
	::	School tuberculin-testing program is extended to include most of state
	::	*May*: Last villages stopped drugs in community-wide INH prophylaxis program
	::	*July*: Rehabilitation Project begins at ANMC, with grant from federal OVR
	::	*August*: 7-H-10 technology for rapid culture of tubercle bacilli is introduced in south-central laboratory
	::	Routine tuberculosis drug-sensitivity testing is instituted by state laboratory
	::	*Late*: Tuberculosis Project Grant from CDC allows organization of "Hot Spot Team" in Alaska
1966	::	25 percent as many reactivations as new cases of tuberculosis
	::	Tuberculosis incidence down 50 percent from 1965
1967	::	Attention first given by Unit of Tuberculosis Control to emphysema, bronchiectasis, and other chronic lung diseases
	::	Estimated 60,000 Alaskans are tuberculin-positive
1968	::	First year with no tuberculosis deaths reported in Alaska
	::	1.6 percent tuberculin reactor rate among school enterers

:: *May*: No pediatric tuberculosis cases hospitalized in Alaska

:: *July*: Community Health Aide Program is officially established

| 1969 | :: Only one-third of new cases reported as infectious, others being healed primary or extrapulmonary |

:: ADHW Unit of Tuberculosis Control becomes Section of Tuberculosis Control and Chest Diseases

:: *Spring*: The Division of Indian Health becomes the Indian Health Service

:: *June*: Rehabilitation Project at ANMC closes

1970
:: ATA becomes "Alaska Tuberculosis and Respiratory Disease Association"

:: *Summer/fall*: Village tuberculosis outbreak at Tanacross

1971
:: Tuberculosis beds in Alaska decline to thirty-one, on a single ward at Anchorage

:: 77 percent of new cases in 1970–71 have had previously positive tuberculin test

:: Emphasis on short hospitalization for new cases

1972
:: A few micro-outbreaks caused by exposure to far advanced open cases

:: Workshops held in smaller communities and hospitals on chronic respiratory disease

:: Inhalation therapist available under contract to ADHW

1973
:: Tuberculosis hospitalization averages less than two weeks

:: Twice-weekly direct chemotherapy is tried in some alcoholic patients

:: *February*: Last tuberculosis ward closes in Alaska, at the Alaska Native Medical Center; Dr. Richard Chao retires

:: *September*: Celebration at Anchorage Westward Hotel to mark the closure of the last tuberculosis ward, sponsored by the Anchorage Service Unit Native Board of Health

1974
:: Majority of new cases of tuberculosis have minimal disease, a situation unique in the US

:: Estimated 2,500 Alaskans, many in bush, have chronic pulmonary disease and pulmonary insufficiency

1976
:: Of those with a previous diagnosis of tuberculosis who later reactivate, two-thirds have had INH at some time

1977
:: Significant increase in drug resistance is noted, suggesting poor compliance in taking drugs

:: *October*: End of follow-up period for INH prophylaxis studies

1978
:: Increase in tuberculin sensitivity is noted among schoolchildren

:: *Summer*: Outbreak of tuberculosis identified in Toksook Bay

1979	::	Call for new statute permitting incarceration for recalcitrant infectious patients
1980	::	50 percent reduction in tuberculosis incidence over previous decade
	::	Continued increase in tuberculin sensitivity among preschool and schoolchildren
1982	::	First AIDS case is reported in Alaska
	::	Tuberculosis outbreak among ICU workers in Fairbanks
1983	::	Legislature passes HB 291 to ensure treatment of noncompliant active tuberculosis cases
1985	::	Significant rise in new cases, especially among Southeast Asian immigrants in Anchorage
	::	First case reported of an Alaskan with both tuberculosis and AIDS
1987	::	Tuberculosis outbreak at Holy Cross
	::	*May 1*: Dr. Fraser retires and is replaced by Dr. John Middaugh
	::	*June*: In-depth review of Alaska tuberculosis program by CDC
	::	*October 1*: Dr. Michael Jones becomes state tuberculosis control officer
1988	::	DOT becomes policy of DPH "whenever possible"
1989	::	Outbreak of drug-resistant tuberculosis at Chevak
1990	::	For period 1988–90, 78 percent of reported cases are Alaska Natives and 12 percent are Asians or Pacific Islanders; 47 percent of all cases are from western Alaska
	::	Large tuberculosis outbreaks on the Pribilof Islands and St. Lawrence Island
1991	::	Outbreaks in Savoonga, Nome, Togiak, and the Pribilofs
1992	::	For the first time, the overall Alaska tuberculosis incidence rate falls below that of the US
	::	Two patients with TB/AIDS reported; four such patients previously reported in Alaska
	::	DPH recommends that all tuberculosis patients at risk for HIV be tested for the virus
	::	*January*: Aplisol found to cause unusually high number of apparent "converters" in Seward
	::	*September*: Anergy testing becomes available in Anchorage
1994	::	Several village tuberculosis outbreaks occur, including Chevak, Hooper Bay, Scammon Bay, Lower Kalskag, and Mt. Village; epidemics continue in the Pribilofs and St. Lawrence Island

	::	*January*: Dr. Jones resigns

1995	::	Tuberculosis outbreaks at Shishmaref and Circle
	::	78 percent of tuberculosis patients in Alaska on DOT
	::	*February*: Second intensive review of tuberculosis program by CDC
	::	*April*: Dr. Beth Funk becomes tuberculosis control officer
	::	*June*: New tuberculosis legislation improves quarantine procedures

1996	::	Major village tuberculosis outbreak involving Levelock, Kokhanok, and Iliamna

1997	::	Over previous five years, 67 percent of all reported cases of tuberculosis were in Alaska Natives and 23 percent in Asian and Pacific Islanders
	::	Over previous five years, 4 percent of tubercle bacillus strains tested in Alaska showed resistance to one or more drugs
	::	Tuberculosis outbreak among NICU workers in Anchorage
	::	41 percent of reported cases of tuberculosis for 1996–97 in Anchorage were foreign-born

1999	::	Anergy testing no longer routinely recommended by DPH
	::	Alaska institutes mandatory reporting of HIV infection

2000	::	Major tuberculosis outbreak in Anchorage
	::	Alaska has highest tuberculosis rate of any state at 17.2/100,000
	::	*June*: Tuberculosis outbreak in Bristol Bay villages
	::	*November*: Unusual number of tuberculin converters at Spring Hill Correctional Institution at Seward

:: Index

Abercrombie, William, 13
acid-fast bacteria (AFB), xxix, 1, 2, 173, 185, 227
active cases: classification of, xxi, 32, 48, 62, 81, 147, 161, 164, 165, 178, 205; new, xxi, 146, 161, 164, 168, 173; statistics on, xi, xxii, 26, 48, 53, 58, 59, 62, 63n2, 69, 72, 76, 77, 81, 85, 89, 135, 147, 148, 163–67, 170–72, 173, 175, 176, 179
Adams, George, 10
adrenal glands: tuberculosis in, xxvii
AIDS. *See* HIV / AIDS
Akiak Native hospital, 23, 40, 49
Alaska: map of, 16; U.S. acquisition of, 11–15
Alaska Crippled Children's Association (ACCA), 69, 90–93, 110, 111, 218
Alaska Department of Health (ADH): AHRC turns over tuberculosis responsibilities to, 144; case finding efforts of, 86; funding for crippled children, 110; funding problems at, 84; laboratory of, 57, 142, 171, 172, 178, 180, 185; legal authority for, 67–68; mental health team of, 117–18; patient treatment cost and, 101; program at Arctic Health Research Center, 139; Seward Sanatorium and, 62, 106–9; takes over administration of ACP, 140; transition to sanatoriums and, 211; tuberculosis control division, 69–70, 72, 93, 102; volunteers and, 91. *See also* Division of Health Education; mobile health units
Alaska Department of Health and Social Services (ADHSS), 187
Alaska Department of Health and Welfare (ADHW), 163
Alaska Federation of Natives, 201, 216
Alaska Health Program, 71
Alaska Native Brotherhood and Sisterhood, 201
Alaska Native health corporations, 170, 172, 176, 179
Alaska Native Health Service (ANHS; PHS), 21–24, 61, 114, 125, 131–32, 154
Alaska Native Medical Center (ANMC; Anchorage, AK): becomes tertiary care general hospital, 217; chest clinic at, 162; decline of tuberculosis at, 155, 166; increasing number of drug-resistant cases at, 178; rehabilitation at, 119–20; sputum analysis at, 163; takes part in TB Committee, 187; tuberculosis outbreak and, 171
Alaska Natives: first report of TB in, 7; forced

acculturation of, 196; health program participation by, 140, 142–43, 146, 148. *See also specific peoples*
Alaska Native Service (ANS; BIA), 58, 94; active case statistics of, 135; AMA surveys and, 85; boarding schools of, 76; military bases transferred to, 114; orthopedic hospitals and, 111; outpatient treatment and, 138; overview of, 49–53; sets daily rate for sanatorium care, 101; Seward Sanatorium and, 107–8; Skagway Sanatorium and, 103–4; transfer of surplus hospital to, 61; tuberculosis beds and, 60, 73; tuberculosis education and, 143
Alaska Native traditional healing, 3–6
Alaska Packers Association, 88
Alaska School Service, 21–23, 36
Alaska's Health, 54, 59, 60, 69, 94
Alaska TB Committee, 53, 187
Alaska Territorial Legislature, 36, 55, 60, 67–68, 70, 117, 155n2
Alaska Tuberculosis and Respiratory Disease Association, 90
Alaska Tuberculosis Association (ATA): beginnings of, 52–55; Christmas Seal fundraising by, 52, 53, 88–90; health education and, 94; improving morale by, 104; praise for work by, 125; rehabilitation program of, 117–20; supplements surgeon salary, 116; tuberculosis survey and, 57
Albrecht, C. Earl: agrees with schoolchildren testing plan, 74; Alaska Health Program and, 71–72; AMA surveys and, 85, 87; ambulatory chemotherapy program and, 136–37; Anchorage Native Hospital and, 121–22; BCG vaccination program and, 82, 84; board of health nominations of, 96n6; Division of Health and, 155n2; Gruening appoints as health commissioner, 68–69; on health of Eskimo soldiers, 51; marine public health unit and, 76; orthopedic hospitals and, 110–11; as Parran survey team member, 123, 136–37; promotes use of Washington state hospitals, 123–24; railway health unit and, 81; sanatorium building and, 70; Seward Sanatorium and, 106, 107–8; on Skagway Sanatorium conditions, 105; speaks at sanatorium closing ceremony, 155; tuberculosis education and, 93, 94; use of military hospital for tuberculosis hospital, 61

Social Security Administration (SSA), 62
social worker, 88, 117, 118, 214
Soloviev, Alexei, 7
Spanish flu (1918–1919), xxxi, 24, 26, 37, 44n51, 55–56
spinal tuberculosis. *See* Pott's disease
spread of tuberculosis, factors favoring: airline travel, 173–74; coughing/sneezing, xxii, 28; crowding, xxix, xxxii, 6, 8, 28, 30, 87, 90, 164, 194, 195, 197, 198; droplet nuclei, xxii, xxiii, xxv; drug resistance, xxi; HIV/AIDS (*see* HIV/AIDS); homelessness, xxi, xxxvi, 169, 174, 175, 181, 186, 187, 197, 198; housing, xxxii, 27, 90, 136, 150, 186, 195; immigration, xxi; immune status, xxii, xxiii, xxv, xxx, 77, 84, 148, 178, 180, 193–95, 198; institutional setting, xxi; malnutrition, xxx, xxxii, 10, 90, 171, 176, 194, 195, 196, 197, 198; milk/meat, xxii, xxix; poverty, xxi, xxx, xxxii, xxxiii, 27, 90; premastication of food, 28, 32; psychological factors, xxviii, 118, 144, 171, 198, 208, 214; sanitation, lack of, 195; singing/talking, xxii; spitting, 28, 31; stress, 171, 193, 197, 198; ventilation, lack of, xxii, 6, 8, 10, 11, 27, 28, 174, 197; war, xxi. *See also* alcohol abuse; nonepidemic diseases
sputum: collection/disposal of, 24, 30–33, 34, 35, 93, 142. *See also* diagnostic tests; signs/symptoms
St. Ann's Hospital (Juneau, AK), 112
St. Lawrence Island, AK, 7, 194; DOT clinics on, 182; epidemic on, 14; living conditions on, 31; new cases on, 173; outbreaks on, 172; pulmonary disease on, 13
statistics, 25–26, 71, 174; active cases, xi, xxii, 26, 48, 53, 58, 59, 62, 63, 69, 72, 76, 77, 81, 85, 89, 135, 147, 148, 163–67, 170–72, 173, 175, 176, 179; converters, 179, 190; death (mortality) rate, xxxi–xxxii, 12–13, 47–49, 63n2, 123, 125, 134, 134, 199, 200, 222–23; deaths, xxi, 9, 26, 47–49, 56, 63n2, 72, 84, 86, 123, 146, 164, 165, 165, 222; hospitalized patients, 58, 76, 104, 108, 139, 144, 154, 165, 166; incidence rate, xxi, 48–49, 63n2, 165, 168, 170, 174, 177, 184, 186, 199, 224–25; new active cases, xxi, 146, 161, 164, 168, 173; reactivations, 161, 167; receiving chemotherapy, 139; receiving home treatment, 154, 165; suspects, 76; total cases, 72, 135, 161, 165–66, 224–25; tuberculin reactors, 135, 139, 148, 167–68, 199; tuberculosis beds, 50, 52, 59, 62, 69, 72, 73, 87, 87, 90, 101, 104, 112, 115, 116, 117, 122, 123, 129n102, 135, 140, 155, 205; waiting list for admission, 81, 89, 117, 123, 126, 136, 139, 143, 153, 154
Stocklen, Joseph B., 84, 133
streptomycin, xxxv, xxxvi, 87, 120–21, 138, 153, 154, 156n16, 177–78, 179, 180, 208
Strong, John F. A., 22, 36–37

surgery, xxxiv–xxxvi, 123, 209; apical resection, 154; bone grafts, 109, 112–13, 216; bronchoscopy, 107; casting, 109, 113, 216; complications of, xxxiv, xxxv; joint fusion, 109, 216; lobectomy, 107, 116, 154, 209; major, 209; minor, 209; phrenic crush, xxxiv, 107, 154, 209; phrenicectomy, xxxiv, 209; plombage, xxxxiv; pneumonectomy, xxxv, 107, 116, 209; pneumonolysis, 209; pneumoperitoneum, xxxiv, 101, 116, 138, 209; pneumothorax, xxvii, xxxiv, 60, 101, 116, 209, 219n9; segmental resection, 154, 209; thoracic, 123; thoracocentesis, 209; thoracoplasty, xxxv, 107, 113, 116, 154, 209; thoracotomy, 154, 209, 217
surplus federal property, 60, 69, 71, 80
Swedish Hospital (Seattle), 111
Swineford, Albert P., 14
Sydenham, Thomas, xxxii
syphilis, 12, 136, 195

Tacoma Indian Hospital, 52
Tanana Native hospital, 38–39, 49, 50, 97n29
tapeworm, 10
teachers: AMA survey and, 85, 86; as chemotherapy aide, 140, 141; death reports by, 56; medical handbook for, 22, 23, 24, 27, 31, 33, 34–35, 40; medical kit for, 22, 143; radio consultation for, 138, 139; recruitment of, late nineteenth century, 21; report on bleeding from lungs by, 13; report on Gambell, 14; report on sanitary conditions, 27, 28–29, 30, 31, 33; resource materials for, 94; of sanitation, 23, 28–29, 33–34; training for, 49; x-raying, 74; x-ray survey and, 80
Territorial Department of Health (TDH): beginnings of, 55–58; post–World War I, 59–60, 62–63
therapeutic pneumothorax, xxxiv
Thomas, George H., 11
Thomas, Lowell Sr., 217
thoracic surgeon, 103, 107, 108, 116
thoracoplasty, 113, 236
Thoreau, Henry David, xxxvii n12
Thygeson, Phillips, 150
tine test. *See* tuberculin testing
Tlingit, 8; benign hemoptysis among, 10, 43n29; consumption among, 13; contact with Russians, 11; living conditions of, 34; Pitcher report on, in Sitka, 14; survey of, 25; traditional healing practice of, 3, 4
tobacco, 27, 28, 32, 195–96, 213
trachoma, 149, 236
treatment methods: Alaska Native, 3–6; ambulatory chemotherapy, 133, 137; ancient, xxxii; bleeding, xxxii; diet/nutrition, xxxiii, 60, 93, 125, 136; directly observed therapy (DOT), xxxvi, 169, 172, 174, 181–82, 184, 185, 186, 187; discipline/routine, xxxiv; drugs (*see* drugs); eighteenth/nineteenth century, xxxii–xxxiii;